The Complete nMRCGP® Study Guide
THIRD EDITION

The Complete nMRCGP® Study Guide
THIRD EDITION

SARAH GEAR

General Practitioner
Cheshire

Radcliffe Publishing
Oxford • New York

Radcliffe Publishing Ltd
18 Marcham Road
Abingdon
Oxon OX14 1AA
United Kingdom

www.radcliffe-oxford.com
Electronic catalogue and worldwide online ordering facility.

First Edition 2004
Second Edition 2006

British Library Cataloguing in Publication Data

A catalogue record for this book is available from the British Library.

ISBN-13: 978 184619 296 8

Typeset by Pindar New Zealand (Egan Reid), Auckland, New Zealand
Printed and bound by TJI Digital, Padstow, Cornwall, UK

Contents

About the author

Dr Sarah Gear graduated in 1995 from Manchester Medical School. She undertook SHO posts followed by the GP vocational training scheme at the North Staffordshire Royal Infirmary in Stoke-on-Trent, qualifying as a GP in August 2001 and successfully gaining the MRCGP® the same year.

In April 2002, she became a principal at her former training practice in Madeley, near Crewe.

Acknowledgements

As with the previous editions, the third edition of the complete nMRCGP® has taken a lot of work to ensure it is as up-to-date as it can be before being published. This new edition would not have been possible without the help of family, friends and colleagues. The medical educational courses that are run both locally and nationally are of huge importance to our continuing professional development, as are the online facilities that we are fortunate enough to be able to access.

Special thanks to Gillian Nineham and her initial belief in the project and to the whole team at Radcliffe for the advice and polite suggestions on how to improve my grammar (which has sometimes left me smiling for days!). Without such dedication I would still be printing off individual work books for circulation. Thank you.

Introduction

In 2007 the Royal College of General Practitioners launched the new MRCGP® as a single route for vocational training to be a General Practitioner. The structure of the exam changed to have three components:
* Applied Knowledge Test
* Clinical Skills Assessment
* Work-based Assessment.

The College website (www.rcgp.org.uk) must be consulted. Even if you have sat the exam before, you must read the rules again – they can change, so don't be caught out.

Part of the groundwork at an early stage is to speak to as many people as possible about their learning techniques and approach for the nMRCGP®. You will find that in most cases people will identify a topic ('learning need') and read around it. Then they might do a Medline search for current review articles or look in *Clinical Evidence* to ensure there has not been some new, revolutionary information that might change the way they would tackle the given subject (i.e. the way they practise).

More enlightened doctors manage to keep up to date with the journals and comics, do their own video analysis and even have a mentor. Thinking about what you want to achieve in general practice from early on in your career will mean you can maximise what you get out of your hospital jobs and training post.

To be a competent GP you need to be well read (a true generalist) and have an open, sensible approach to acquiring knowledge that will fill in any gaps. You need to be able to work as part of a team (you will be part of the primary healthcare team, not to mention the doctor-patient aspect), and you need to be open to differing ethical and cultural ideas and beliefs. That's all just for starters!

In this book I have covered the main medical topics that are fundamental to general practice. The book is not meant to provide comprehensive coverage of aetiology, pathophysiology, investigations and treatments – quite the opposite. I assume if you aren't up to speed and need to recap, you will be able to access this information easily. I have incorporated current treatment issues, National Service Frameworks, the latest research, questions, etc. The information is all clearly referenced and the issues are not clouded by my personal opinions – the whole point to postgraduate learning is to formulate your own opinions. Having said that, where it seemed important to do so, I have included the opinions of published authors from the journals.

All this is to save you the colossal amount of time that you would otherwise need to prepare for the exam.

Finally, it is important to remember the following.

◆ You don't need to know everything (you cannot possibly).
◆ Learning is easier if what you are learning is topical/relevant.
◆ It is not how much you know, but how you apply that knowledge, that matters.
◆ There is no value in being able to regurgitate study notes. You will do better if your understanding is practical.
◆ Hot topics form only a small part of the exam, be it MRCGP® or summative assessment.
◆ You generally do not need to quote specific references.

Sarah Gear
September 2008
gear@doctors.org.uk

How to use this book

Probably the worst thing you could do at this stage is to try and plough through the book from beginning to end – you would never make it, and even if you did, you would be unlikely to remember much of it.

Use the book as a starting point, a guide or for summing up to ensure that you are as well read as you think you are. Flick through and get a handle on the layout and what is included. No doubt there will be parts you know inside out – so don't be tempted to spend too much time here, move on. Scribble comments and questions, highlight text, use Post-it notes, or completely deface it. Do whatever you like, but make sure it works for you.

As you go through the different sections, think not only of possible questions the examiners might set, but also how you would explain the various issues if you had to teach the subject. Write down the questions you come up with and use them for revision. Try some mind-mapping for more complicated topics.

Consider the online facilities that you can access free of charge, such as BMJ Learning (www.bmjlearning.com), and doctors.net modules (www.doctors. org.uk). Such facilities can make the difference between thinking you know something you have skim-read, and really knowing the answers. Information from these sources is well written and peer reviewed before being published.

Each part of the exam-style questions explains what is involved. All answers are comprehensive but not exhaustive. As you get used to the techniques and increase your knowledge, there will be points that you feel are important which I have not included – keep them as part of your answer.

No book will ever cover everything you need to know, but this one encompasses a huge amount. I hope you find it an indispensable guide to both your GP registrar year and the nMRCGP®.

General practice is a fantastic career and the MRCGP® has always been a worthwhile exam to work for. You will gain an incredible amount from it if you are willing to put in the time and effort.

Enjoy and good luck!

Part 1

Clinical

Cardiovascular

Hypertension
This is bread-and-butter general practice, and you must know these guidelines. With a prevalence of around 11% you would expect to see this every day of your working life.

British Hypertension Society Guidelines 2004
J Hum Hypertens 2004; 18: 139-85 and *BMJ* 2004; 328: 634-40 (summary)
The British Hypertension Society (BHS) published a 2004 update of previous guidelines (1989, 1993 and 1999). The guidelines state that the main determinant of benefit from blood pressure-lowering drugs is the achieved blood pressure rather than the choice of therapy.

Summary of BHS Guidelines
- Start antihypertensive treatment in patients with:
  - a sustained systolic BP greater than or equal to 160 mmHg
  - a sustained diastolic BP greater than or equal to 100 mmHg.
- Start antihypertensive treatment in diabetic patients who have:
  - systolic BP greater than or equal to 140 mmHg
  - diastolic BP greater than or equal to 90 mmHg.
- Treat borderline blood pressure (140–159/90–99 mmHg) if there is target organ damage, cardiovascular disease, diabetes or a 10-year cardiovascular disease risk ≥ 20% (this is equivalent to the CHD risk of around 15%).
- Optimal BP targets in non-diabetics are:
  - systolic BP less than 140 mmHg
  - diastolic BP less than 85 mmHg.
- The minimum acceptable control for audit purposes is 150/90 mmHg, and for patients with diabetes, chronic renal disease and established cardiovascular disease (CVD) it is 130/80 mmHg.
- Give non-pharmacological advice to all hypertensives (and borderline hypertensives).
- Consider statins to reduce cardiovascular risk in:
  - primary prevention, where the 10-year cardiovascular risk factor is greater than or equal to 20%
  - secondary prevention, where high blood pressure is complicated by CVD (irrespective of the base-line total cholesterol).
- Optimal cholesterol lowering should reduce the total cholesterol by 25% (or LDL-cholesterol by 30%), or achieve a cholesterol < 4.0 mmol/L (or LDL-cholesterol less than 2.0 mmol/L) – whichever is the greater reduction.

✦ Consider aspirin (75 mg/day), when the BP is controlled (< 150/90 mmHg) in:
  • primary prevention if over 50 years of age with a 10-year CVD risk ≥ 20%
  • secondary prevention of ischaemic cardiovascular disease.

The guidelines are based on the HOT Trial, summarised below.

National Institute for Health and Clinical Excellence. *Hypertension: management of hypertension in adults in primary care: NICE clinical guideline 34*. London: NIHCE; June 2006 www.nice.org.uk/CG034
NICE and the BHS differ mainly in their approach to drug treatments. The BHS suggest that triple therapy would be a combination of an ACE inhibitor (A), calcium-channel blocker (C) and diuretic (D), with beta-blockers being used for patients who do not respond to or who are intolerant of other medication.

In 2006 the BHS collaborated with NICE to update the recommendations for the pharmacological management of hypertension.

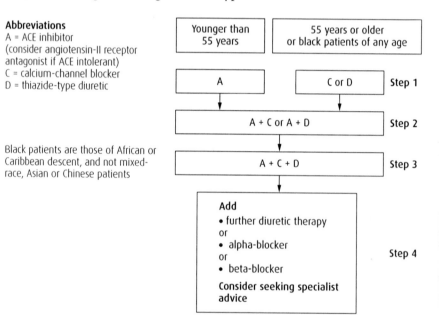

FIGURE 1.1 Choosing drugs for patients newly diagnosed with hypertension (NICE 2006).

Effects of intensive BP lowering and low dose aspirin in patients with hypertension: principal results of the Hypertension Optimal Treatment (HOT) randomised trial
Lancet 1998; 351: 1755–62
This trial included 18 790 patients in 26 countries (with a follow-up of 3.8 years on average). It looked at outcomes in terms of major cardiovascular events.

Felodipine (a calcium-channel antagonist) was the baseline therapy.

The lowest incidence of major cardiovascular events, a 30% reduction, occurred at a mean achieved diastolic blood pressure of 83 mmHg. For diabetes, the lowest incidence was found at a BP less than 80 mmHg.

Daily addition of aspirin 75 mg reduced the risk of myocardial infarction by 36% in men, in well controlled hypertension.

Anglo-Scandinavian Cardiac Outcome Trials – BP-lowering arm (ASCOT-BPLA)
Lancet 2005; 366: 895–906

This trial has attracted a huge amount of attention, as up until this publication no trial had found an antihypertensive regime that was better than a thiazide and beta-blocker combination (for morbidity, mortality and cost-effectiveness).

It was a randomised controlled trial of 19 257 patients (aged 40–79 years) with hypertension and at least three additional risk factors (not including patients who had recently had a myocardial infarction, stroke or angina). The patients were randomised to receive either atenolol (and a thiazide if needed) or amlodipine (and perindopril if needed).

The primary end points (non-fatal myocardial infarction and fatal coronary heart disease) showed no significant difference; however the amlodipine group found:

- fewer patients developing new-onset diabetes (5.9% vs. 8.3%; HR 0.70, 95% CI 0.63–0.78 and a NNT 41)
- a significantly better outcome in secondary end points – including cardiovascular mortality and strokes (NNT 116 and 101 respectively).

This trial helps to build on our current knowledge on the cautious use of beta-blockers as first line therapy, the conclusion reached by a Cochrane Review published on the subject in 2007. For people already well controlled on beta-blockers it was not recommended that these be stopped, as it is recognised from other meta-analyses that the control of blood pressure itself is the most important factor in protecting against cardiovascular disease.

Major outcomes in high-risk hypertensive patients randomised to ACEI or Ca-channel blockers vs. diuretics: the antihypertensive and lipid-lowering treatment to prevent heart attack trial (ALLHAT Trial)
JAMA 2002; 288: 2981–97

This multicentre randomised controlled trial involving 42 418 patients aged over 55 years confirmed the above meta-analysis. It was concluded that the most important factor in reducing risk and mortality is reducing the blood pressure, not the actual drug used.

Blood-pressure measuring devices

Most sphygmomanometers in general practice are not serviced and calibrated. That could mean GPs misclassify patients. The need for recalibration has been emphasised by the BHS since 1986.

Following a report by the Medicines and Healthcare Products Regulatory Agency warning that oscillometric devices were often inaccurate, the Government has recommended:

+ safety procedures, such as spillage kits, be maintained where mercury devices are used
+ CE-marked oscillometric devices should not be assumed to be suitable for diagnosis of hypertension
+ alternative devices should be used where oscillometric devices are unsuitable (e.g. arrhythmias)
+ aneroid devices should be checked regularly
+ the NHS must only purchase devices that meet MHRA standards.

Hypertension guideline recommendations in general practice: awareness, agreement, adoption and adherence
Br J Gen Pract 2007; 57: 948-52

It is known that around three-quarters of patients are not treated to target in general practice. This study surveyed 401 general practitioners, of whom 99% were aware of the guidelines on statin therapy but only 43% adhered to them. Three-quarters (77%) were aware that blood pressure should be checked on both arms but only 30% agreed with the recommendation.

The study concluded that lack of awareness was seldom a problem but that where GPs did not agree with guidance they were unlikely to apply it, even if given financial incentive.

Half of all people over 60 years have hypertension. Several age-specific studies have provided evidence about treating hypertension in the elderly. BHS Guidelines state drug treatment is of proven benefit up to 80 years of age. Once started, it should be continued. If hypertension is diagnosed after the age of 80 years, the decision whether to treat should be based on the clinical picture. A recent trial on hypertension in the very elderly (HYVET) has been stopped early. Initial reports were that over-80s benefit from blood pressure reduction in the same way as younger people do.

Further learnings from the European Working Party on Hypertension in the Elderly (EWPHE) study: focus on systolic hypertension
Cardiovascular Drug Therapy 1991; 4 Suppl: 1249-51

In this study of 840 patients aged over 60 years and with BP > 160/90 mmHg, thiazide vs. placebo produced a significant reduction in cardiovascular mortality and death from myocardial infarction.

Cardiovascular disease risk assessment

Individuals are at increased risk of developing CVD if they are smokers, hypertensive, diabetic, or have dyslipidaemias. It is also known that obesity, increased waist : hip ratio, increased alcohol consumption, family history and ethnicity all increase an individual's risk. Preventing CVD could be argued to be one of the most important tasks for GPs.

Absolute risk is the probability of developing CHD (non-fatal myocardial infarction or coronary death) over a defined period of time. It can be estimated using risk assessment charts. These help us to explain risks to the patient, which in turn empowers the patient to make informed choices on available options. The information from the charts should not replace clinical judgement.

Most risk assessment tools are based on complex mathematics from the Framingham studies. They are for use in *primary prevention*. They are not for use with patients who have existing diseases that already put them at high risk such as CHD, diabetes, stroke, atherosclerotic disease, familial hypercholesterolaemia, inherited dyslipidaemia or renal dysfunction (including diabetic nephropathy).

The original Framingham study (named after a town in Massachusetts) was published in 1971, having looked for over 14 years at the lipid profiles and coronary heart disease risks of 2282 men and 2845 women. Since then a number of spin-off studies relating to CHD have been published. The main concern surrounding the use of Framingham models is that they are based on affluent white patients and there is no consideration of ethnicity, family history or socioeconomic groupings. For this reason, NICE is considering a review of all risk assessment charts currently used.

Framingham, SCORE and DECODE risk equations do not provide reliable cardiovascular risk estimates in type 2 diabetes
Diabetes Care 2007; 30: 1292–4

The 10-year fatal CVD event rate was 7.4% in the United Kingdom Prospective Diabetes Study (UKPDS). Framingham gave an absolute risk of 5% (an underestimation of 32%), SCORE overestimated the risk by 18% and DECODE gave an acceptable estimate of 6.6%. Both SCORE and DECODE overestimated the five-year risk.

Although we tend to treat patients with diabetes in a secondary prevention bracket the study discussed the need for diabetes-specific risk calculators.

The accuracy of the Framingham risk-score in different socioeconomic groups: a prospective study
Br J Gen Pract 2005; 55: 838–45

This study looked at 12 304 men and women with complete risk-factor information and found that there was a relative underestimation of cardiovascular risk (by up to 48%; 95% CI 0.48–0.56) for manual participants, compared to 31% in non-manual. It concluded that the Framingham study underestimated risk in a poor socioeconomic cohort (an area not previously documented).

Joint British Societies coronary risk prediction chart

This chart was produced by British Cardiac, Hypertension, Hyperlipidaemia and Diabetic Associations. It distinguishes between diabetics and non-diabetics, men and women and smokers and non-smokers. The graphs then depend upon systolic blood pressure, total cholesterol : HDL ratio and a person's age. It can be found in the *British National Formulary* and *MIMS*.

SCORE

This is a project based on the meta-analysis of 12 studies in Europe (involving 250 000 people), as it is thought that the risk assessment tables based on Framingham overestimated the CHD risk in certain subgroups. Individual risk charts will be tailor-made for a specific population.

Problems with tables

These risk assessment tables have all been valuable. They have given us a place to start ongoing evaluations and have helped us work out levels of treatment. However, no system is perfect. Some of the main concerns with the use of risk assessment tables are listed below.

◆ Tables usually calculate a 10-year risk and this becomes inaccurate with blood pressure and life style changes over time, so you need to re-assess periodically.
◆ They can be time consuming to include opportunistically in a consultation (despite IT facilities).
◆ They do not always take into account ethnicity (which can increase the risk by around 1.5).
◆ They underestimate the risk if there is a strong family history of CHD below 65 years of age, or hyperlipidaemia (in these cases it is thought you need to increase the risk estimate by a factor of 1.5).

New risk scoring systems (QRISK and ASSIGN) have been developed and validated, and are in the process of being rolled out.

QRISK

QRISK is a new score that includes a measure of social deprivation as a risk factor (through a postcode-linked deprivation index). Source data for QRisk was obtained from around 1.28 million primary care patients. The data also include family history of heart disease in a first degree relative under 60 years; being on blood pressure treatment; body mass index; and usual risk factors (age, gender, smoking status, systolic blood pressure and total cholesterol : HDL ratio).

Derivation and validation of QRISK a new cardiovascular disease risk score for the United Kingdom: prospective, open cohort study
BMJ 2007; 335: 136

This paper brought together the evidence that QRISK probably gives more appropriate risk assessments for the UK population. Working on the principle that more than a 20% risk of developing cardiovascular disease over a 10-year period was high risk, it found 8.5% of the UK population aged 35–74 (as opposed to 13% with Framingham and 14% with ASSIGN, the new alternative being used in Scotland) were in this category.

Other risk factors in cardiovascular disease

In February 2007 the British Heart Foundation investigated novel risk indicators (homocysteine, C-reactive protein (CRP) and fibrinogen). To be clinically valuable they must be reliably quantifiable and must help predict more accurately the risk of developing coronary heart disease. At present there is insufficient evidence to use any of these indicators.

Homocysteine

Homocysteine is an amino acid that stimulates platelet aggregation and thrombus formation (hence atherosclerosis). It is produced as a breakdown product from the animal protein we digest (methionine). In 2002, the British Cardiac Society presented research showing that elevated homocysteine levels (greater than 12 mmol/L) doubled the risk of a second coronary event.

High homocysteine levels in the general population are mainly due to insufficient folate and vitamin B concentrations (hence the role of folic acid in the polypill). However, there is not enough evidence to recommend homocysteine levels as part of the routine CHD risk assessment.

Guidelines from the International Atherosclerosis Society recommend screening in high risk patients (this is not agreed by the National Screening Committee). If the levels are checked and are found to be raised, treatment with diet or 400 µg folic acid should be initiated and the test repeated after three months. If the levels are still raised, higher doses of folate, vitamin B6 and vitamin B12 are advocated.

CRP

This is a non-specific marker of inflammation.

A CRP concentration greater than 3 mg/L may indicate the need for intensive treatment to reduce cardiovascular risk. US guidelines suggest case selection and use for patients with a 10-year CHD risk of 10–20%.

Fibrinogen

Fibrinogen is a blood-clotting factor that in high levels is hypothesised to be a marker for CVD.

Nitric oxide

Nitric oxide has been looked at for many years to try to understand its role in endothelial function and repair. The first dietary supplement was launched in 2005, supporters advocating its use as a primary preventative measure.

Vitamin D

Circulation 2008; 117(4): 503–11

Lack of vitamin D may be linked to cardiovascular disease (and poorer prognosis in some cancers) after adjusting for the usual risk factors.

Coronary heart disease

National Service Framework for Coronary Heart Disease

www.dh.gov.uk

This was launched in March 2000 as a follow-on from the White Paper *Saving Lives: Our Healthier Nation*, in which CHD was set out as a priority. It is a 10-year plan that aims to reduce death from CHD and stroke in people up to 75 years of age by 40% by 2010, and emphasises the need to provide structured systematic care.

Since the launch of the framework, statin prescribing has doubled.

There are 12 standards that highlight these priorities:

+ smoking cessation advice
+ CHD register in primary care
+ rapid assessment chest pain clinic
+ faster treatment for myocardial infarction and improved secondary prevention
+ more heart operations/revascularisation.

Standards affecting mainly primary care

+ Standard 2, concerning smoking cessation
+ Standards 3 and 4, which cover secondary prevention followed by primary prevention
  * establish comprehensive CHD register for audit purposes
  * develop protocols and guidelines (these need to be agreed at practice level, PCGT and across primary, secondary and tertiary care).
+ Standard 11, concerning heart failure and palliative care for people with CHD. GPs are responsible for arranging appropriate investigations to confirm diagnosis and offering appropriate treatment.

Workload issues include identifying patients and maintaining registers; regular audit (every three months); practice time (meetings, clinics, following protocols and guidelines, etc.); and treating the patient/pharmacology.

Coronary Heart Disease *Shaping the Future* – Progress Report 2006

This report compared figures from 2000 to 2005.

+ Smoking reduced from 28% to 24% of the population.
+ Estimated number of lives saved with statins increased from 2900 to 9700.
+ Percentage of people given thrombolysis within 30 minutes of arrival at hospital increased from 38% to 83%.

Secondary prevention of coronary heart disease in older patients after the national service framework: population based study

BMJ 2006; 332: 144-5

This study looked at men and women aged 60–79 years in 1998–2001 with established coronary heart disease. Data were collected at two time points (from 817 men and 465 women in 1998–2001; and 857 men and 548 women in 2003). It was found that statin uptake and the use of combined drug treatment in elderly men and women increased markedly (from 34% to 65% and from 48% to 67% respectively). There was still room for further improvement in the use of beta-blockers and ACE inhibitors.

If GPs are to be held accountable then they need adequate staffing with appropriate training.

Interestingly, *Health Statistics Quarterly* (www.nationalstatistics.gov.uk) gives weight to the argument that GPs do not need Government guidance to keep their practice up to date. Prescribing habits had changed appropriately prior to the publication of the NSF (as was seen with ACE inhibitors in congestive cardiac failure).

Myocardial infarction: secondary prevention

National Institute for Health and Clinical Excellence. *Myocardial infarction: secondary prevention: NICE clinical guideline 48.* London: NIHCE; 2007

www.nice.org.uk/nicemedia/pdf/CG48NICEGuidance.pdf

The guideline suggests taking each of the following into account.

+ Lifestyle:
  - dietary advice should recommend having 7 g omega-3 oils a week (not β-carotene or antioxidant supplements) and encourage a Mediterranean-style diet
  - alcohol consumption should be within the current recommended limits (14 units a week for women and 21 units a week for men)
  - encourage physical activity and offer smoking cessation advice
  - encourage achievement and maintenance of a healthy weight.
+ Cardiac rehabilitation should be offered to all patients who are stable.
+ Drug therapy – after an MI all patients should be offered a combination of: ACE inhibitor, aspirin (and clopidogrel for 12 months in the case of non-ST-segment elevation acute coronary syndrome), beta-blocker and statin.

✦ Drug therapy – after an MI more than 12 months ago ACE inhibitors, statins and aspirin should be continued if tolerated. Beta-blockers, if started post-MI, should be continued; otherwise do not start unless the patient is at increased risk of a further cardiovascular event.

Heart failure

Pode-Wilson described heart failure in 1997 as:

> . . . a complex clinical syndrome characterised by abnormalities in left ventricular function, neurohormonal regulation, exercise intolerance, shortness of breath, fluid retention and reduced longevity.

✦ Prevalence is 3–20 per 1000 among the general population.
✦ Prevalence is 100 per 1000 if over 65 years of age.
✦ Afro-Caribbeans aged over 65 years are at 2.5 times greater risk than the general population.

Heart failure is not a diagnosis. It can include features of impaired left ventricular function or reduced cardiac output, seen in a number of conditions. You need to consider causes such as ischaemic heart disease, hypertension, arrhythmias, cardiomyopathy, valvular heart disease and so on, as this will help you deliver the correct management plan. There is poor correlation between symptoms and signs when comparing the echocardiographic findings to the degree of impairment. SIGN (www.sign.ac.uk/pdf/qrgchd.pdf) published guidance on heart failure in 2007 (Guidance 95), which considers diagnosis and management options. These guidelines are not summarised here as they are similar to NICE, but they are worth considering as part of your research.

Heart failure has been targeted by Standard 11 of the NSF, as it is known that we under-diagnose and under-treat heart failure. It highlights the need for correct diagnosis and appropriate investigation.

Chronic heart failure

National Institute for Health and Clinical Excellence. *Management of chronic heart failure in adults in primary and secondary care: NICE clinical guideline 5.* **London: NIHCE; 2003**
www.nice.org.uk/nicemedia/pdf/CG5NICEguideline.pdf
This is a comprehensive guide for heart failure in the following areas:
✦ diagnosis
  • a 12-lead ECG and/or BNP (or NTproBNP) are recommended. If one or more is found to be abnormal then echocardiography is recommended
  • other recommended tests include chest x-ray, urea and electrolytes, haemoglobin, glucose, thyroid function tests, etc.
✦ treatment

- ACE inhibitors are recommended for left ventricular systolic dysfunction (LVSD)
- beta-blockers should be started in LVSD after ACE inhibitors and diuretics, regardless of whether symptoms persist
- monitoring
  - clinical states, including cardiac rhythm, cognitive and nutritional status should be assessed
  - review of medication
  - urea, electrolytes and creatinine
- referral and approach to care
- supporting patients and carers
- anxiety and depression
- end of life issues.

Diagnosis

The European Society of Cardiology's guidelines for diagnosis of heart failure include the following:

- *Essential:* symptoms – shortness of breath, swollen ankles, fatigue – and objective evidence of cardiac dysfunction at rest
- *Non-essential:* response to treatment directed towards heart failure.

New York Heart Association (NYHA) grading of dyspnoea or angina

Grade	Criteria
1	Symptoms occur only on severe exertion; almost normal lifestyle possible
2	Symptoms occur on moderate exertion; patients have to avoid certain situations (e.g. carrying shopping up stairs)
3	Symptoms occur on mild exertion; activity is markedly restricted
4	Symptoms occur frequently, even at rest

Diagnostic accuracy

It is known (Finland report and the ECHOES study) that 60–80% of people with a diagnosis of heart failure may not have consistent features on echocardiography.

Barriers to accurate diagnosis and effective management of heart failure in primary care: qualitative study

BMJ 2003; 326: 196–200

This study identified three reasons why GPs had difficulty in diagnosing and managing heart failure.

- Uncertainty about clinical practice:
  - diagnostic process – third heart sound, raised jugular venous pulse especially in obese patients

- availability and use of echocardiography services
- treatment issues.
♦ Lack of awareness of relevant research evidence.
♦ Influences of individual preferences and local organisational factors.

Despite the lack of diagnostic accuracy there have been some studies that found the diagnosis made by hospital physicians was equally inaccurate.

If we were to refer everyone for echocardiography the system would be overwhelmed. It has been suggested that we refer patients whose ECG or CXR are abnormal. Interestingly, the NSF has stated that open access Echo should be available to all GPs by April 2002. Resources for this have not been available in all areas and in some areas the service has been scaled back as it has been underused.

Natriuretic peptides

Brain natriuretic peptide (BNP) and N-Terminal pro-BNP (NTproBNP) are found at high levels in patients with impaired left ventricular systolic function (due to increased pressure or volume overload of the myocardium). As yet there are conflicting studies related to practical use, as there is a low positive predictive value (other factors that increase BNP are age, renal failure, drugs such as beta-blockers or ACE inhibitors). A role may develop for their use in helping to determine who to send for echocardiography as well as for monitoring treatment.

Treatment of heart failure

NICE reviewed treatment in their 2003 guidance, and the Drugs and Therapeutics bulletin also published a review in April 2000.

Diuretics

These are essential for symptomatic management (first line treatment). Their long-term effect on mortality is not known and it would be unethical to conduct a randomised controlled trial given the known benefits of treatment.
♦ Potassium-sparing diuretics, e.g. amiloride.
♦ Spironolactone (competitive aldosterone inhibitor).

Both the RALES and the EPHESUS trials have shown improved mortality and morbidity values with treatment.

The effect of spironolactone on morbidity and mortality in patients with severe heart failure. RALES Trial (Randomised Aldactone Evaluation Study)
NEJM 1999; 341: 709–17
In this study 1663 patients with NYHA grade 4 who were already on an ACE

inhibitor and a loop diuretic (i.e. severe heart failure) were randomised to either spironolactone 25 mg/day or placebo.

An improved mortality rate (a reduction in the risk of death of 30%) was seen when spironolactone was used to block aldosterone receptors in addition to standard therapy. Hyperkalaemia was uncommon if a low dose was used (25 mg/day).

ACE inhibitors

Trials have consistently shown prolonged survival, reversal of left ventricular hypertrophy and a reduced need for hospital admission due to left ventricular dysfunction when patients were on ACE inhibitors.

The results of the HOPE Study (Heart Outcomes Prevention Evaluation Study) suggest that everyone with heart failure without contra-indications should be on an ACE inhibitor.

The number needed to treat (NNT) for one year to prevent one death (quoted in different papers) is as follows:
* 74 if using ACE inhibitors alone
* 29 if using ACE inhibitor and a beta-blocker.

An International Survey of the Management of Heart Failure in Primary Care was presented in September 2001. A total of 1000 GPs was questioned, and it was found that 90% were aware of the benefits of ACE inhibitors, 90% were sending patients for ECGs and 80% were sending patients for chest x-rays. About one-third referred patients for echocardiography (services were thought to be inadequate). Although ACE inhibitors were being used they were being used at inadequate doses. Only 19% of GPs were starting beta-blockers, and only 30% of patients under the age of 70 years with heart failure were receiving them.

Reassuringly, as GPs our knowledge of heart failure is quite high and we are starting to get success with ACE inhibitors, but we need to promote beta-blockers in a similar way.

Listed below are brief summaries of the relevant trials.
* CONSENSUS I 1987 (Co-operative North Scandinavian Enalapril Study): this study showed decreased mortality (with 20 mg enalapril bd) after a follow-up period of one year. This was in severe heart failure (NYHA grade 4).
* SOLVD 1991 (Study of Left Ventricular Dysfunction): this study showed benefits with enalapril 10 mg bd (with a follow-up period of four years). SOLVD-P confirmed that progression of the disease was slowed even if the patient was asymptomatic.

The following trials support the use of ACE inhibitors after myocardial infarction.

◆ SAVE 1992 (Survival and Ventricular Enlargement Trial): this found that long-term administration of captopril reduced the risk of fatal and non-fatal stroke by 21% (95% CI 5–35).

◆ AIRE 1993 (Acute Infarction Ramipril Efficacy Study): ramipril was given to 1014 patients (out of 2006 for randomisation) following an acute myocardial infarction. There was an observed risk reduction of all causes of mortality by 27% in the ramipril group (95% CI 11–40).

◆ TRACE 1995 (Trandalopril Cardiac Evaluation Study): trandalopril was seen to reduce mortality and progression to heart failure (1749 were randomly assigned to receive trandalopril). The benefit was seen as early as 30 days into the treatment.

Beta-blockers

Beta-blockers are thought to work by their effects on the renin-angiotensin system and anti-arrhythmic properties in all degrees of heart failure. Over 20 randomised controlled trials involving 20 000 patients have been conducted. They have found that the NNT (to prevent one death over one year) is 29 if beta-blockers and ACE inhibitors are both used.

Beta-blockers are indicated only in moderate heart failure secondary to ischaemia (confirmed by echocardiography). They should be started slowly and titrated. Below is a brief summary of the main trials.

◆ CIBIS (Cardiac Insufficiency Bisoprolol Study): the results were not significant, but the trend was towards improvement in survival.

◆ CIBIS II: bisoprolol was superior to placebo for mortality and morbidity (32%). The trial was stopped early because the results were so dramatic.

◆ CAPRICORN: this study found that carvedilol was superior to placebo for mortality and morbidity following myocardial infarction. The trial was stopped early.

◆ COPERNICUS: this study found that carvedilol improved mortality even in severe heart failure.

◆ SENIORS: nebivolol improved mortality in elderly patients. However patients over 75 years gained less benefit.

Angiotensin II receptor antagonists

The following randomised controlled trials have found positive results.

◆ ELITE: (Evaluation of Losartan in the Elderly): this tolerability study of losartan vs. captopril in patients over 65 years suggested there was a benefit to patients who could not tolerate ACE inhibitors.

◆ ELITE II: losartan proved not to be superior to captopril with regard to survival. There was a confirmed better tolerability of losartan in this trial of 3152 patients.

◆ Val-HeFT: in this trial of 366 patients who were not on ACE inhibitors, valsartan was used as an additional treatment. There was a significant reduction in all causes of mortality (by up to 33% if patients had not already been receiving an ACE inhibitor).

* CHARM: in this study candesartan was used in a double blind, randomised controlled trial of 7599 patients. It was found that good adherence to medication was associated with a lower risk of death by 15% ($p = 0.011$).
* VALIANT: this study randomised 14703 patients to receive captopril, valsartan or both. It found that valsartan was as effective as an ACE inhibitor in patients with left ventricular systolic dysfunction after myocardial infarction (i.e. the outcomes were not statistically different between the two groups).

Digoxin

It is known that digoxin prevents clinical worsening of heart failure and gives improvement of symptoms. The two main trials that found this to be the case were:

* RADIANCE (Randomised Assessment of Digoxin on Inhibitors of ACE) and
* PROVED study (Prospective Randomised Study of Ventricular Failure and the Efficacy of Digoxin).

One trial has found no reduction in mortality.

* DIG (Digoxin Investigators Group): this trial of 6800 patients with heart failure but no atrial fibrillation found no decrease in mortality, but there was a reported symptomatic improvement in patients.

Vasodilators

* V-HeFT I and II: Hydralazine and isosorbide dinitrate vs. placebo (I) or Enalapril (II): There was an improved mortality rate with these drugs, although this was not as good as the improvement seen with enalapril (i.e. this is an alternative in renal failure patients).

Multidisciplinary approaches to nutrition, patient counselling and education

There have been six randomised controlled trials of highly selected patients looking at the multidisciplinary approach to care. These showed reduced hospital admission rates, better education and improved quality of life.

Randomised controlled trial of specialist nurse intervention in heart failure
BMJ 2001; 323: 715–8
This trial showed that home-based intervention from nurses can reduce admission. This is thought to be due to education, treatment and regular contact. This

is interesting in light of the recent community matron posts that have been introduced.

Exercise and heart failure

A great deal of attention is given to exercise therapy, across all chronic disease groups, looking at improvement in quality of life, exercise tolerance and hopefully reduced morbidity and mortality. The British Heart Foundation has produced several fact sheets around exercise (www.bhf.org.uk/factfiles). The current advice (for fit healthy people) is 30 minutes of exercise a day. In people with limitations, exercise should be within these limitations.

Exercise training meta-analysis of trials in patients with chronic heart failure (ExTraMATCH Collaboration)
BMJ 2004; 328: 189–92

Meta-analysis of randomised controlled trials gives no evidence that properly supervised medical training programmes for patients with heart failure are dangerous. There is clear evidence of an overall reduction in mortality rate.

Public awareness of heart failure in Europe: first results from SHAPE
Eur Heart J 2005; 26(22): 2413–21

This first part of the SHAPE study showed that, of the 7958 lay people completing the survey, only 3% could correctly identify heart failure from a description of typical signs and symptoms.

Part of the study design included a survey of 378 GPs in the UK (due to be published) which found that only 20% regularly used beta-blockers, 36% started heart failure treatment either alone or in combination with a diuretic (the lowest rate of any country in the study), and that three-quarters of GPs were diagnosing heart failure by signs and symptoms alone.

Cardiac Rehabilitation British Heart Foundation Factfile 09/2000

The aim is to restore the patient to the best possible function after acute coronary syndrome and to minimise the risk of recurrence.

Cardiac rehabilitation improves risk, morbidity, mortality and psychosocial outcome. However, it needs to be an individual programme rather than prescriptive, and it needs to have a multidisciplinary approach. Several studies have shown the programmes are cost-effective (both medically and socially).

The National Service Framework for CHD recommends cardiac rehabilitation as part of secondary prevention within the NHS Trust.

It is thought that cardiac rehabilitation can reduce mortality by 20–25%.

Omega-3 Fatty acids

It has been known since the 1970s that omega-3 fish oils protect against coronary heart disease. The mechanism of action is not fully understood. NICE is currently recommending that patients are prescribed omega-3 oils post infarction for up to four years, although from a recent check on its site it looks as though this is undergoing further review.

Omega-3 fatty acids and cardiovascular disease – fishing for a natural treatment
BMJ 2004; 328: 30–5 (Clinical Review)
This review summarises the topic, including trials, two of which are below.

Study	Intervention	Absolute risk reduction	NNT
DART 1989	Fish meal or fish oil capsule twice a week	3.7%	27
GISSI 1999	Fish oil (EPA + DHE 0.85 g/d)	2%	50

Omega-3 fatty acids for cardioprotection
MayoClin Proc 2008; 83: 324–32
This study looked at 32 000 patients from three large controlled trials. They were randomised to receive omega-3 fatty acid supplements containing docosahexaenoic acid (DHA) and eicosapentaenoic acid (EPA) or to the control group. The study showed reductions in cardiovascular events of 19–45% suggesting that intake, whether from dietary sources or fish oil supplements, should be increased (aiming for 1 g/d for those with known coronary artery disease and at least 500 mg/d for those without disease). Two meals of oily fish per week can provide 400 to 500 mg/d.

Lipids and statins in cardiovascular disease
Around 55% of the UK population has a total cholesterol greater than 5.5 mmol/L. In 25% it is greater than 6.5 mmol/L, and in 5% it is greater than 7.8 mmol/L.

Serum cholesterol levels can vary by up to 20% through the course of the day (current guidelines are based on the sample being taken while the patient is fasting).

Despite guidelines and all the research done in this area there are still areas where thoughts are changing, such as primary prevention with statins for men and women over 69 years of age. As yet the evidence of benefit is not thought to be certain.

Primary prevention evidence
Treatment is advised (BHS and NICE) if the 10-year cardiovascular risk is greater than 20%. If the risk is 10–20%, you need to take local advice in terms of resources, although such patients are at a moderately high risk of developing cardiovascular problems and may benefit from treatment. The number needed to treat (to prevent one death over five years) is 69.

Treatment in primary prevention is difficult despite risk assessment tools, especially when you consider potential cost. Diet and secondary causes should always be looked at in the first instance.

- AF/TexCAPS (Air Force/ Texas Coronary Atherosclerosis Prevention Study): primary prevention study comparing placebo vs. lovastatin 20–40 mg. The study was of 5608 middle-aged males (997 females were included) with a 7-year follow-up. There was a 34% decrease in new events; this became evident after six months of treatment.
- WOSCOPS (West of Scotland Coronary Prevention Study): primary prevention in high risk male patients. There was a 22% decrease in mortality and a 25% decrease in coronary events.
- ASCOT (Anglo-Scandinavian Cardiac Outcomes Trial): this trial looked at adding atorvastatin to antihypertensive treatment in patients with a normal cholesterol level. It found a 30% reduction in myocardial infarction and stroke. The trial was stopped two years early and there are huge financial implications for the NHS.

National Institute for Health and Clinical Excellence. *Statins for prevention of cardiovascular events: NICE quick reference guideline.* **London: NIHCE; 2006**
www.nice.org.uk/nicemedia/pdf/TA094quickrefguide.pdf
This is quite straightforward guidance stating that patients with a cardiovascular risk of 20% or over should be offered statin treatment.

Lipid modification guidance is currently under way and expected to be published later in 2008.

Secondary prevention evidence

- 4S Study (Scandinavian Simvastatin Survival Study)
  This was a triple blind Scandinavian study (94 centres) of 4444 patients aged 35–70 years (81.4% of whom were male) with coronary heart disease (angina or myocardial infarction). Only 37% were on aspirin and 57% were on beta-blockers. It compared placebo vs. 20 mg simvastatin and there was a follow-up of 5.4 years.

  There was a decreased number of coronary events (42% reduction in mortality; RR 0.58; CI 0.46–0.73), and a decrease in cardiovascular mortality (35%; RR 0.65; CI 0.52–0.8).
- LIPID (Long Term Intervention with Pravastatin in IHD)
  In this study, 9000 patients with ischaemic heart disease were randomised to either placebo or pravastatin. There was a 25% decrease in mortality, cardiac events and procedures (six-year follow-up). A trial follow-up in 2002 reinforced the initial findings.
- CARE (Cholesterol and Recurrent Events Trial)
  Post-myocardial infarction patients were treated with pravastatin or placebo.

There was a five-year follow-up. There was a 22% decrease in mortality, 33% decrease in CHD, and a 20–31% decrease in stroke.

◆ MRC/BHF Heart Protection Study 2002

This was a randomised trial (20 536 people including 2000 who were at increased risk of cardiovascular disease, and 3000 people with diabetes but no history of cardiovascular disease) of simvastatin and antioxidant supplementation (vitamin E, C and β-carotene). It found randomisation to vitamins had no effect on vascular (or other) disease, but appeared safe. It found that simvastatin 40 mg (as compared to placebo) was associated with a reduction in all causes of mortality of 14% ($p < 0.001$), despite 15% stopping therapy because of side effects. It also found a 17% reduction in vascular deaths ($p < 0.0001$) with no significant effect on non-vascular deaths.

Statin treatment (alongside lifestyle advice) should be offered to all patients with atherosclerotic disease to reduce cholesterol to less than 5 mmol/L (this will become 4 mmol/L) or by 30%, whichever is the greater reduction.

The number needed to treat (NNT) to prevent one death over five years is 16. (Another NNT quoted is 91 over two years.)

Ezetimibe

This is a new cholesterol-lowering drug option. It works as a selective inhibitor of intestinal cholesterol absorption and can be used in addition to a statin to achieve cholesterol target (once statin is at the maximum dose, or if a statin is not tolerated). There are limited data so far.

National Institute for Health and Clinical Excellence. *Ezetimibe for the treatment of primary (heterozygous-familial and non-familial) hypercholesterolaemia: NICE quick reference guideline.* **London: NIHCE; 2007**
www.nice.org.uk/nicemedia/pdf/TA132QRGFINAL.pdf
Advocated use of ezetimibe:

◆ monotherapy, where a patient is intolerant of statin
◆ add-in therapy if targets are not met when taking maximum (tolerated) dose of statin.

Role of plant stanols and sterols

A low-fat, high-fibre diet with five portions of fruit and vegetables (although we understand that more is probably beneficial) has been advocated for many years. Plant stanols are naturally occurring but have come to our attention with the launch in the supermarkets of Benecol and Flora Pro-active (1 teaspoon a day is the maximum needed for cholesterol-lowering effects). Phytosterols and stanols compete with cholesterol for intestinal absorption, lowering serum cholesterol concentrations.

Moderately elevated plant sterol levels are associated with reduced cardiovascular risk – LASA study

Atherosclerosis 2008; 196: 283–8

One current thought is that elevation of plant sterols in the circulation may reduce coronary heart disease. This study was designed to look at the association. Over 65 years, 1242 people (in the Longitudinal Aging Study Amsterdam (LASA)), were looked at. High plasma concentrations of a marker plant sterol, sitosterol, were associated with reduced risk for coronary heart disease (OR 0.78, CI 0.62–0.98, $p < 0.05$). The study concluded that plant sterols could have neutral or even protective effects on the development of coronary heart disease.

Cardiovascular disease and antiplatelets

Aspirin has been advised for primary and secondary prevention of cardiovascular disease in high-risk patients for many years. Although not completely supported by evidence, healthy patients use it for many reasons, including to reduce the risk of bowel cancer and Alzheimer's disease.

Aspirin works by blocking cyclo-oxygenase, which then has the knock-on effect of reducing platelet aggregation (through reduction in thromboxane A2 and prostacycline). Clopidogrel inhibits platelet aggregation by interacting with the platelet ADP receptor.

The *MeRec Bulletin* July 2005 (volume 15) gave an excellent overview of options and recommendations for the use of antiplatelets in primary and secondary prevention. It can be summarised as follows:

- primary prevention
  - low dose aspirin (75 mg/day) should be considered in all patients over 50 years with a 10-year cardiovascular risk greater than 20%
  - clopidogrel and MR-dipyridamole are not indicated or licensed for primary prevention.
- secondary prevention
  - low dose aspirin (75 mg/day) is recommended for indefinite use following a myocardial infarction and in people with symptomatic peripheral arterial disease
  - MR-dipyridamole (200 mg twice daily) plus aspirin (75 mg/day) is recommended for a period of two years after an ischaemic stroke or TIA, from the most recent event
  - clopidogrel (75 mg/day) is a suitable alternative to aspirin (or aspirin plus dipyridamole post-stroke) where aspirin is not tolerated (even with a proton-pump inhibitor) or contra-indicated
  - clopidogrel (75 mg/day) plus aspirin (75 mg/day) for a period of 12 months should be considered in patients with a non-ST-segment-elevation acute coronary syndrome who are at moderate to high risk of a further

myocardial infarction or death. Thereafter treatment should revert to aspirin (75 mg/day).

Aspirin dose for the prevention of cardiovascular disease: a systematic review
JAMA 2007; 297: 2018-24

This review looked at aspirin dose, efficacy and safety. The meta-analysis looked at trials involving 5228 patients and found no evidence to support use of aspirin doses above 75–81 mg a day.

Aspirin 'resistance' and risk of cardiovascular morbidity: systematic review and meta-analysis
BMJ 2008; 336: 195-8

This was a meta-analysis of 20 studies including 2930 patients, to try to establish why some patients do not benefit from aspirin. A total of 810 patients (28%) were resistant to aspirin (based on thromboxane A2 in relation to platelet haemostasis or other suitable assay). This group was found to be at greater risk of death, acute coronary syndrome, failure of intervention and new cerebrovascular events.

Incidence of death and acute myocardial infarction associated with stopping clopidogrel after acute coronary syndrome
JAMA 2008; 299: 532-9

This study found a prothrombotic effect in patients who had just stopped taking clopidogrel, with heart attack and death peaking at 90 days, the duration of clopidogrel treatment having no effect. Of the 3137 patient group, death or AMI occurred in 17.1% (n = 268) with 60.8% (n = 163) of events occurring during 0 to 90 days, 21.3% (n = 57) during 91 to 180 days, and 9.7% (n = 26) during 181 to 270 days after stopping treatment with clopidogrel. A number of suggestions have been forthcoming following publication of the study: leaving people on clopidogrel (although this would have financial implications), a gradual reduction in dose, or a temporary bridging with a higher dose of aspirin.

The polypill

It was proposed by Wald and Law, in 2003, that the polypill would be a medication containing six ingredients: a statin, aspirin, folic acid and three antihypertensives (all at half strength). Initial thoughts were that it should be given to everyone over the age of 55 years (with or without existing cardiovascular disease) without screening, the aim being to reduce the risk of ischaemic heart disease events by up to 88% and stroke by up to 80%. This would be achieved by reducing four risk factors: blood pressure, platelet function, lipid and homocysteine concentrations.

There have been no new papers of any great significance on this subject. Although reducing blood pressure, reducing cholesterol and using aspirin are thought to have a beneficial effect (especially in those aged over 55) there are on-going concerns about the use of this across a population. Questions arise, such as whether this would mean people would be less likely to come for a blood pressure checkup; whether it would create missed opportunities for health promotion; and the risk of side effects.

Revisiting Rose: strategies for reducing coronary heart disease
BMJ 2006; 332: 659-62

This is an excellent paper on preventative healthcare, with an accompanying editorial. It discusses the point that strategies currently used work on the principle that the risk is widely distributed, whereas large national samples show that those at risk are only a modest proportion of the population. The authors looked at updating Rose's work using three different strategies:

✦ population health strategy – lowering cholesterol in the entire population
✦ single raised risk factor strategy – treating if the cholesterol is greater than 6.2 mmol/L
✦ high baseline risk strategy – treating those with increased risk.

Wald and Law had expressed the opinion that CHD could be reduced by 80% if men and women over 55 took the polypill, but this is probably unlikely as adherence and response to treatment differs and is difficult to assess. Population health strategies should focus on population risk using the best available methods.

Atrial fibrillation (AF)

AF is the most common tachydysrhythmia diagnosed on ECG. It is important to diagnose, as it may be the first sign of heart disease and is an important risk factor for strokes. There is no known cause in 20–30% of cases; however the majority of cases are associated with hypertension or structural valvular disease.

The prevalence of AF is 1.5% up to 60 years of age, increasing to 8% at 90 years of age. The annual risk of stroke (from emboli from the left atrium) increases from 6.7% in the 50–59 year age band to around 36% in the 80–89 year band.

The NICE guidance gives an excellent overview of treatment with algorithms of different options.

Anticoagulation

In discussing this, it is important to differentiate between atrial fibrillation (sustained or paroxysmal) with or without valve problems, and patients being warfarinised prior to cardioversion. It is important to consider rate control as well as rhythm.

Many trials have shown that warfarin is superior to aspirin (for both primary and secondary prevention) at reducing thromboembolism in non-rheumatic AF by up to 68% (compared with 28%). However these studies are generally based on patients in secondary care with higher risks; the selected/excluded patient groups have been chosen quite strictly and have been well monitored. Most of the studies compared either aspirin or warfarin to placebo.

Warfarin has also been compared with aspirin and clopidogrel in combination and has been found to be superior and to have less risk of bleeding.

National Institute for Health and Clinical Excellence. *Atrial fibrillation: the management of atrial fibrillation: NICE clinical guideline 36.* London: NIHCE; 2006
www.nice.org.uk/nicemedia/pdf/CG036niceguideline.pdf

Aguilar MI, Hart R, Pearce LA. Oral anticoagulants versus antiplatelet therapy for preventing stroke in patients with non-valvular atrial fibrillation and no history of stroke or transient ischaemic attacks. *Cochrane Database Syst Rev.* 2007 Jul 18; (3): CD006186
This reports on eight randomised trials of 9598 patients looking at warfarin vs. aspirin (75 to 325 mg/day) and a mean follow-up of 1.9 years/patient.

Adjusted-dose warfarin and related oral anticoagulants reduce stroke, disabling stroke and other major vascular events for those with non-valvular AF by about one-third when compared with antiplatelet therapy. Oral anticoagulants reduced all stroke (odds ratio (OR) 0.68, 95% confidence interval (CI) 0.54–0.85); ischaemic stroke (OR 0.53, 95% CI 0.41–0.68); and systemic emboli (OR 0.48, 95% CI 0.25–0.90). Disabling or fatal strokes (OR 0.71, 95% CI 0.59–1.04) and myocardial infarctions (OR 0.69, 95% CI 0.47–1.01) were substantially but not significantly reduced by oral anticoagulants. Vascular deaths (OR 0.93, 95% CI 0.75–1.15) and all-cause mortality (OR 0.99, 95% CI 0.83 to 1.18), were similar with these treatments.

Intracranial haemorrhages (OR 1.98, 95% CI 1.20–3.28) were increased by oral anticoagulant therapy.

Aspirin and warfarin
www.nice.org.uk/nicemedia/pdf/CG036niceguideline.pdf
It is not clear whether certain groups of patients (following myocardial infarction or a stent implant) may get an additional therapeutic effect using both warfarin and aspirin, or whether the increased risk of bleeding outweighs the benefits.

This was also discussed in the MeRec No.28 in terms that, although it could be considered in those at high risk of having a thromboembolism, it would need to be put in the context of the increased risk of bleeding.

Combined aspirin-oral anticoagulation therapy compared with oral anticoagulation therapy alone among patients at risk for cardiovascular disease
Arch Intern Med 2007; 167: 117-24
This study looked at ten randomised trials (4180 patients) followed up over at

least three months: five studies in mechanical valves, two in atrial fibrillation, two with coronary heart disease and one primary prevention study.

Overall there was a reduction in arterial thromboembolism (including myocardial infarction, unstable angina and stroke) with combined therapy (NNT 40). There was a greater incidence of bleeding for combined therapy.

Don't add aspirin for associated stable vascular disease in a patient with AF receiving anticoagulation
BMJ 2008; 336: 614–15

This discusses the evidence for and against adding aspirin. The thought that aspirin would be beneficial has been based on the concept of antiplatelets working on the platelet-rich thrombus (white clot) whilst warfarin works on the fibrin-rich thrombus (red clot). Despite this theory, there is no solid supporting evidence that addition of aspirin reduces stroke and vascular events. It does, however, increase the risk of bleeding.

Screening

Screening is currently being considered as an option in an attempt to reduce the risk of strokes. Almost without realising, we selectively screen patients with every blood pressure we take, pulse we feel, heart we listen to and ECG we perform. The study below looked at formalising the process.

Screening versus routine practice in detection of AF in patients aged 65 or over: a cluster randomised controlled trial
BMJ 2007; 335 (7616): 383–6

This study randomised 14 802 patients to either an intervention practice or a control practice. The follow-up was over a 12-month period.

The intervention group was then further randomised to either systematic screening with ECG or opportunistic screening with a pulse check, followed by an ECG if this was irregular. No screening took place in the control practices.

Rates of new cases of atrial fibrillation were:
- intervention practice
  - 1.62% in the systematically screened group
  - 1.64% in the opportunistically screened group
- control practice
  - 1.04% (as compared to an average of 1.63% in the intervention practices, a difference of 0.59%, CI 0.2–0.98).

The paper summarised that the preferred method was opportunistic screening (which brings us back to what we do on a daily basis).

Stroke

Stroke is defined as a sudden loss of neurological function (for which there is no other cause than a vascular one) lasting for more than 24 hours. A transient ischaemic attack (TIA) lasts less than 24 hours.

- The incidence of stroke is 2 in 1000 (double this in 45–84 year olds).
- It is the third most common cause of death in the UK and the greatest single cause of disability, affecting 130 000 people per year.
- Around 80% of all strokes are ischaemic.
- Six months after the event, 50% of patients are physically dependent on others.
- The incidence of TIA is 0.4 in 1000 (the future risk of stroke is 10% in the first year and 5% thereafter).
- There is a 1–2% risk of a myocardial infarction following TIA.

A simple score (ABCD) to identify individuals at high early risk of stroke after TIA
Lancet 2005; 366: 29–36

Deciding which patients need emergency assessment following a TIA is an important part of our initial management in general practice (although the gold standard is that all should be investigated within seven days) and this article outlines a simple scoring system to assist decision making.

The criteria used were:

ABCD	Meaning	Question	Score
A	Age	< 60 years	0
		> 60 years	1
B	Blood Pressure	Systolic >140 mmHg and/or diastolic >90 mmHg	1
C	Clinical features	Unilateral weakness	2
		Speech disturbance, no weakness	1
		Other	0
D	Duration of symptoms	60 minutes	2
		10–59 minutes	1
		< 10 minutes	0

A score greater than 5/8 was predictive (in up to 24% of the 190 patients) of a subsequent stroke within seven days of a TIA.

Interestingly, the system does not use smoking history/pack years; nor, as it is part of the initial assessment, does it include cholesterol.

Standard Five – Stroke
Older People's National Service Framework

The outcome for stroke patients is better, and their stay is usually shorter, if cared for by specialist teams in stroke units.

Standard Five specifically states:
+ people who are thought to have had a stroke should have access to diagnostic and specialist stroke services
+ subsequently they, and their carers, should participate in a multidisciplinary programme of secondary prevention and rehabilitation (e.g. speech therapy, occupational therapy, physiotherapy, social services, district nurse support, etc).

National Stroke Strategy

The Department of Health has set a target to reduce the death rate from stroke and cardiovascular disease by 40% in people aged less than 75 years. The development of the strategy included six key areas.
+ Public awareness and prevention – recognising emergency admission to hospital along with primary and secondary preventative measures.
+ TIA Services – rapid access to diagnostics and treatment.
+ Emergency response – recognition that early treatment improves outcome.
+ Hospital stroke care – by specialist stroke units.
+ Post-hospital stroke care – rehabilitation in the community with long term services where needed.
+ Workforce – ensuring development of skills to allow implementation of the strategy.

Targeting risk factors in primary and secondary prevention
Hypertension

Hypertension accounts for up to 50% of ischaemic strokes.

The British Hypertension Society guidelines state that hypertension persisting more than one month after a stroke should be treated (other sources state from two weeks). Stroke risk can be reduced by up to 40% if the diastolic BP is reduced by 6 mmHg or the systolic BP is reduced by 10–12 mmHg (irrespective of whether the BP is elevated or not).

Role of blood pressure and other variables in the differential cardiovascular event rates noted in the Anglo-Scandinavian Cardiac Outcomes Trial - blood pressure lowering arm (ASCOT-BPLA)
Lancet 2005; 366(9489): 869–71

This showed significantly lower rates of stroke in the amlodipine regime versus the atenolol regime. The significance was not fully understood and may be statistical rather than a real finding in this group of patients.

Heart Outcomes Prevention Study (HOPE)
NEJM 2002; 347: 145-53

This was a ramipril study showing a 32% decrease in stroke incidence in patients with controlled blood pressure. It made the case for all patients having an angiotensin converting enzyme inhibitor irrespective of their blood pressure.

Antiplatelet drugs
National Institute for Health and Clinical Excellence. *Clopidogrel and modified release dipyridamole in the prevention of occlusive vascular events: NICE technology appraisal 90.* **London: NIHCE; 2005**
www.nice.org.uk/nicemedia/pdf/TA090guidance.pdf

It is recommended after an ischaemic stroke or TIA:
- dipyridamole and aspirin be used in combination for two years after the most recent event; thereafter (or if dipyridamole is not tolerated) aspirin should be used
- clopidogrel be used for patients who are intolerant of aspirin.

Give dipyridamole with aspirin instead of aspirin alone to prevent vascular events after ischaemic stroke or TIA
BMJ 2007; 334: 901

This is an interesting article on changing our practice in medicine, specifically in relation to prescribing both aspirin and dipyridamole for patients following a stroke or TIA, as this reduces the risk for vascular events by a fifth as compared to prescribing aspirin alone. The discussion is focused around the European stroke prevention study (ESPS-2) and the European/Australasian stoke prevention in reversible ischaemia trial (ESPRIT), both of which show that there is a reduction in vascular events by using aspirin with dipyridamole.

Medium intensity oral anticoagulants versus aspirin after cerebral ischaemia or arterial origin (ESPRIT): a randomised controlled trial
Lancet Neurol 2007; 6(2): 115-24

This was an international, multicentre trial where 2739 patients were randomly assigned after a TIA or minor stroke to either anticoagulants or aspirin. Anticoagulants were compared with the combination of aspirin and dipyridamole (200 mg twice daily) and there was a mean follow-up of 4.6 years. A primary outcome event (death from a vascular cause, non-fatal stroke or myocardial infarction or major bleeding) occurred in 99 (19%) patients on anticoagulants and in 98 (18%) patients on aspirin. Oral anticoagulants (target INR range 2.0–3.0) were not found to be more effective than aspirin for secondary prevention after transient ischaemic attack or minor stroke of arterial origin.

Anticoagulation in atrial fibrillation

Atrial fibrillation increases the risk of stroke six fold.

Warfarin was previously the drug of choice for prevention of stroke in AF. Several randomised controlled trials confirmed the benefit and low complication rate (0.4%). The number needed to treat to prevent one stroke was 11.

Systematic review of long term anticoagulation or antiplatelet treatment in patients with non-rheumatic AF
BMJ 2001; 322: 321-6

This review found no added benefit in *non-rheumatic AF*. Previous meta-analyses had not included these trials.

There were 3298 patients (thought to be too low a number, as around 5000 are needed).

Individual trials were small and used slightly different international normalised ratios to monitor warfarin.

Forty-five per cent of patients were more likely to bleed on warfarin (even within the controlled setting of trial). It was concluded that there was no obvious benefit to using warfarin.

Cholesterol

Statins are indicated as part of a secondary prevention treatment plan for patients following a stroke or TIA. Guidance on statin use for primary prevention includes patients with a 10-year coronary heart disease risk of 20%.

The Heart Protection Study
Lancet 2002; 360: 7-20

This study of the treatment of high-risk CHD looked at treatment of high-risk CHD patients with simvastatin and found that simvastatin reduced the incidence of stroke by up to 25%.

The Stroke Prevention by Aggressive Reduction in Cholesterol Levels (SPARCL) investigators. High dose atorvastatin after stroke or TIA
NEJM 2006; 355: 549-59

This study compared atorvastatin 80 mg to placebo in 4731 patients over a 4.9-year follow-up period. It found that there was a reduction in further TIA and other cardiovascular events (by 1.9%, $p = 0.05$) although this was slightly offset by an increased risk in haemorrhagic stroke.

Carotid endarterectomy

If there is a symptomatic stenosis, the benefit of surgery relates to the degree of stenosis. This is classified as mild–moderate–severe (Cochrane Review 2003).

Carotid endarterectomy for asymptomatic carotid stenosis reduces the risk of stroke by 30% over three years (Cochrane Review 2005).

See also www.eGuidelines.co.uk for information based on the Royal College of Physician's Guidelines for stroke management (published 2002). Their most recent publication is Stroke Transfer Care (August 2005), which takes you through care and rehabilitation in primary care.

Smoking

Smoking is the number-one preventable cause of ill health (120 000 deaths/year).

- One in four adults in the UK smokes (13 million in total in the UK).
- The cost to the NHS is £1500 million/year.
- Seventy per cent of smokers want to stop (National Statistics 2000).
- Smoking cessation by someone with angina may decrease their chances of having a myocardial infarction by up to 50%.
- Smoking data accounts for 87 of the quality indicator points in the GMS contract (2004).

Since 1 July 2007 there has been a ban on smoking in enclosed public places and work places (including company cars in some instances).

Some useful smoking cessation websites are:

- www.quit.org.uk
- www.click2quit.com

1998 White Paper Smoking Kills

In this framework for the NHS on smoking cessation, funding was initially guaranteed only in New Health Action Zones before being rolled out nationally.

It was recommended that practitioners should:

- assess smoking 'at every opportunity'!
- advise patients to stop smoking
- provide accurate information
- recommend nicotine replacement therapy (NRT)
- refer patients to specialist services as necessary
- follow up patients.

February 2000 Royal College of Physicians initiative on 'Nicotine Addiction in Britain'

The study suggested:

- Government should provide access to evidence-based smoking cessation service
- NRT is effective and should be available by NHS prescription
- GPs give brief advice at least once a year – if there is a positive response they should refer to a smoking cessation clinic.

Intervention	Success rate at 1 year
Brief opportunistic advice from GP	2%
Face-to-face behavioural support from specialist	7%
Nicotine gum	5%
Zyban (300 mg/day)	9%
Behavioural support in clinic with NRT or Zyban	13-19%

Managing smoking cessation
BMJ 2007; 335: 37

This clinical review looks at published evidence and gives a good review.

Despite the concern that there is little enough time in a consultation, what we say to our patients in that time has been shown to make a difference. It considers the treatments available and nicotine replacement therapy. Buprenorphine and varenicline are considered first line (also advocated by NICE guidance), nortriptyline would be second line.

National Institute for Health and Clinical Excellence. *Brief interventions and referral for smoking cessation in primary care and other settings: NICE public health intervention guidance 1.* London: NIHCE; 2006
www.nice.org.uk/nicemedia/pdf/SMOKING-ALS2_FINAL.pdf

This guidance summarised such interventions as offering opportunistic advice, discussion, negotiation and encouragement, usually taking 5–10 minutes; and outlined four recommendations.

+ Everyone who smokes should be advised to quit, unless there are exceptional circumstances.
+ People should be asked how interested they are in quitting.
+ We should take the opportunity to encourage people to quit at every consultation and refer to services to help them. Where patients are unable to use these services they should be offered pharmacotherapies.
+ Nurses in primary care should also be recommending smoking cessation.

Smoking Cessation Action in Primary Care Taskforce (SCAPE) – Launched September 2001

The aim of this initiative was to encourage GPs and practice nurses to maintain the impetus of smoking cessation services.

+ It suggests the 30-second approach:
  - do you smoke?
  - would you like to stop?
  - would you like my help to stop?

The aim is to catch people at the right point of the cycle of change to help them engage with services.

- A major concern of GPs (in a survey published by SCAPE in May 2001) is workload implications.
- With regard to smoking cessation, 93% of GPs thought it was 'the best thing you could do for their health'.
- Around 91% of GPs put off advising patients to stop because of time pressures.

Mortality among never-smokers living with smokers: two cohort studies 1981–4 and 1996–9
BMJ 2004; 328: 988–9
This New Zealand study followed two cohorts for three years, looking at mortality. They found that in adults who had never smoked but who had exposure to second-hand smoke in the home, there was an increased mortality (around 15%) compared to never-smokers who lived in a smoke-free environment.

Diabetes

The prevalence of diabetes in the UK is 3% (10% in those over 65 years of age).
- There are 33 000 deaths per year due to diabetes.
- Life expectancy is reduced by up to 20 years in type 1, and 10 years in type 2 diabetes.
- Seventy per cent of mortality in diabetes is related to cardiovascular disease.

Diabetes is a complex multisystem disease. For effective management you need, preferably, a co-ordinated patient-centred approach with set standards and a computerised register. It is a common disease, the incidence of which is estimated to rise by 25% over the next decade due to the aging population, obesity, sedentary lifestyle and other factors. St. Vincent's declaration, ratified by the WHO regional committee for Europe in 1991, set aspirations and goals for reducing the impact of diabetes.

Diagnosis
The criteria for diagnosis were agreed by the World Health Organisation in June 2000.
- *Diabetic symptoms* with random venous glucose concentration greater than 11.1 mmol/L, or fasting BM greater than 7.0 mmol/L, or 2 hr BM greater than 11.1 mmol/L after 75 gm glucose tolerance test.
- *No symptoms* – do not diagnose on a single glucose measurement, but do a repeat plasma test (same values apply as above).

Patients should be classified according to pathological type (i.e. type 1 or 2) and then by stage (i.e. insulin dependent or not).

The implications of these changes are that more people will be diagnosed as being diabetic (most will be diet controlled). Hopefully, long-term complications will be reduced but in the meantime the workload for primary care will be substantial.

Research presented at the European Association for the Study of Diabetes in September 2001 emphasised that even the new WHO guidelines on oral glucose tolerance test (OGTT) (for those with plasma glucose 6.1–6.9 mmol/L) would miss up to 20% of people with impaired glucose tolerance and recommended that OGTT be performed at 5.0–6.9 mmol/L. Even using this range, 11% of diabetes would go undetected.

National Service Framework for Diabetes (2003 Delivery Strategy)
www.dh.gov.uk/en/Publicationsandstatistics/Publications/PublicationsPolicyAndGuidance/DH_4003246

The document states that 'all adults with diabetes will receive high quality care throughout their lifetime, including support to optimise the control of their blood sugar'.

It includes 12 standards in nine areas of diabetic care.

1 Prevention of type 2 diabetes:
  • Multiagency approach to reduce the number of people who are inactive, overweight and obese.
  • Physical education and a balanced diet need to be promoted from childhood.
2 Identification of people with diabetes:
  Follow up of those at increased risk – gestational diabetics, known family history, ischaemic heart disease, obesity and ethnicity.
3 Empowering people with diabetes:
  • Has been shown to reduce blood glucose and improve quality of life.
  • Could involve structured education, personal care plans and patient-held records.
4 Clinical care of adults with diabetes:
  Would include management of diabetes, hypertension, smoking cessation, all aimed at improving measurements and quality of life.
5 Clinical care of children with diabetes:
  Similar high quality care as with adults. It would also include physical, psychological, intellectual, educational and social development needs.
6 Clinical care of young people with diabetes:
  As above.
7 Management of diabetic emergencies:
  Diabetic ketoacidosis (DKA), hyperosmolar non-ketotic syndrome (HONK) and hypoglycaemia.

8 Care of people with diabetes during admission to hospital:
   Outcome could be improved by better liaison between diabetes team and ward
   staff.
9 Diabetes and pregnancy:
   Policies will be developed for women with pre-existing diabetes and those who
   develop diabetes to help achieve blood pressure control before and during
   pregnancy.
10, 11 and 12 – Detection and management of long-term complications:
   - Regular surveillance for long-term complications.
   - Effective treatment and investigation for complications.
   - Integrated health and social care.

Effective diabetes care: a need for realistic targets
BMJ 2002; 324: 1577-80 (Education and Debate)
Aggressive treatment of hyperglycaemia, dyslipidaemia and hypertension as well
as the regular use of antiplatelet agents has been advocated in type 2 diabetes.

Current targets are attainable in only 50–70% of individuals.

Targets are often impractical and involve so many drugs that the patient will
not comply with treatment. Individually tailored targets are needed and their
effectiveness will be shown by improvement in diabetic clinics.

Training in flexible intensive insulin management to enable dietary freedom in people with type I diabetes: dose adjustments for normal eating (DAFNE) RCT
BMJ 2002; 325: 746-9
This secondary care study from the UK looked at 169 adults with type 1 diabetes
with moderate or poor glycaemic control. It was found that at six months the
group that had been given training that promoted dietary freedom had a better
quality of life, better glycaemic control (HbA1C mean 8.4% compared to 9.4% in
non-trained) and the number of hypoglycaemic episodes was no worse.

The DAFNE programme offers a week-long intensive training course in small
groups working with specialist nurses and dietitians. The course costs £500 and
is awaiting consideration by NICE.

The new treatment framework for diabetes can be summarised as follows:
- tools of intensive management are presented as a means to increase freedom
  in a patient's life
- the focus is on developing an insulin regimen that is flexible and fits into the
  demands of life
- the implicit message is that you can have good diabetes control without
  having to yield control of your life to diabetes.

Type 2 diabetes
www.nice.org.uk/nicemedia/pdf/CG66NICEGuideline.pdf

Management of blood glucose
+ HbA1C should be measured 2–6 monthly and may be above 6.5%; the guidance advised against pursuing highly intensive management of <6.5%.
+ Weight loss (5–10% if obese) and physical activity should be encouraged if the patient is overweight.

Management of blood pressure and lipids
+ If there is no ischaemic heart disease an annual risk assessment should be made using the UKPDS risk engine. If the risk is greater than 20% over 10 years then a statin should be started to reduce the cholesterol below 4.0 mmol/L.
+ Blood pressure should be checked yearly; add treatment if it is greater than 140/80 mmHg and lifestyle changes have not improved the blood pressure (130/80 if renal, eye or cerebrovascular disease).
+ Aspirin should be started in patients over 50 with a blood pressure <145/90 mmHg, and those under 50 who have significant other cardiovascular risks.

Joint British Societies 2 suggested targets
Heart 2005; 91 (suppl5): v1–v52
+ Glycated haemoglobin less than 6.5%.
+ Blood pressure less than 130/80 mmHg.
+ Total cholesterol less than 4.0 mmol/L.
+ Aspirin therapy.

HbA1C <7.0 What is the Evidence?
(NICE 2008 is aiming for 6.5%, the Quality and Outcomes Framework (QOF) 7.5%)

Although we aspire to good glucose control there are often practical problems with the medication and lifestyle, as well as the risk of hypoglycaemic episodes.

Safety of tight glucose control in type 2 diabetes
BMJ 2008; 336: 458–9

This editorial considers the glucose-lowering arm of the ACCORD trial, looking at people at risk of cardiovascular disease with type 2 diabetes. It has been stopped 18 months early because of safety concerns. Intensively lowering glucose to less than 6% increased the risk of death compared with the less intensive treatment (7–7.9%). This was in contrast to the ADVANCE trial, which showed the opposite (although in a smaller group of patients).

Glycaemic Control and type 2 Diabetes: the Optimal Haemoglobin A1C targets. A guidance statement from the American College of Physicians

Ann Intern Med 2007; 147(6): 416–22

This is an evaluation based on the various guidelines recommending:

- to prevent microvascular complications of diabetes, the goal for glycaemic control should be as low as is feasible without undue risk for adverse events or an unacceptable burden on patients
- treatment goals should be based on a discussion of the benefits and harms of specific levels of glycaemic control with the patient
- a haemoglobin A1C level less than 7% based on individualised assessment
- further research to assess the optimal level of glycaemic control, particularly in the presence of comorbid conditions.

Diabetes Control and Complications Trial (DCCT)

NEJM 2000; 342: 381–5 (the long-term FU publication)

A total of 1441 patients was followed over a period of 6.5 years while they received either intensive treatment or conventional treatment. Intensive treatment improved microvascular and neuropathic complications. These improvements correlated with decreased HbA1C levels. The intensive treatment group did have more hypoglycaemic episodes (so this would be a less favourable approach in children younger than 13 years and adults older than 70 years).

UK Prospective Diabetes Study 33 (UKPDS 33)

Lancet 1998; 352: 837–53 and 854–65

The UKPDS is a large ongoing study of type 2 diabetes involving around 5000 patients. It was set up in 1977. It looked at newly-diagnosed diabetics and treated them with diet for three months. If their HbA1C remained elevated they were entered into the trial.

   Findings:

- intensive treatment (average HbA1C 7% over the first 10 years) reduced the frequency of microvascular end points
- in overweight patients with non-insulin dependent diabetes, metformin and dietary improvement reduced the risk of diabetes-related end-points by 32%, and diabetic deaths by 42%
- blood pressure control of less than 150/85 mmHg reduced microvascular complications and diabetic-related deaths (there were similar findings in HOT Study, where blood pressure was reduced to <130/80 mmHg)
- around 50% of diabetics had early signs of complications at time of diagnosis (this raises the importance of screening).

UKPDS 35

BMJ 2000; 321: 405–12

Each 1% reduction in HbA1C was associated with risk reduction of 21% for diabetic end-points; 21% related to diabetic deaths; 14% for myocardial infarction and 37% for microvascular complications.

The case against aggressive treatment of type 2 diabetes: critique of UKPDS

BMJ 2001; 323: 854–8

UKPDS grew out of the author's interest in the use of basal rather than post-prandial glucose. The first report was published in 1983. During the course of the study, length of follow-up has changed and end points have been redefined. The study is not blinded, the statistical analyses used have been questioned and the changes have not been in keeping with scientific principles.

Hypertension in diabetes

Around 70% of adults with type 2 diabetes have hypertension and more than 70% have raised cholesterol levels.

British Hypertension Society (BHS) guidelines based on the HOT Trial, 2000

* Start treatment if blood pressure is greater than 140 mmHg systolic or greater than 90 mmHg diastolic.
* Aim for a blood pressure 130/80 mmHg or 125/75 mmHg if there is proteinuria (this is more tight than the NICE guidance).
* Less than 30% of cases respond to monotherapy.
* *Do not forget* non-pharmacological treatment.

UK Prospective Diabetes Study 36 (and 49)

BMJ 2000; 321: 412–19

In type 2 diabetes the risk of diabetic complications is strongly associated with raised blood pressure. Any reduction in BP is likely to reduce the risk of complications. The lowest risk seen is in those diabetics with a systolic BP less than 120 mmHg.

Intensive BP control is at least as important (if not more so) than intensive blood glucose control.

For systolic blood pressure, each 10 mmHg decrease is associated with a risk reduction of 12% for any complications related to diabetes (15% for deaths related to diabetes, 11% for myocardial infarction and 13% for microvascular complications).

Trials

There are many more trials showing the clinical benefit of blood pressure lowering in reduction of risk (below is listed a small selection). Reference BHS, NICE and your local guidelines if you would like to look into references for a more comprehensive understanding of the trials that underpin the guidance.

◆ Hypertension Optimal Treatment (HOT) randomised trial

Effects of intensive blood pressure lowering and low dose aspirin in patients with hypertension: principal results of the HOT trial
Lancet 1998; 351: 1755-62

The results showed low rates of cardiovascular events if raised blood pressure was lowered. There were benefits of lowering diastolic blood pressure to 82.6 mmHg and there was a 50% decrease in major cardiovascular events with a target diastolic of 80 mmHg in diabetics compared to 90 mmHg.

Acetyl salicylic acid reduced major cardiovascular events, especially myocardial infarction. There was no effect on incidence of stroke or fatal bleeding and non-fatal major bleeds were twice as common.

◆ HOPE and Micro-HOPE (Health Outcomes Prevention Evaluation)

Effects of Ramipril on cardiovascular and microvascular outcomes in people with diabetes mellitus
Lancet 2000; 355: 253-59

A total of 3577 diabetic patients aged 55 years and over were randomised to ramipril 10 mg/day or placebo and then vitamin E or placebo.

Ramipril had a beneficial effect on cardiovascular events (which decreased by 25 to 30%) and on overt nephropathy in people with diabetes. The benefit was greater than that attributable to the decrease in blood pressure.

Vasculoprotective and renoprotective effects of ramipril in diabetics were seen.

Obesity in diabetes

In 1973, following research by Sims, the phrase 'diabesity' was introduced, emphasising the link between diabetes and obesity.

Up to 80% of type 2 diabetes is due to obesity (BMI greater than 27 kg/m²). The duration of obesity is significant. Weight loss improves morbidity (UKPDS 7).

Diet, lifestyle and the risk of type 2 diabetes mellitus in women
NEJM 2001; 345: 790-7

A total of 84 941 female nurses aged 30–55 years were followed from 1980 to 1996. An important risk factor was a BMI greater than 35 kg/m². Poor diet, minimal exercise, smoking and abstinence from alcohol were all associated with significant risk of developing diabetes. So it is no great surprise that lifestyle is a key risk.

Cholesterol and diabetes

The NICE guidance being reviewed recommends:

+ annual assessment of cardiovascular risk
+ starting statins (simvastatin 40 mg) if over 40 years (unless risk using the JBS tables is less than 20% over 10 years)
+ if triglycerides are greater than 4.5 mmol/L, treat with a fibrate (after excluding secondary causes).

Effect of lowering LDL cholesterol substantially below current recommended levels in patients with coronary heart disease and diabetes: the Treating to New Targets (TNT) study

Diabetes Care 2006; 29: 1220–6

This study randomised 1501 patients to either 10 mg or 80 mg atorvastatin (follow-up 4.9 years). There were significant differences between the groups in favour of atorvastatin 80 mg, observed for time to cerebrovascular event (0.69 [0.48–0.98], $p = 0.037$) and any cardiovascular event (0.85 [0.73–1.00], $p = 0.044$). No significant difference was found for adverse events or persistent elevations in liver enzymes. The study concluded that for patients with CHD and diabetes, intensive therapy with atorvastatin 80 mg reduced the rate of major cardiovascular events by 25%, compared with atorvastatin 10 mg.

Other trials

Heart Protection Study

Lancet 2003; 361: 2005–16

+ LDL cholesterol reduction of 1% reduced cardiac deaths by 25%.

Collaborative Atorvastatin Diabetes Study

Lancet 2004; 364: 685–96

+ Atorvastatin in type 2 diabetics (primary prevention) reduced the risk of major vascular events by 37%.

Aspirin in diabetes

Given the cardiovascular risk seen in diabetes, aspirin has become considered to be a 'guardian drug'. Diabetes UK (www.diabetes.org.uk) recommends offering 75 mg aspirin to people over 30 years of age in the following groups of diabetic patients:

+ known cardiovascular disease
+ dyslipidaemia (total cholesterol greater than 5 mmol/L)
+ raised blood pressure (greater than 140/80 mmHg) once it is controlled
+ microalbuminuria or albuminuria
+ family history of coronary heart disease
+ smoker

- overweight (BMI greater than 25 kg/m^2)
- Indo-Asian backgrounds
- diabetic retinopathy.

It is also recommended that aspirin is offered for all diabetic patients over 50 years (younger if diabetes has been diagnosed for more than 10 years).

Self-monitoring of blood glucose in diabetes
Drugs and Therapeutics Bulletin (DTB) 2007; 45(9): 65-9
This topic was addressed because of the huge cost of glucose sticks to the NHS. Fluctuations in blood glucose can be significant and not always linked to symptoms. Monitoring, especially when using insulin, can be a way of regulating and timing intake. Monitoring is not thought to be of benefit if patients are not acting on the results or interpreting them correctly. Diabetes UK advised (and DTB concurs) that in patients not using insulin, blood glucose monitoring may be useful as a supplement in certain situations (e.g. patients experiencing hypoglycaemia). Where insulin is used, monitoring 3–4 times a day enables better titration of insulin dose.

In pregnant women a seven-point testing approach may be needed because of greater fluctuations and unpredictability. NICE does support the use of home monitoring as part of integrated self-care.

Impact of self monitoring of blood glucose in the management of patients with non-insulin treated diabetes: open parallel group randomised trial
BMJ 2007; 335(7611): 132
This trial was structured to determine whether self-monitoring, either alone or with instruction, was more effective than usual care for improvement of glycaemic control in NIDDM. A total of 453 patients (mean age 65.7 years) was followed for three years.

The outcome measure was HbA1C at 12 months and this showed that at 12 months the differences between the three groups were not statistically significant ($p = 0.12$). Their conclusions were that self-monitoring with or without instruction did not improve glycaemic control.

Glitazones/thiazolidinediones
These drugs enhance the effects of insulin in adipose tissue and skeletal muscle by acting as ligands that regulate gene expression (i.e. they reduce the body's resistance to insulin).

An increased incidence of cardiac failure has been seen with rosiglitazone when used with insulin. It has also been linked to an increase in fracture risk. Pioglitazone has been licensed for use with insulin in the USA and both have been approved for monotherapy. It is recommended that liver function tests are checked prior to starting treatment and then at two-monthly intervals for the first year, stopping the drug if the liver enzymes rise three times the normal level or if the patient becomes jaundiced. NICE recommends their use second-line and in combination with either metformin or a sulphonylurea.

Secondary prevention of macrovascular events in patients with type 2 diabetes in the PROactive study (PROspective pioglitAzone Clinical Trial In macroVascular Events): a randomised controlled trial
Lancet 2005; 366(9493): 1241-2
A total 5238 patients with type 2 diabetes and evidence of macrovascular disease (i.e. high-risk patients) were randomised to either pioglitazone or placebo. Pioglitazone improved HbA1C by 0.8% (on average) and reduced all causes of mortality, non-fatal myocardial infarction and stroke.

Effect of rosiglitazone on the risk of myocardial infarction and death from cardiovascular causes
NEJM 2007; 356(4): 2457-71
This meta-analysis of 42 trials involved 27 843 patients (mean age 57 years) with relatively poor control (HbA1c of 8.2%). Odds ratio in the rosiglitazone group for myocardial infarction was 1.43, statistically significant (95% CI 1.03–1.98; $p = 0.03$) for cardiovascular deaths. There was a trend towards the rosiglitazone group but this was not significant ($p = 0.06$).

Although a safety alert was issued after this trial, many felt the study was flawed, based on incomplete evidence, and the alert premature. The PROACTIVE study produced some results indicating that pioglitazone may not have the same effect.

Rosiglitazone evaluation for cardiovascular outcomes – an interim analysis
NEJM 2007; 357(1): 28-38
This was an unplanned interim analysis given the publication outlined above. A total 4447 NIDDM patients with poor control were randomised to receive add-on therapy of either rosiglitazone or metformin or a sulphonylurea. The mean follow-up was 3.75 years.

After the inclusion of end points, the hazard ratio was 1.11 (95% CI 0.93–1.32). There were no statistically significant differences between the rosiglitazone group and the control group for myocardial infarction or death from cardiovascular causes. There were more patients with heart failure in the rosiglitazone group than in the control group (hazard ratio, 2.15; 95% CI 1.30–3.57).

Meglitinides/prandial glucose regulators
These are amino acid derivatives that are licensed for use with metformin in type 2 diabetes, where better control is needed, or where patients experience hypoglycaemia when treated with sulphonylureas.

The drugs are 'glucose responsive', so induce insulin release when the patient eats, by acting on the pancreatic beta-cells to stimulate a rapid, short-lasting release of insulin to a level dependent on the glucose concentration, i.e. where there is a post-prandial rise in glucose. This is thought to be beneficial where the patient has an erratic lifestyle (e.g. junior doctors).

As stimulation is not over 24 hours the endocrine function should be preserved.

Glucose tolerance and mortality: comparison of WHO and American Diabetes Association diagnostic criteria. DECODE Study Group
Lancet 1999; 354: 617–21

This study of 18 048 men and 7316 women over 30 years of age looked at risk of death according to different diagnostic glucose categories. There was a follow-up of 7.3 years.

It found that fasting glucose alone did not identify risk of death associated with hyperglycaemia. Mortality increased with increasing two-hour glucose (i.e. post-prandial spike).

Dipeptidyl peptidase-4 inhibitors (DPP-4 inhibitors)

This is a new class of oral hypoglycaemics that stop breakdown of incretin (an intestinal hormone that stimulates insulin release in response to food). Sitagliptin and vildagliptin are currently under investigation. Exenatide is also under investigation. This is a drug that simulates the effect of incretin when injected.

Efficacy and safety of sitagliptin added to ongoing metformin therapy in patients with type 2 diabetes
Curr Med Res Opin 2008; Jan 11 (Epub ahead of print)

This was a multinational, randomised, placebo-controlled, parallel-group, double-blind study of 190 non-insulin dependent type 2 diabetic patients. Sitagliptin was found to reduce HbA1C (by 1%), fasting glucose and two-hour post-prandial glucose at 18 and 30 weeks, all with statistical significance $p < 0.001$. It was also found to be well tolerated.

Screening for diabetes

It is estimated that in 2030 half the UK population will be diabetic, and already up to half of the people with type 2 diabetes have vascular complications at the time of diagnosis.

Mass population screening would be costly and inefficient, with low specificity, as less than 1% of undiagnosed cases were revealed by a British Diabetic Association study in 1994. Many organisations have published arguments for a targeted approach to high risk groups (e.g. obesity, family history of diabetes, ethnic groups, patients who have had gestational diabetes or impaired glucose tolerance, or hypertension).

Diabetes UK recommends opportunistic screening for those at high risk of diabetes and, slowly, research into oral glucose tolerance testing is adding weight to the argument.

Should we screen for type 2 diabetes? Evaluation against National Screening Committee Criteria
BMJ 2001; 322: 986-8

This discussion paper looks at the role of the National Screening Committee in evaluating a screening programme for type 2 diabetes.

It argues as follows:
* benefits of early detection and treatment of undiagnosed diabetes have not been proved
* disadvantages of screening are important and should be quantified
* universal screening is not merited, but targeted screening may be justified
* clinical management of diabetes should be optimised before a screening programme is considered.

No agreement was reached on how targeted screening could be achieved. A further report is expected.

Psychological impact of screening for type 2 diabetes: controlled trial and comparative study embedded in the ADDITION (Cambridge) randomised controlled trial
BMJ 2007; 335: 486-9

This trial over 15 practices (10 trial and 5 control) looked at 7380 adults. It examined the effect of screening on anxiety and depression, worry about diabetes and self-rated health. It found limited psychological impact on patients. Those who screened positive were found to have poorer general health, higher anxiety, higher depression rates and higher worry about diabetes, although effect sizes were small.

The editorial accompanying this paper explains there is insufficient evidence to advocate either mass or targeted screening.

Miscellaneous
Acarbose
Acarbose for prevention of type 2 diabetes mellitus: the STOP-NIDDM RT
Lancet 2002; 359: 2072-7

People with impaired glucose tolerance treated with acarbose are 25% less likely to develop type 2 diabetes than are those on placebo. It was concluded that acarbose could be used either as an alternative or in addition to lifestyle changes in patients with impaired glucose tolerance.

Vitamin D

Intake of vitamin D and risk of type 2 diabetes: a birth cohort study
Lancet 2001; 358: 1500-3

In this longitudinal study, conducted between 1966 and 1997, a total of 10 366 children were looked at. Those who were given vitamin D (irrespective of dose) had a lower rate of type 2 diabetes.

The study suggests ensuring infants get at least the RDA of Vitamin D.

Vaccine

Beta-cell function in new-onset type 1 diabetes and immunomodulation with a heat shock protein (DiaPep277): a randomised, double-blind, phase II trial
Lancet 2001; 358: 1749-53

DiaPep277 is the first drug to successfully halt the immune system's destruction of pancreatic beta cells. However, the intervals at which the vaccine should be given are not known. Phase III trials are in progress.

Insulin needs after CD3 antibody therapy in new-onset type 1 diabetes
NEJM 2005; 352(25): 2598-608

This study of 80 people in Belgium showed that the monoclonal antibody preserved the remaining beta-cells in newly diagnosed diabetics. Patients diagnosed early would be ideal candidates for this type of treatment – opening again the debate on the need for a screening programme.

Inhaled insulin

The first inhaled insulin to be launched is Exubera. The inhalation into the nose delivers a dry powder to the lungs which enables the relatively large insulin molecule to be absorbed. The role of this insulin will be similar to that of short-acting insulin. It would not be suitable for smokers, people with lung disease, women who may become pregnant or, initially, children.

Islet cell transplant

In the UK London and Oxford have specialist laboratories to process islet cells from donors to develop a national transplant service. This is in the very early developmental stage.

Drugs for prevention of diabetes

This is an ongoing area of research and it is not recommended that we prescribe. Metformin has long been recognised for its ability to help weight loss (although this is not a licensed use).

Waking up from the DREAM of preventing diabetes with drugs
BMJ 2007; 334: 882–4

This analysis considers metformin, troglitazone (no longer available), and angiotensin-converting enzyme inhibitors and receptor blockers. As the title suggests, although there was some evidence for the effectiveness of these drugs (mainly for metformin), because of the risk of harm lifestyle adjustment is still recommended as the number one intervention.

The DREAM study (Diabetes Recall And Management System) looked at patients with impaired glucose tolerance or fasting glucose and randomised them, one of the arms being to rosiglitazone. It was found that, although there was a small increase in heart failure, it reduced the risk of diabetes over three years (only 11.6% of the patients developed diabetes compared to 26% in the placebo arm).

Chronic kidney disease

www.renal.org

The introduction of the quality and outcome framework has led most of us in primary care to focus on estimated glomerular filtration rates (eGFRs) and to look at chronic kidney disease (CKD) before there are changes in the creatinine. We routinely dip urine for protein and microalbumin, but having eGFRs reported on all our renal results has meant we are in effect screening these cohorts for renal disease more actively than ever in the past. As CKD is an independent risk factor for vascular disease and increases mortality and morbidity, this is going to be an area of our routine work that can only expand.

Stage	Description	eGFR (mL/min/1.73 m²)
1	Kidney damage (dip positive for protein, microalbumin or blood) with normal or increased eGFR	> 90
2	Kidney damage with mild decrease eGFR	60–89
3	Moderate decrease eGFR	30–59
4	Severe decrease eGFR	15–29
5	Kidney Failure	< 15 or dialysis

The estimated glomerular filtration rate

As up to 50% of renal function is usually compromised before any increase in creatinine is seen, the eGFR allows us to identify issues to enable us to take action, sooner. The gold standard for renal function is inulin clearance. This

is costly and time consuming, and is certainly not practical for primary care numbers. Fortunately, there is an automatic calculator we can use on www.renal.org. The calculation of eGFR is based on:
+ age
+ sex
+ ethnicity
+ creatinine.

$$eGFR = 186 \times \left(\frac{Creatinine}{88.4} \right)^{-1.154} \times [age^{-0.203}] \times [0.742 \text{ (if female)}] \times [1.21 \text{ (if black)}]$$

Problems that may give misleading eGFRs include:
+ there are laboratory variations
+ any reading greater than 90 will not be exact, as the test is not accurate in extremes
+ the result may be falsely low if performed following a high-protein meal (i.e. a fasting sample is best)
+ if the patient is elderly or has extreme body mass, the reading may be inaccurate
+ must be stable (over three months).
   It is important not to interpret eGFRs out of context.

Glomerular filtration rate
BMJ 2006; 333: 1030–1
This is the accompanying editorial to the paper published on page 1047 (*BMJ* 2006; 333: 1047) that looked at different screening strategies aimed at identifying patients with low GFRs. The study found that screening people with hypertension, diabetes or patients aged 55 years or more was the most effective strategy, with the number needed to screen for finding one case being 8.7. The conclusion was that case finding should actively continue.

New results from the modification of diet in renal disease study: the importance of clinical outcomes in test strategies for early chronic kidney disease
QJM 2008; January 14
The modification of diet in renal disease study (MDRD) led to the eGFR formula used today. This is not the same as the Cockroft-Gault equation, which estimates creatinine clearance.
   This 10-year follow-up of the MDRD patients looked at the results of four tests of kidney function measured at base line as predictors of long-term clinical outcome. Neither method showed an advantage over creatinine measurement. Cystatin C looked more promising than the other tests (including eGFR). This is an initial report. Further analysis of the data is ongoing.

Effects of statins in patients with chronic kidney disease: meta-analysis and meta-regression of randomised controlled trials
BMJ 2008; 336: 645–51

This meta-analysis of 30 144 patients (pre-dialysis and transplant patients) looked at the benefits vs. the harm with statin treatment. It found that although lipid concentration was reduced and cardiac outcomes improved, all causes of mortality showed no improvement. It concluded that the role of statins in primary prevention was uncertain and the reno-protective effect of statins was also uncertain.

Gastrointestinal tract

Dyspepsia

This is defined as 'chronic or recurrent pain, or discomfort, centred in the upper abdomen'. It is a symptom, not a diagnosis.

Gastro-oesophageal reflux disease (GORD) is the term used to describe reflux of gastric contents into the oesophagus causing symptoms such as dyspepsia.

◆ Annually 40% of adults will have dyspepsia.
◆ Five per cent will consult their GP.
◆ One per cent will be referred for endoscopy.
◆ Of those having endoscopy 40% will have a non-ulcer dyspepsia, 40% will have GORD, 13% will have an ulcer and 3% will have a gastric carcinoma.

There is a huge amount of literature published on gastro-oesophageal reflux, *Helicobacter pylori*, ulcer and non-ulcer dyspepsia. We suggest referencing the following for the most up to date information:

◆ NICE guidelines (*see* below)
◆ Guidelines – summarising guidelines for primary care
   www.eguidelines.co.uk
◆ Clinical evidence at www.clinicalevidence.com

National Institute for Health and Clinical Excellence. *Dyspepsia: Management of dyspepsia in adults in primary care: NICE clinical guideline 17.* London: NIHCE; 2004.
www.nice.org.uk/nicemedia/pdf/CG017NICEguideline.pdf

An important part of initial assessment in primary care is determining if there are any ALARM features (Anaemia, weight Loss, Anorexia, Refractory problems, Melaena or swallowing problems) or an acute gastrointestinal bleed that warrants urgent investigation.

The following have been identified as priorities:

- referral for endoscopy
- interventions for uninvestigated dyspepsia
- interventions for gastro-oesophageal reflux disease
- interventions for peptic ulcer disease
- interventions for non-ulcer dyspepsia
- reviewing patient care
- *Helicobacter pylori* testing and eradication.

Helicobacter pylori

H. pylori is a gram negative bacterium that colonises the stomach. It seems to have an aetiological role in gastric and duodenal ulceration, gastric lymphoma, gastric cancer and colorectal adenoma (*J Gastroenterology* 2005; 4099: 887–93). Its exact role in these conditions (and coronary heart disease) is unclear.

It affects 20% of people under 40 years of age and 50% of people over 60 years.

Re-infection in adults is rare (less than 1% per year) so eradication is almost curative.

RCT of effects of *H. pylori* infection and its eradication on heartburn and gastro-oesophageal reflux: Bristol helicobacter project
BMJ 2004; 328: 1417

This study showed that 1558 *H. pylori* positive people, with and without gastro-oesophageal reflux disease, showed no difference between eradication treatment and placebo after two years. The eradication treatment was neither beneficial nor harmful.

There is still no real conclusion as to whether to eradicate in *H. pylori* positive individuals who have non-ulcer dyspepsia, as more recent work seems to confirm that even after eradication there is an increased mortality.

Management

In cases of confirmed ulcers, eradication speeds healing and reduces recurrence (NNT = 2). This is not the case in GORD (NNT = 17). Most guidelines suggest that it is not necessary to test for *H. pylori* if there is a known duodenal ulcer, but to treat empirically and investigate if there are ALARM symptoms or if the patient does not improve.

Triple regimen is more successful than the double. There is no difference between the different triple regimens, and one week is as successful as two weeks.

Non-invasive tests for *H. pylori*

- *Serology:* this does not distinguish between old and active infection (IgG antibodies can remain in the circulation for up to nine months after eradication), i.e. 50% of positives could be false positives. At present this is a suboptimal test and not recommended. Its sensitivity is 60–85%. Specificity is 80%, depending upon which paper you read.

◆ *Carbon-13 urea breath test:* urea is hydrolysed by *H. pylori* urease to carbon dioxide and ammonia. The specificity and sensitivity are 95% and positive predictive value 88%. It is easy to use in primary care (but does still have to be sent to the laboratory for analysis). It should not be used whilst taking antacids/proton pump inhibitors because this causes false negative results in some cases. The test becomes negative once *H. pylori* is eradicated. It is more expensive than serology but it reduces the need for endoscopy, so is more cost effective in the long run.

◆ *Stool antigen detection test:* this is usually a monoclonal test (polyclonal tests are less sensitive). The specificity and sensitivity are up to 95%, positive predictive value is 84% and you now only need a pea-sized piece of stool. It is not known whether positive tests should ultimately lead to endoscopy to look for secondary pathology.

◆ Stool antigen tests should not be performed within two weeks of taking PPIs or antibiotics.

Invasive test/endoscopy

Histology: has a sensitivity and specificity greater than 90%.

Although it is more invasive and expensive, it is preferable to empirical treatment. It decreases drug consumption, the number of visits to the doctor, and sick leave for two years after endoscopy compared to the year before; and patients are generally more satisfied with the treatment. The symptomatic outcome (endoscopy vs. empirical treatment) is similar in the two groups.

Coeliac disease

www.pcsg.org.uk/

Coeliac disease is a gluten-sensitive enteropathy, histologically an inflammatory picture, which affects the small bowel. As part of the base-line investigation three different antibodies can be looked for: antigliadin antibody, anti-endomysial antibody and anti-transglutaminase antibody.

Adult coeliac disease

BMJ 2007; 335: 558–62

This is a clinical review of interest. It tabulates conditions known to be associated with coeliac disease, including dermatitis herpetiformis, recurrent aphthous ulcers, iron deficiency anaemia and irritable bowel.

Prevalence is 0.5–1% internationally and delay to diagnosis can be 4.5–9 years.

Banbury Coeliac Study
BMJ 1999; 318: 164-7

This study was set up to determine the under-diagnosis of coeliac disease. In the study, 1000 patients were tested for endomysial antibody (other antibody tests could include gliadin and reticulin). Thirty of these were positive with a positive biopsy result; 15 out of 30 patients presented with anaemia and 25 out of 30 presented with non-gastrointestinal symptoms. The study found that only around 20% of patients with coeliac disease are currently being diagnosed.

Prevalence of coeliac disease in dyspeptic patients
Arq Gastroenterol 2005; 42(3): 153-6

This study looked at 142 patients being investigated for dyspepsia. Thirty patients were found to have patterns suggestive of coeliac disease, a prevalence of 1.4% in this study group (patients with irritable bowel are also known to have a higher prevalence).

The study suggested considering serological assays in this group of patients.

GPs can prescribe gluten-free foods to patients with coeliac disease or dermatitis herpetiformis but must endorse the prescription 'ACBS' (According to Borderline Substance Act), otherwise the script may be queried or rejected. Compliance to a gluten-free diet has been shown to improve with medical follow-up. The British Society of Gastroenterology suggests that this is done yearly.

Long term complications of coeliac disease include small bowel lymphoma and osteoporosis (up to 50%). The Primary Care Society for Gastroenterology guidelines suggest a DEXA scan at the time of diagnosis and a repeat after the menopause for women, or at 55 years for men. If a fragility fracture occurs at any age then a scan should be done.

The Coeliac Society produces an annual food list of gluten-free products, which is available to members (www.coeliac.co.uk).

The Department of Health advises prophylactic immunisation against *Pneumococcus* in coeliac disease patients over two years of age due to the risk of hyposplenism.

Enzyme treatment

Prolyl endonuclease is an enzyme that has been found to degrade proteins and the amino acid proline (which makes up approximately 20% of gluten), even at low pH. Although this is purely experimental at the moment, it is thought that in the future it may allow coeliac patients to eat gluten-containing foods.

Colorectal cancer

◆ Lifetime incidence of colorectal cancer is 5%.
◆ In the UK 16 000 people die each year from colorectal cancer.
◆ Of people with bowel cancer, 5% have more than one cancer.

◆ Eighty-five per cent of colorectal cancers occur in patients over 60 years of age.

◆ Around 90% of cases are diet related and 10% are genetic (*GUT* 2000; 46: 746–8).

Role of the GP

◆ Identify high-risk patients – early detection improves the five-year survival.

◆ Provide detailed counselling and information about causes of colorectal cancer.

◆ Promote lifestyle issues that may prevent colorectal cancer (eat five portions of fruit and vegetables a day, take 30 minutes of brisk exercise daily, stop smoking and maintain a BMI 18.5–25 kg/m² throughout life).

Screening for bowel cancer

www.cancerscreening.nhs.uk/bowel/

It is estimated that a 10-year screening programme would prevent 5000 new cases and 3000 deaths a year in the UK.

The Government made clear its commitment to screening for bowel cancer in the NHS Plan (2000), and the Colorectal Screening Pilot study began looking at faecal occult bloods (FOBs) and flexible-sigmoidoscopies as an option, building on original studies from Nottingham and Denmark. Screening with faecal occult bloods (FOBs) could potentially reduce mortality from bowel cancer by 15%.

In October 2004 the Health Secretary announced that the National Screening Programme for bowel cancer will be rolled out to both men and women over 60 years of age from April 2006. This will be a phased plan and will be underpinned by £37.5 million of funding.

Home testing kits will be sent, every two years, to men and women registered with a GP. They will have to collect a sample from three separate bowel movements within two weeks and then send the kit back (by post) to the laboratory.

If the results are positive, patients will be offered a colonoscopy (this will be a separate route to the two-week cancer referrals) through the local screening centres.

Faecal occult blood (Cochrane Review 1998)

◆ Low sensitivity and specificity (tumour needs to be bleeding) in the range of 50–60%.

◆ Most extensively studied screening test for colorectal cancer.

◆ False positives with red meat and vegetables rich in peroxidase.

◆ Several large randomised controlled trials have shown that FOB screening is feasible.

Flexible sigmoidoscopy

+ Can detect 80% of colorectal cancers.
+ Only detects cancers up to the splenic flexure (50% of cancers are proximal).

Population screening for colorectal cancer

DTB 2006; 44(9): 65–8

This gives a good review of trials published around the various screening methods, as well as the UK Screening Pilot. It concludes that FOBs can reduce mortality from colorectal cancer, whereas the same outcome benefit is not known for either flexible sigmoidoscopy or colonoscopy.

Role of aspirin

There is increasing evidence that aspirin protects against development of colorectal cancer, but its use as a chemoprotective agent is not yet advocated for the general population.

Effect of aspirin on long-term risk of colorectal cancer: consistent evidence from randomised and observational studies

Lancet 2007; 369(9573): 1603–13

This study looked at two large trials with 20-year follow up (as colorectal adenomas often take at least 10 years to develop). Aspirin 500 mg for five years; 300 mg or 1200 mg for one to seven years and placebo were considered. It concluded that 300 mg of aspirin for five years or longer was protective against colorectal cancer, with a latency of 10 years. Side effects and risk of bleeding would need to be further evaluated before this was recommended.

Respiratory disorders

Asthma

+ The National Asthma Campaign estimates 5.4% of the population has asthma.
+ New diagnoses in children rose from 4% to 10% from 1964–89.
+ Around 1500 deaths per year are due to acute exacerbations of asthma.
+ The annual cost of asthma to the NHS is £700 million (this does not include the economic cost of working days lost).
+ Children exposed to antibiotics *in utero* are thought to be more likely to develop asthma (by up to 43%), hay fever (by up to 38%) and eczema (by up to 11%). However this has been shown in only one study.

Asthma diagnosis started to increase in the second half of the twentieth century. Although BTS guidelines (due to be updated in 2008) have been successful, asthma is still under-diagnosed and under-treated.

A recent Government inquiry into asthma deaths concluded that many could have been prevented by more proactive GP care. It cited the following problems:

* under-use of primary care services
* under-prescribing of oral steroids
* inadequate use of peak expiratory flow meters (PEFR).

It also found only 12 % of those who had died had attended a practice asthma clinic in the year before death.

Some recent work has looked at the use of nitric oxide (NO), and pilot studies have found that patients with low NO levels have better asthma control and lung function.

Improvement in quality of clinical care in English general practice 1998–2003: longitudinal observational study

BMJ 2005; 331(7525): 1121

This study looked at asthma (as well as coronary heart disease and type 2 diabetes).

Recording of smoking advice, peak flow and asthmatic symptoms had all improved. The score (as a measure of improvement) rose from 60.1% to 70.3% in asthma patients.

Scottish Intercollegiate Guidelines network/BTS Asthma Guidelines

Thorax 2003; 58 Suppl 1

www.brit-thoracic.org.uk

These guidelines, updated from the 1995 guidelines, amended in 2004 and further updated in 2007 (for full review in 2008), aim to achieve accurate diagnosis and symptom control quickly by stepping up treatment and then stepping down treatment when control is good.

2007 Update to the British Guideline on the management of asthma

* Steroid replacement in children on more than 800 mcg per day of beclomethasone (or equivalent) should be included as part of the management plan.
* Ciclesonide (new inhaled corticosteroid) is not placed, as it is felt there is not adequate safety data.
* Advises practitioners that higher doses of inhaled corticosteroids may be needed in smokers.

- Doubling the dose of inhaled steroid at the time of an exacerbation (in adults) has not been shown to be effective.
- There is a new section on Anti-IgE monoclonal antibody (omalizumab), although it is not yet possible to place this in the step-wise guidelines for control of asthma.

The guidelines are broken down into recommendations for adults; children aged 5–12 years; and children younger than five years. They suggest that there should be a method of identifying poorly controlled asthmatics so that they can be asked to come in for review or chased up if they fail to attend, as there is a higher mortality in this group of patients.

Organisation of care
All practices should have a list of people with asthma.

Review
- This should be routine, with a standard recording system.
- It should include inhaler technique, PEFR, current treatment, morbidity and a personal asthma action plan (PAAP).
- It should be audited regularly.
- The best results are seen with nurses who have been trained in asthma management.

The following three questions should be asked.
1 Do you have difficulty sleeping because of your asthma?
2 Have you experienced your asthma symptoms during the day?
3 Has your asthma interfered with your usual activities?

Accessibility, clinical effectiveness, and practice costs of providing a telephone option for routine asthma reviews
Br J Gen Pract 2007; 57: 714-22
Initially, GPs were able to offer telephone consultations (especially for patients who were well controlled and working, and so unable to attend in normal hours) to fulfil the QOF requirements. This then became frowned upon, despite good uptake and with no suggestion that it compromised patient care.

In this trial in Whitstable, Kent, asthma patients receiving care were randomised to either a telephone encounter (554), face-to-face consultation (659) or usual care (515) over a 12-month period. Morbidity was the same in each of the three groups. Cost for telephone consultation was less than cost for a face-to-face review. The study concluded that, as well as being cost-effective, telephone consultations increased review rates, and enhanced patient enablement and confidence with management.

Personal asthma action plans
+ These should be customised and written.
+ They should be offered to all patients with asthma.

Acute exacerbations
+ In-patients should be on specialist units.
+ Discharge should be a planned and supervised event. It may take place as soon as clinical improvement is apparent.

Targeting care
Identify groups at risk. They include:
+ children with frequent upper respiratory tract infections
+ children over five years of age with persistent symptoms
+ asthmatics with psychiatric disorders or learning disability
+ patients who are using large quantities of beta-2 agonists.

Main additions in the 2004 update
+ Medication: inhaled steroids should be introduced in milder cases and the dose should be titrated.
+ Helping those with asthma to help themselves: patients should be offered education. Prior to hospital discharge they should be given an individual action plan.
+ Organisation and delivery of care: primary care services – patients should have a regular structured review.

A further addition in 2005 was the question whether symptoms improved when the patient was away from work. If there was a suggestion of work-related asthma then patients should be referred.

Self-management plans for asthma
Since the revised 2003 BTS/SIGN guidelines, increasing importance is being placed on patients having the education and the confidence to manage their own asthma, enabling them to live a symptom-free life, detecting and treating their exacerbations early. Personal action plans are intended for use by patients over 12 years of age.

Self-management plans reduce exacerbations, hospital admission rates and time off work. Although many asthma patients think their asthma is well managed, their symptoms (hence quality of life) could be improved. However, the use of self-management plans is still suboptimal.

Written action plans for asthma: an evidence based review of the key components
Thorax 2004; 59(2): 94–9

This study looked at 26 randomised trials and found that improved health outcomes were seen if the action plan:

◆ was based on a personal best peak flow reading
◆ used two to four action points based on symptoms or lung function
◆ included recommendations for inhaled and oral corticosteroid use.

Long acting beta-2 agonists
MIASMA (Meta-analysis of increased dose of inhaled steroid or addition of salmeterol in symptomatic asthma)
BMJ 2000; 320: 1368–73

Lung function was higher in patients who received salmeterol rather than steroids. Symptom-free days and nights were more frequent with salmeterol and rescue-free day and nights higher with salmeterol. There were fewer exacerbations with salmeterol and the severity was less in those who did have an exacerbation.

Leukotriene-receptor antagonists

These are derived from arachidonic acid, the precursor of prostaglandins. By preventing prostaglandin release, they reduce bronchoconstriction, mucus secretion and oedema.

Improving asthma control in patients suboptimally controlled on inhaled corticosteroids and long acting beta-2 agonists: addition of montelukast in an open-label pilot study
Curr Med Res Opin 2005; 21(6): 863–9

This is a real-life observational study of 313 Belgian patients already taking inhaled corticosteroids and long-acting beta-2 agonists but who were inadequately controlled.

It was found that 78.6% of the patients reported an improvement of their asthma with addition of montelukast.

Chlorofluorocarbons (CFC)-free inhalers

This is again topical, as beclomethasone inhalers are all to become CFC-free between now and 2010.

◆ CFCs have implications for the depletion of the ozone layer.
◆ They can be used as a propellant in metered-dose inhalers (MDIs).
◆ CFC-free MDIs have been available since 1995 in the UK and are now being widely used.
◆ Hydrofluoroalkane (HFA) compounds are being used in preference. Their safety profile is similar to CFCs.

Breathing exercises

The Butekyo method is a breathing technique developed by a Russian physician who believes that a significant amount of asthma is caused by hyperventilation. In the UK, the method can be taught by a trained physiotherapist.

As yet there is no reliable body of evidence to indicate whether breathing exercises work to reduce symptoms of asthma (Cochrane 2001), although it would make sense if they did.

Other issues

The use of tumour necrosis factor (TNF) blockers is being trialled, alongside usual treatment, for brittle asthmatics. Also being considered is an injection called omalizumab (a protein that blocks the immune response to allergens), which could prevent severe allergy-related asthma attacks. It would be administered by injection every two to four weeks.

NICE has recently published guidance on the use on inhaled corticosteroids in both adults and children. It recommends the option of a combination inhaler, based on therapeutic need and the likelihood of treatment adherence. There is concern expressed in the GP media that as NICE hasn't backed this as a treatment preference, some PCTs may continue with their restrictions on its use.

Risk assessment of asthma patients
TENOR risk tool predicts healthcare in adults with severe- to difficult-to-treat asthma
Eur Resp J 2006; 28(6): 1145-55

This is a validated (2821 adult patients) risk tool to predict those patients with asthma who are at highest risk. Patients received a score out of 18 (based on age, steroid bursts, ethnicity, FEV1; as well as other factors based on history, BMI and sex). Those scoring 5 to 7 points were up to 3.5 times more likely to be admitted to hospital or seen in Accident and Emergency compared to those scoring less than 4.

Chronic obstructive pulmonary/airways disease

Chronic obstructive pulmonary disease (COPD) has recently been recognised as a systemic disease. The systemic symptoms of muscle weakness and weight loss seem to relate poorly to lung function. Hence lung function should be only one of the tools we use to assess disease severity and progression.

British Thoracic Society (BTS) definition

'A chronic slowly progressive disorder characterised by airflow obstruction that does not change markedly over several months. Most of the lung function is fixed, although some reversibility can be produced by bronchodilator (or other) therapy.'

♦ COPD causes around 26 000 deaths per year (respiratory disease is now the biggest killer in the UK).

♦ It is responsible for 400–1000 per 10 000 consultations in general practice.

♦ Risk factors include smoking, pollution, occupation (cadmium and coal related), lower social classes, genetic factors and chronic under-treatment of asthma.

The BTS guidelines were published in 1997 and aimed to improve diagnosis and management (*Thorax* 1997; 52 Suppl 5: S1–28). GOLD has also published COPD guidelines at www.goldcopd.com.

It is thought (following a recent publication in *Chest* 2005; October) that the UK BTS guidelines may miss 1.5% cases of COPD when compared to use of the European Respiratory Society guidelines (the difference being that BTS guidelines are fixed and ERS guidelines are weighted for gender).

National Institute for Health and Clinical Excellence. *Chronic obstructive pulmonary disease: Management of chronic obstructive pulmonarydisease in adults in primary and secondary care:* **NICE clinical guideline 12. London: NIHCE; 2004.**
www.nice.org.uk/nicemedia/pdf/CG012_niceguideline.pdf
This is available for reference, and the summary is probably more concise than the BTS for ease of everyday use and reference. A new National Service Framework is also being developed (it is anticipated that GPs will be asked to screen high-risk groups).

Diagnosis of COPD

This is suggested by symptoms and established by objective measurements using spirometry, with a chest x-ray to exclude other pathologies.

Spirometry is the most reliable means of confirming a diagnosis and assessing severity and reversibility. A trial of steroids (30 mg prednisolone for two weeks, or six weeks beclomethasone 1000 µg per day), following baseline spirometry, is recommended in looking for reversibility. Reversibility is an increase of FEV1 by 15% *and* 200 ml above the base line.

In October 2001, *GP News* looked at the potential savings that could be made identifying COPD patients on asthma registers and withdrawing inhaled steroids (following data presented at the 11th European Respiratory Society Conference).

Steroid use in COPD

Inhaler and steroid use, amounts and best combinations for symptom control and to reduce disease progression are always under debate. A validation study (*Respir Med* 2007; 101: 1313) of 749 randomly selected patients found that 90% of patients taking medication for their COPD do so based on trials for which they would not have been eligible. Many studies have suggested that inhaled corticosteroids reduce exacerbation and improve health.

The prevention of chronic obstructive pulmonary disease exacerbations by salmeterol/ fluticasone proprionate or tiotropium bromide
Am J Resp Crit Care Med 2008; 177(1): 19–26

The INSPIRE trial looked at 1323 patients with severe COPD and found that although the number of exacerbations was similar, those on salmeterol/ fluticasone were more likely to need antibiotics while those on tiotropium tended to be treated with steroids. The fact that the drugs may have different and possibly synergistic effects is leading to an interesting debate that may lead to the development of a triple inhaler.

TORCH study: Towards a revolution in chronic obstructive pulmonary disease health
Salmeterol and fluticasone proprionate and survival in chronic obstructive pulmonary disease
NEJM 2007; 356: 775–86

This study was a three-year, randomised, double-blind study in 6112 patients with COPD. It looked at the effects of combined salmeterol/fluticasone (50/500 µg) as compared to placebo, salmeterol or fluticasone.

Salmeterol/fluticasone reduced moderate to severe exacerbations, but not exacerbations requiring hospitalisation, compared with salmeterol alone. Patients in the group on fluticasone alone were more likely to have pneumonia (number needed to harm = 17).

The study quotes the NNT 4 to prevent one exacerbation in one year and NNT 32 to prevent one hospitalisation in seretide vs. placebo (probably not the best comparison).

Smoking cessation

This reduces the rate of decline in lung function (*BMJ* 1977; 1: 1645–8). Legislation in the UK means that people are no longer allowed to smoke in public places and work areas (including company cars).

Environmental tobacco smoke and risk of respiratory cancer and chronic obstructive pulmonary disease in former smokers and never smokers in the EPIC prospective study
BMJ 2005; 330: 277–80

This was a prospective study of 303 020 people who had never smoked or who had stopped smoking at least 10 years ago, and who provided information about environmental tobacco smoke. Controls were matched for sex, age, smoking status and country of recruitment. Over a seven-year follow-up period the whole cohort had an increased risk of events (hazard ratio 1.30, 95% CI 0.87–1.95).

The study concluded that environmental tobacco smoke was a risk factor for respiratory diseases, especially in ex-smokers.

Long-term oxygen therapy (LTOT)

In hypoxaemic patients, LTOT prolongs life.

Patients with cyanosis and cor pulmonale should be considered for LTOT assessment.

LTOT should be considered if PaO_2 is less than 7.3 kPa. It is important to ensure that it does not cause carbon dioxide retention. Oxygen should be prescribed for 15 to 20 hours per day.

MRC Trial
Lancet 1981; 1(8222): 681-6
This trial showed that five patients would need to be treated for five years to avoid one death (NNT 5). Treatment involved administration of 15 hours oxygen per day. The difference was evident only after 500 hours.

Domiciliary oxygen for COPD
Cochrane Database Syst Review 2005 October 19; 4: CD001744
Six randomised controlled trials were identified. They found long-term oxygen therapy improved survival of patients with severe hypoxaemia (arterial PaO_2 less than 55 mmHg).

Smoking and home oxygen therapy – a preventable public health hazard
J Burn Care Res 2008; 29(1): 119-22
This study looked at patients in a burns unit in America, who had continued to smoke while on home oxygen. A total of 14 patients (10 male) with facial burns, who had been smoking and using nasal oxygen, were seen. Of the seven patients who survived, only one had stopped smoking following the injury. The study concluded that there needs to be specific guidelines in these instances and consideration should be given to testing saliva for cotinine (a nicotine breakdown product).

Self management plans for COPD
The principles follow the same lines as for asthma management plans.

Self-management reduces both short- and long-term hospitalisation in COPD
Eur Resp J 2005; 26(5): 853-7
This Canadian study of 191 patients who had been hospitalised with an exacerbation of their COPD involved a randomised issuing of the self-management programme 'Living with COPD' versus standard hospital care. At two years the intervention group showed a reduction from 26.9% to 21.1% in cases of hospitalisation.

N-acetylcysteine

This is a mucolytic agent with antioxidant properties that has been found to reduce the exacerbations of COPD (NNT 6). It may also slow the rate of decline in lung function.

New developments in the treatment of COPD: comparing the effects of inhaled corticosteroids and N-acetylcysteine
J Physiol Pharmacol 2005; 56 suppl 4: 135–42

The results of this complicated study showed that inhaled corticosteroids improved lung function in COPD. The N-acetylcysteine group showed a reduction in inflammatory markers.

Pulmonary rehabilitation

It has been shown to reduce symptoms, increase mobility and improve quality of life. It will become an increasing part of the holistic care approach we should have as GPs.

Exercise can reduce the risk of relapses that require hospital admission by 50% (*Thorax* 2003; 58: 100–5).

Pulmonary rehabilitation and the BODE index in COPD
Eur Resp J 2005; 26(4): 630–6

The BODE index integrates body mass index, airflow limitation (forced expiratory volume in one second), dyspnoea and a six-minute walking distance. It predicts mortality in COPD. A total of 246 patients was divided into groups of those who had received pulmonary rehabilitation and those who had not. BODE worsened by 4% over 12 months in those with no rehabilitation. Mortality in this group was 39%. BODE improved by 19% following rehabilitation, but returned to the original baseline after two years. Mortality in this group was 7%. It is thought that the BODE index change after pulmonary rehabilitation may provide valuable prognostic information.

Long-acting anticholinergics

Tiotropium is a once-daily maintenance dose for COPD that has been shown to improve FEV1 against placebo, salmeterol and ipratropium.

Prevention of exacerbation of COPD with tiotropium, a once-daily inhaled anticholinergic bronchodilator: a randomised trial
Ann Int Med 2005; 143(5): 317–26

This was an American study of 1829 patients with moderate to severe COPD.

Tiotropium, after six months, was found to reduce exacerbations (there were 27.9% as compared to 32.3% in the placebo group).

Osteoporosis

There is a higher risk of osteoporosis in COPD (compared to asthma), even when patients have not had long-term steroid treatment (*Chest* 2003; 122: 1949–55). The cause of this is not completely understood, although multisystemic effects, poor nutrition and lower testosterone levels probably all contribute to the effect.

Tuberculosis

Tuberculosis (TB) is caused by *Mycobacterium tuberculosis* and affects nine million people, with two million deaths a year worldwide. Where we work will determine whether we see TB or whether we just see an occasional letter telling us about a patient being in contact with a case diagnosed on the ward.

The Annual Report from the Health Protection Agency 2007 (www.hpa.org.uk/) outlines the data below, emphasising that the rate has not dropped since 2005 and remains higher than at any other time since 1987.

◆ There are currently 8000 cases a year in England (rate 14.0 per 100 000).
◆ The majority of cases are seen in 15–45-year-olds.
◆ Seventy-two per cent of cases are seen in non-UK born.
◆ Resistance to at least one first-line drug is seen in 7.7% of cases.

Research into a TB vaccine as part of the ongoing drive to control and eliminate the disease is looking at:
◆ replacing the current BCG with an improved version either by introducing genes (recombinant BCG30) or delivering it orally
◆ boosting existing BCG
◆ developing an attenuated strain of tuberculosis.

National Institute for Health and Clinical Excellence. *Tuberculosis: Clinical diagnosis and management of TB and measures for its prevention and control: NICE clinical guideline 33.* **London: NIHCE; 2006.**
www.nice.org.uk/CG033
This was published by NICE in 2006 and outlines a comprehensive care pathway of screening, testing, treating and vaccinating for TB.

Influenza

It is estimated that flu causes 2000–4000 deaths per year in the UK, mainly from December to March. It is known that 10–20% of the American population will show serological conversion each year, whether or not they are symptomatic. All through the influenza season the Health Protection Agency publishes a weekly report.

Immunisation

Immunisation of those at high risk of serious illness from influenza reduces hospital admissions and deaths. Immunisation can reduce mortality by up to 40% (up to 70% in repeated vaccination), and respiratory illness by up to 50%.

In October every year there is a marvellous influenza immunisation campaign run by primary care, the aim being to reduce morbidity and mortality. Current work is looking into the role of children in transmission of the virus, as well as how the illness affects them. They may be part of new inclusion groups in future campaigns that are sent out yearly by the Chief Medical Officer (CMO).

The Department of Health's flu campaign targets all people over 65 years and all people over six months of age in the following risk groups:
+ all high-risk groups (cardiovascular disease, diabetes, immunosuppression and chronic diseases, including chronic liver disease)
+ all those in long-stay residential and nursing homes, as well as other long-stay facilities
+ people who are the main carer for an elderly or disabled person whose welfare may be at risk if their carer falls ill (added 2005)
+ immunisation of healthcare workers (as part of what is called 'prudent winter planning')

CMO immunisation programme 2005 targets

+ A minimum target of 70% in those over 65 years of age. The World Health Organisation has set targets of 85% to be achieved by 2010 (alongside this the GP contract sets out percentages needing to be achieved in certain disease areas).
+ NHS employers should offer the vaccination to employees directly involved in patient care through the occupational health service, not their own GPs (unless they have been specifically contracted). Vaccines for staff should not be obtained at the expense of vaccine for the high-risk groups.

A number of different articles in the *British Journal of General Practice* found variously that patients who decline flu vaccine:
+ consider influenza a mild disease
+ hope they won't get flu
+ doubt the effectiveness of the vaccine
+ fear the side effects of the vaccine and that it will give them flu
+ lack campaign awareness
+ are apathetic
+ are unable to attend for immunisation (e.g. housebound or in residential care)
+ find the timing of immunisation clinics inconvenient
+ lack information about the vaccination.

Influenza immunization uptake and distribution in England and Wales using data from the general practice research database 1989/90–2003/04
J Public Health 2005; Oct 5

Major changes to the influenza vaccination programme were introduced in 1998 and 2000 (immunisation of elderly patients became age-related rather than risk-related). This review examined groups by age and medical risk. Vaccine uptake among high-risk individuals over 65 years of age increased from 36.7% in 1989/90 to 72.1% in 2003/04.

Vaccine uptake among high-risk individuals under 65 years increased from 10.8% in 1989/90 to 24.3% in 2003/04. This is still well below satisfactory levels. It will be interesting to see the follow-through from implementation of the new contract.

Effectiveness of influenza vaccine in community-dwelling elderly
NEJM 2007; 357(14): 1373

Resulting from concern that short-term studies may provide misleading pictures of long-term benefits, this study considered the effectiveness of influenza vaccine from 20 cohorts (713 872 person-seasons) of community-dwelling elderly over 10 flu seasons. Vaccination was associated with a 27% reduction in the risk of hospitalisation for pneumonia or influenza (adjusted odds ratio, 0.73; 95% CI 0.68–0.77), and a 48% reduction in the risk of death (adjusted odds ratio, 0.52; 95% CI 0.50–0.55).

Antiretroviral treatment for influenza

The neuraminidase inhibitors inhibit the replication of influenza A and B. They should be started within 48 hours of symptoms and are designed to complement the vaccination programme. Amantadine has been available since the 1970s, but is effective only against influenza A. If there is an influenza pandemic, of whatever strain, these drugs will be part of our management. It is not yet clear if they have a significant role to play in prophylaxis.

NICE 58 (Feb 2003) Guidance in the use of zanamivir, oseltamivir and amantadine

Advice for treatment: recommended for at-risk adults who can start treatment within 48 hours of the onset of symptoms of an influenza-like illness.

Advice for prevention: should be used if influenza A or B is circulating in the community, for people over 13 years of age in the following groups:
+ those in an at-risk group who have not had a flu jab this season, or had one too recently to have developed good protection
+ those who have been in close contact with someone with flu-like symptoms.

People in the latter category could start taking oseltamivir within 48 hours of contact.

Oseltamivir in the management of influenza
Expert Opin Pharmacother 2005; 6(14): 2493-500

A worldwide influenza pandemic could cause 20–40 million deaths. This report states that the World Health Organisation has recommended stockpiling oseltamivir for such an occasion, as it not only reduces severity and duration of symptoms, complications and mortality, but has also been shown to be effective against the circulating strain H5N1 (bird flu).

Comparison of elderly people's technique in using two dry powder inhalers to deliver zanamivir: randomised controlled trial
BMJ 2001; 322: 577-9

Delivery of zanamivir was as a dry powder through a diskhaler. The study concluded that most elderly people (i.e. one cohort deemed to be at high risk) were unable to use the inhaler device, so treatment with the drug was unlikely to be effective unless this delivery system could be improved.

Pandemic framework

The Department of Health has issued a pandemic framework (www.dh.gov.uk/pandemicflu) advising that:

♦ antiretrovirals are stockpiled to cover half of the UK population (currently 25%)
♦ there will be phone line support for primary care with direct access to antiretrovirals (GPs seeing only cases with complications) to aid rapid diagnosis and treatment.

The framework highlights secondary bacterial infections and advises antibiotics should be considered for adults with co-morbid diseases who are worsening or not improving over 48 hours.

Preparing for the pandemic
BMJ 2006; 332: 783-6

It is not known when the pandemic will occur or what strain will be the cause, but given that it has been over 40 years since the last outbreak it will not come as too much of a surprise when it happens. This edition of the *BMJ* had several articles looking at contingency plans, guidelines, lessons to be learnt from other outbreaks (such as AIDS, BSE, foot and mouth disease and SARS). It stresses the importance of clear lines of communication and accountability, and explores human behaviour. It suggests some practices are not always in the best interest of the population as a whole (for example, bulk buying may compound shortages if a pandemic was to affect people working in the distribution and supply of the pharmaceuticals).

The H5N1 strain of influenza

This has received much interest. This is a type of avian flu that has been known about for over 10 years. H7N2 is another strain that is less pathogenic. Since 2003 there have been 351 confirmed cases reported, of whom 219 (62%) have died. Although the numbers are small, the proportion of deaths is extremely concerning and reflects the virulence of the strain. A lot of work has been done to examine whether a strain of H5N1 could be incorporated into the current influenza vaccine, replacing the strain of lower virulence.

Pneumococcal vaccine

This is a one-off vaccination (re-vaccinate after 5 to 10 years if antibody levels are likely to have declined). It can be given at the same time as the influenza vaccination but at different sites.

The Department of Health Pneumococcal Immunization Programme was introduced in August 2003 as an all-year-round campaign. The age of eligibility for vaccination has gradually been reduced.

Current target groups (April 2005) include:
- all people over 65 years of age
- at-risk groups, from the age of two months (the main difference to the flu programme is that asthma is not included unless the patient needs frequent oral corticosteroids)
- individuals with cochlear implants
- individuals with the potential for cerebrospinal fluid leaks
- children under five years who have had a previously invasive pneumococcal disease.

Older people

National Service Framework for Older People

Although this was published in March 2001 (www.dh.gov.uk/en/Publications andstatistics/Publications/PublicationsPolicyAndGuidance/DH_4010161) it is retained in this edition of this book because it is important and because ageism is a political hot potato. The framework is an action plan to improve health and social services for older people wherever they live. It focuses on:
- rooting out age discrimination, which is believed to happen due to problems in society, education and the use of resources

◆ patient-centred care
◆ promoting older people's health and independence/an active life
◆ management of specific clinical conditions, with timely access to specialist care.

The eight standards are listed below.
1 Root out age discrimination – providing care on the basis of clinical need alone.
2 Person-centred care – treating patients as individuals. Planning for a single assessment process with integrated provision of services. GPs will be involved mainly in the contact assessment.
3 Intermediate care – to enable early hospital discharge and to prevent premature or unnecessary admission to long-term residential care.
4 General hospital care – delivered through appropriate specialist care, by staff with the skills to meet the needs of the elderly.
5 Stroke – the NHS will take action to prevent strokes (primary and secondary); and it will provide treatment by specialist stroke services with a multidisciplinary programme of secondary prevention and rehabilitation.
6 Falls – the NHS and councils will take action to prevent falls and reduce resultant fractures or other injuries. Advice will be provided through specialised falls services.
7 Mental health in older people – there will be access to integrated mental health services (for patients and carers).
8 Promotion of health and active life in older age.

As well as the standards listed above, there are five other major projects under way to improve quality, availability and consistency of services.
◆ Changes in long-term care funding, including availability of NHS nursing care.
◆ Expansion of intermediate care (and community equipment) services.
◆ Establishment of Care Direct to provide comprehensive information and ease of access to health, housing, social care and social security.
◆ Various initiatives (retirement health check, flu immunisations) to help older people stay healthy.
◆ Use of Section 31 of the Health Act 1999 to promote joint working between NHS and Social services.

Progress will be overseen by the NHS Modernisation Board and the Older People's Taskforce.

The Department of Health will publish the *Information Strategy for Older People*, which is due out later this year and will describe how GPs will be supported in achieving this.

Parkinson's disease

Parkinson's disease (PD) affects over 100 000 people in the UK. NICE guidelines were published for the diagnosis and management of this condition.

National Institute for Health and Clinical Excellence. *Parkinson's disease: Diagnosis and management in primary and secondary care: NICE clinical guideline 35.* **London: NIHCE; 2006**
www.nice.org.uk/nicemedia/pdf/cg035niceguideline.pdf

The priorities are summarised as:
+ referral to an expert for accurate diagnosis
+ regular expert review and access to specialist nursing care
+ access to physiotherapy, occupational therapy and speech therapy
+ palliative care.

Pharmacologically, the guidelines consider various drug treatments for both early and later PD. They do not advocate a specific treatment, but rather recommend discussion of the short- and long-term benefits and drawbacks, so enabling decisions to be made in partnership. Avoid withdrawing medication suddenly (e.g. drug holidays or reduced absorption due to surgery), as this may cause acute akinesia or neuroleptic malignant syndrome.

Surgery

NICE has also published guidance on deep brain stimulation for PD.

Bilateral subthalamic nucleus (STN) or globus pallidus interna (GPi) stimulation may be used in patients who fit certain criteria, including being levodopa responsive.

Non-motor features of PD

+ Depression
  This is common in up to 50% of cases of Parkinson's disease. It is thought to have neurobiological manifestations rather than being a purely emotional response to the disease (*J Neurol Neurosurg Psychiatry* 1999; 67: 492–6).
  NICE recommends that we have a low threshold for diagnosis.
+ Dementia
  It is recognised that Parkinson's patients have an increased risk of developing dementia. Acetylcholinesterase inhibitors have been used successfully, but further research has been recommended.

Prognosis of PD: risk of dementia and mortality: Rotterdam study
Arch Neurol 2005; 62(8): 1265-7

This study found that the risk of dementia was greater if patients carried the APOE epsilon allele. The dementia risk was also dependent on disease duration.

♦ Sleep disturbance

Poor sleep may improve with sleep hygiene. Restless legs syndrome should be considered. Patients with sudden onset of sleep need to take care with driving.

♦ Autonomic disturbance

This includes urinary dysfunction, weight loss, constipation, erectile dysfunction, excessive sweating, orthostatic hypotension and sialorrhoea.

Parkinson's disease Clinical Review
BMJ 2007; 335: 441-5

This is a comprehensive and useful review looking at differential diagnosis of tremor, practical applications of treatment options, management of psychosis in PD and the roles of professionals. Although there was a degree of criticism in other papers about GPs being excluded from the NICE guidelines, this review helps put us firmly in the picture – the main challenge being to keep abreast of developments.

Safety and tolerability of gene therapy with adeno-associated virus-borne GAD gene for PD: an open label phase 1 trial
Lancet 2007; 369(9579): 2056-8

Phase 1 human trials are under way. This trial looked at 11 men and one woman, all with severe PD. The gene was transferred to a virus, which was then injected into the subthalamic nucleus region. One patient found his movements had improved by 65%.

Although this is looking at only one genetic mutation in PD, results so far are encouraging.

Falls

♦ Falls are the leading cause of accidental death in people over 75 years of age; treatment of fractures alone cost the NHS £1.7 billion per year (DoH 2003)

♦ Every year 33–50% of people over 65 years of age suffer a fall (the percentage increases with age); of whom 20% will need medical help and 10% will have sustained a fracture.

♦ The current blood pressure targets seem to be causing an increase in falls due to postural hypotension and medication.

How can we help older people not fall again? Implementing the Older Person's NSF Falls Standard Six
Department of Health 2003

This is a comprehensive overview of reasoning and evidence behind current thinking around fall prevention, as well as the evidence behind the case for funding a fall prevention strategy locally. NICE has produced guidelines to support the Government.

National Institute for Health and Clinical Excellence. *Falls: the assessment and prevention of falls in older people: NICE clinical guideline 21.* London: NIHCE; 2004.
www.nice.org.uk/nicemedia/pdf/CG021NICEguideline.pdf

One of the most important things to understand in this document is how you would offer a multifactoral assessment of falls by assessing:

+ fall history: gait, balance, mobility and muscle weakness
+ osteoporosis risk
+ visual and cognitive impairment
+ urinary incontinence
+ home hazards, including footware and rugs
+ cardiovascular examination and medication review.

Promoting health and function in an aging population
BMJ 2001; 322: 728-9

This article is still one of the better reviews looking at the evidence for strategies to promote health and function. It concludes that it is necessary to take into account social, mental, economic and environmental determinants of health in old age. Most health benefits can be gained from regular physical activity of moderate intensity. Substantial gains could be made by promoting health and fitness throughout life.

GPs should:

+ review repeat prescriptions
+ consider physiotherapy referral
+ consider occupational therapy referral to reduce home hazards
+ consider a joint meeting with the relevant primary healthcare team members for individual cases
+ consider asking if there have been any falls in the past twelve months at routine reviews.

Falls assessments

There are a number of reasons we are not doing this:

+ patients don't tell us they have fallen/slipped
+ GPs don't know how to do it
+ GPs are seeing people at surgery, not at home
+ GPs forget or run out of time.

The SLIPS Project (www.slipsonline.co.uk) is an integrated care pathway developed to help assess falls. There are three pathways, depending on who sees the person who has had a fall:

+ basic screen – anyone
+ general screen – any trained health, social or voluntary provider
+ specialist screen – in specialist falls service.

The following should be considered:
+ does the person who fell know why he/she fell – was there LOC?
+ are there environmental elements? – if so, consider occupational therapy
+ was the patient able to get up? – if not, consider physiotherapy
+ are the falls recurrent or unexplained? – consider specialist falls referral
+ don't forget to review medications, blood pressure, eyesight and footwear.

Dementia

Dementia is a chronic deterioration of intellect and personality.
+ Around 5% of people over 65 years of age have some form of dementia.
+ Around 20% of people over 80 years of age have some form of dementia.
+ Sixty per cent of cases of dementia are thought to be an Alzheimer's type, accounting for 340 000 cases in the UK.
+ One in seven elderly people with dementia is in residential care.
+ It is important to diagnose dementia early and to identify the type of dementia, to improve care and reduce morbidity for our patients and their carers.

The Mental Health Foundation has published a report, *Tell me the Truth*, which reveals that most people who develop dementia are not usually told what is wrong with them. It is this information that, although initially difficult to accept, helps patients to understand the changes in themselves and helps them to adapt.

The Alzheimer's Society website is comprehensive, informative and useful for professionals, patients and families: www.alzheimers.org.uk.

Dementia – NICE and Social Care Institute for Excellence November 2006
www.nice.org.uk/nicemedia/pdf/CG042NICEGuideline.pdf

The guideline considers Alzheimer's disease, dementia with Lewy bodies (DLB), frontotemporal dementia, vascular dementia and mixed dementias. It covers diagnosis, assessment, principles of care (with a view to promoting independence), treatments, end-of-life challenges and support for carers.

Risk factors and prevention

For primary prevention, general population screening is not recommended and preventative treatments such as statins, HRT, Vitamin E and NSAIDs are not advised.

In rare cases Alzheimer's is inherited via the AD gene. There are also connections to the APOE gene, but no useful diagnostic or prognostic test is yet available. NICE recommends offering referral for genetic counselling in familial cases of dementia such as autosomal dominant Alzheimer's disease or frontotemporal dementia, and cerebral autosomal dominant arteriopathy with subcortical infarcts and Huntington's disease.

For secondary prevention, it is recommended that arteriovascular risk factors are targeted, as they are also risk factors for dementia. Smoking, alcohol excess, obesity, hypertension and raised cholesterol levels are all important.

Diagnosis and assessment

The clinical cognitive assessments recommended are the Mini-Mental State Examination (MMSE), General Practitioner Assessment of Cognition, 6-item Cognitive Impairment and the 7-minute screen. Blood tests routinely include biochemistry, haematology, thyroid function tests and vitamin B_{12} and folate levels.

If imaging is required, request this through the specialist service. Referral at an early stage is recommended (this is also recommended in the National Service Framework for Older People).

Treatment of dementia

- *Non-pharmacological:* in the initial stages this is geared towards support for patients and their families.
- *Pharmacological:* three cholinesterase inhibitors have been licensed in the UK for mild to moderate Alzheimer's disease: donezipil, rivastigmine and galantamine. It is recommended that these be started if the MMSE is 10–20/30, i.e. for moderate dementia. Although the drugs' costs can amount to around £1000/year it is thought the costs may ultimately be offset by delaying the need for residential care. It is of interest that in the initial draft of the guidance it was recommended that these treatments should no longer be available on the NHS because of lack of effectiveness. This met with a great deal of resistance and the final guidance was revised. The effects of the medication should be reviewed by the specialist team starting care.

Interventions for non-cognitive symptoms and behaviour

- *Non-pharmacological:* following early assessment to identify potential causes, holistic therapies such as aromatherapy, massage and animal-assisted therapies are suggested.
- *Pharmacological:* it is suggested that antipsychotics (contra-indicated in DLB) and acetylcholinesterase inhibitors are only used if there is severe distress or risk of harm to the patient or others. Be aware of the increased risk of cardiovascular events with the use of antipsychotics.

Palliative and end-of-life care in dementia

Information on end-of-life care is available at www.endoflifecare.nhs.uk. It is recommended that this approach is adopted from diagnosis until death to enable patients to die with dignity.

Support for carers

Assessments of carers should seek to identify psychological distress and impact on the carer. Care plans and support as well as psychological therapy should be offered.

Effectiveness of acetylcholinesterase inhibitors: diagnosis and severity as predictors of response in routine practice

Int J Geriatr Psychiatry 2006 Aug; 21(8): 755-60

This Oxfordshire-based four-year study looked at the monitoring of cholinesterase inhibitor prescribing. A Mini-Mental State Examination (MMSE) improvement of two or more points was defined as a 'cognitive response'. Medication was prescribed for 1322 patients and outcome data were available for 1250. Subsequently, 939 patients were reassessed after a mean of 120 days. The finding that cognitive, but not clinical, response was more likely in those with moderate dementia than in those with mild dementia accords with the findings from randomised studies in the January 2006 revision of the NICE Appraisal Consultation Document.

Dementia: still muddling along?

Br J Gen Pract 2007 Aug; 57(541): 606-7

Professors Iliffe and Manthorpe wrote an insightful article focusing on the reasons GPs should use the dementia guidelines. Firstly, incidence is increasing (the estimated annual cost of dementia in the UK (1998) was £5.5 billion). Secondly, dementia is now included in the QOF. Thirdly, public expectations about dementia and treatments are changing, so we may have more people presenting early. And fourthly, we are a fundamental part of the NHS in implementing new treatments and moving medicine forward.

The same authors wrote a review article for *GP Clinical* in July 2007, bringing attention to the PAID acronym for the management of problems related to dementia.

P Physical problems, like pain, may trigger behavioural change.
A Activities of others are annoying or frightening to the patient.
I Intrinsic features of dementia are appearing, like wandering.
D Depression underlies the behaviour change, or there are delusions/psychotic symptoms.

Miscellaneous factors and Alzheimer's disease (AD)
Other treatments for Alzheimer's disease

* *Selegiline and Vitamin E:* treatment with either was found to slow progression of the disease. The Cochrane Review 2000 found selegiline was better than placebo at improving cognitive function, behavioural disturbance and mood.

◆ *Vitamin C and Vitamin E for Alzheimer's disease: Ann Pharmacother* 2005; 39: 2073–9 concluded that vitamin C and E supplements do not have the supporting evidence to be recommended for use in Alzheimer's disease.

◆ *Ginkgo biloba* (40 mg three times daily): one systematic review (of eight randomised trials) reported that *Ginkgo biloba* improved cognitive function and was well tolerated in patients with Alzheimer's disease (*Clin Drug Invest* 1999; 17: 301–8)

◆ *Reality orientation:* this involves presenting information designed to reorientate a person in time, place and person. It may be a notice board giving day, date and time, or a member of staff reorientating patients at each contact. *Clinical Evidence* found one systematic review of small RCTs that showed improvement in cognitive function and behaviour compared to no treatment.

None of the above treatments are recommended by NICE.

Exercise
Leisure-time physical activity at midlife and the risk of dementia and Alzheimer's disease
Lancet 2005; 4(11): 705–11

This was a study of 1239 people aged 65 to 79 years of age that found exercising at least twice a week was associated with a 50% lower relative risk of dementia and 60% lower risk of Alzheimer's disease. This was especially so (once adjusted for other factors) in carriers of the APOE gene.

Diet

Diet is a difficult topic, as good nutrition is linked with so many other lifestyle issues and attitudes. It is hard to deny that a healthy diet is good for you; and the social interaction of meal times may be presumed to be similarly so.

Lifestyle-related factors in predementia and dementia syndromes.
Expert Rev Neurother 2008 Jan; 8(1): 133–58

This paper looked at observational studies from Italy. In older subjects healthy diets, antioxidant supplements, the prevention of nutritional deficiencies, and moderate physical activity could be considered the first line of defence against the development and progression of predementia and dementia syndromes. However, in most cases, these were only observational studies, and results are awaited from large multicentre randomised clinical trials.

Driving and dementia
www.dvla.gov.uk/media/pdf/medical/aagv1.pdf

Having dementia doesn't mean that a patient is unsafe to drive. The loss of the ability to drive affects independence, especially in rural parts of the country. It is not the

GP's role to formally assess fitness to drive; that is the DVLA's responsibility. However we do have to:

◆ inform the patient that he/she must contact the DVLA and his/her insurance provider
◆ complete the medical report requested by the DVLA, if there is consent
◆ consider whether a patient is fit to drive while awaiting assessment
◆ inform the DVLA if we consider there is a danger to the patient or others.

Driving and dementia
BMJ 2007; 334: 1365–9

This was a clinical review article. Crash data published found that the risk was acceptably low for three years after the onset of dementia, by which time most patients would have stopped driving.

How to assess capacity to make a will
BMJ 2007; 335: 155–7

This was written with legal input. Due to an increasing number of wills that are contested after a testator's death, solicitors are asking doctors to certify testamentary capacity (capacity for making a will) in certain cases. There is a useful summary box on tests for capacity. The testator must be capable of understanding:

◆ the nature and effect of making a will
◆ the extent of his/her estate
◆ the claims of those who might expect to benefit from the will (both those included and excluded).

The testator should not have a mental illness that influences the testator to make bequests that he/she would otherwise not have made.

Our role as doctors is to satisfy ourselves of the capacity and understanding of the testator and to record these findings (known as the 'golden rule'). The solicitor will detail the legal tests, we assess (writing answers verbatim) and then check the extent of the estate and previous wills with the solicitors.

The Mental Capacity Act 2005
www.opsi.gov.uk/ACTS/acts2005/ukpga_20050009_en_1

Revised from 1983; came into force 1 October 2007.

The definition of a mental disorder is 'any disability or disorder of the mind or brain whether permanent or temporary which results in an impairment or disturbance of mental functioning'. Not only is the definition broad, but also it concerns an emotive subject where patients and public have preconceived ideas, especially with regard to loss of rights. The reformed Act goes some way towards addressing difficult issues but it is important to remember there is a distinct difference in treating mental disorders and exercising social control.

A New Mental Health (and Public Protection) Act was first published in 1959. The main issues were that decisions on involuntary treatment for mental disorders became primarily a matter for doctors. In 1983 limits to medical discretion were set out.

The key issues with regards to mental health are listed below.
- Risk of patients to themselves and others
  - care and treatment provided should reflect the best interest of the patient.
- Simpler template for formal assessment
  - assessment will be conducted by two doctors and an approved social worker (no change)
  - the template will be set out in a formal care plan which must be of 'direct therapeutic benefit' or address the management of 'behaviours arising from the disorder'
  - after 28 days will have to be reauthorised by the Mental Health Tribunal (a new independent body)
  - it will be followed by a care and treatment order applicable in both civil and criminal justice which will be made by the Mental Health Tribunal or by a court.
- Care and treatment in the community
  - care and treatment orders may apply to patients outside hospital
  - there will be contingency plans, if patients refuse to take their medication in the community, to prevent patients becoming a risk to themselves and others.
- Safeguards
  - there is entitlement to free legal service
  - there is a statutory obligation for care plans.
- The Mental Health Tribunal is an independent body taking advice from the clinical team, patients, independent experts and other agencies. It is also concerned with long-term use of compulsory powers. It may exceptionally reserve the right not to accept the clinical supervisor's decision to discharge a patient if there is serious risk of harm to others.
- The New Commission for Mental Health has responsibilities for maintaining formal powers and looking after people subject to care and treatment orders.

Assessing lack of capacity is a fundamental part of the Act. A person is regarded as lacking in capacity if he or she is unable to:
- understand and retain information to enable them to make a decision
- consider the information
- communicate their decision.

This is in keeping with the GMC guidance on consent in that, for it to be valid (i.e. a decision to consent) it must be informed, competent, uncoerced and continuing.

Mental Capacity Act 2005
BMJ 2007; 335: 989
This editorial sets out the ethos behind the Mental Capacity Act, affirming that it is intended to protect people who lack capacity and encourage them to participate in decisions. Every adult is assumed to be capable until that assumption is displaced.

If certain conditions are met, it explains, doctors are protected from civil and criminal liability when treating people who lack capacity. This does not provide a defence against a claim of negligence.

Changing Minds: Every Family in the Land
This was a five-year campaign organised by the Royal College of Psychiatrists in 1998 to combat the stigmatisation of people with anxiety disorders, severe depression, dementia, schizophrenia, eating disorders, or drug and alcohol dependencies.

Mental Illness: Stigmatisation and Discrimination within the Medical Profession is a report targeted at professionals as part of the campaign.

In 2001 the WHO published the first global profile of mental health services, which concluded that in most countries mental health is not taken seriously.

Mental health

National Service Framework for Mental Health (September 1999)
- At any one time one in six adults suffers from a mental illness (mainly anxiety or depression).
- One in 250 people have a psychotic illness, e.g. schizophrenia or bipolar affective disorder.
- Nine in 100 people that consult their GP with a psychiatric problem will be referred to specialist services.
- Mental health is one of four target areas in *Saving Lives: Our Healthier Nation.*
- There is a specific target to reduce suicide by 20% by 2010.
- The Framework fleshes out policies in the White Paper, *Modernising Mental Health Services.*
- An investment of £700 million in Mental Health Services was planned over the next three years.

The National Service Framework has five main areas and seven standards.

Mental Health Promotion (Standard 1)

Health and Social Services should:
+ promote mental health for all
+ combat discrimination against individual groups.

Primary Care and Access to Services (Standards 2 and 3)

Any service users who contact their Primary Care Trust (PCT) with a common mental health problem should:
+ have their mental health needs identified and assessed
+ be offered effective treatments, and referral if required.

Any individual with a common mental health problem should:
+ be able to have 24-hour contact with social services
+ be able to use NHS Direct for first-level advice.

Effective Services for People with Severe Mental Illness (Standards 4 and 5)

All mental health service users on a care programme should:
+ receive care which prevents or anticipates crisis and reduces risk
+ have written care plans that include action to be taken in a crisis, as well as GP advice if the patient needs additional help; and these should be regularly reviewed by the core co-ordinator
+ be able to access services 24 hours a day, 365 days a year.

Each service user who is assessed as requiring a period of care away from their home should:
+ have access to an appropriate bed
+ be placed as close to home as possible
+ receive a copy of a written after-care plan on discharge.

Caring About Carers (Standard 6)

All individuals who provide regular and substantial care for a person on a care programme approach should:
+ have an assessment of physical and mental needs annually
+ have their own written care plan.

Preventing Suicide (Standard 7)

All standards 1 to 7, and in addition:
+ supporting local prison staff in preventing suicide among prisoners
+ ensuring the competence of staff
+ developing local systems for suicide audit.

The overall performance will be assessed at national and local level in a number of ways:

- long-term improvement in psychological health of the population, as measured by the National Psychiatric Morbidity Survey
- reduction in suicide rates
- prescribing data
- access to psychiatric services and therapies
- experience of users
- reduction in emergency admissions.

Although this framework was welcomed, general opinion being that it was workable and clearly set out, an editorial opinion (*BMJ* 2002; 324: 61–2) pointed out discrimination issues in that it covered people up to 65 years of age only; and that it did not cover bipolar affective disorder.

Admission under compulsion

This is only to be used where the patient is suffering from a mental disorder and cannot be persuaded to enter hospital voluntarily. It is never to be done lightly. Keep comprehensive notes. Acceptance by the receiving hospital is necessary.

Section 2 (Assessment)

- Should be used where possible (Section 4 may be more appropriate in General Practice).
- Applied for by an approved social worker or nearest relative.
- Supported by two doctors (one of whom must be section 12 approved and one with knowledge of the patient). The two doctors need to examine the patient within five days of each other.
- The maximum length of stay is 28 days.

Section 3 (Admission and treatment)

- Application is based on two medical recommendations.
- Length of stay is six months initially, typically following on from a section 2.

Section 4 (Emergency in the community)

- The maximum length of admission is 72 hours.
- It is applied for by an approved social worker or nearest relative.
- It is supported by one doctor, who should have previous knowledge of the patient if possible. Both individuals must have seen the patient within 24 hours.

Suicide prevention strategy for England

www.dh.gov.uk/Publicationsandstatistics/Publications/PublicationsPolicyAndGuidance/
DH_4009474
www.nimhe.org.uk

- Around 5000 people take their own lives each year.
- Suicide is the most common cause of death in men less than 35 years of age.
- Risk factors include the following:
  - male
  - living alone
  - unemployed
  - alcohol and drug misuse
  - mental illness.

The strategy was written to support the target set by the White Paper, *Saving Lives: Our Healthier Nation* and the NSF for Mental Health.

The aim is to reduce death from suicide by at least 20% by 2010.

The goals of the programme are as follows:

- to reduce risk to key high risk groups
- to promote mental wellbeing in the wider population
- to reduce availability and lethality of suicide methods
- to improve reporting in the media of suicide behaviour
- to promote research on suicide prevention
- to improve monitoring of progress.

Anyone who self-harms requiring admission should have a follow-up visit by Community Mental Health Teams within one week. Such patients should not be issued with repeat medication lasting more than two weeks.

Implementation will fall to the National Institute for Mental Health in England.

A qualitative study of health seeking and primary care consultations prior to suicide
Br J Gen Pract 2005; 55(516): 503–9

Half, or more, of people who take their own life do not consult a doctor the month before their death. Members of family and immediate social networks may play a key role in determining whether or not suicidal individuals seek help.

RCT of acute mental health care by a crisis resolution team: the north Islington crisis study
BMJ 2005; 331: 599–602

This study found that mental health crisis resolution teams can reduce hospital admissions.

Depression

+ The annual incidence of depression is 8–12%.
+ The economic cost in the UK is £8 billion each year (*BMJ* 2006).
+ The rate of depression in nursing/residential homes is 22–33% (*The New Generalist* 2005).

DSM-IV diagnostic scale

Five of the following options should be present over a two-week period for the diagnosis of major depression (a score of 5–6 is moderate depression):
+ One of the following
  • depressed mood or irritability
  • loss of interest or pleasure
+ And three or four of these, to make a total of five
  • appetite or weight loss
  • sleep loss/change in sleep pattern
  • psychomotor agitation or retardation
  • fatigue/loss of energy
  • worthlessness or guilt
  • poor concentration
  • recurrent suicidal thoughts/thoughts of death.

The above criteria are useful in differentiating between low mood and clinical depression. In chronic depressive illness (dysthymia), be aware that patients may not meet DSM-IV criteria but could still benefit from drug treatment in the short term. We can improve identification of depression (it is estimated that we miss up to 50% of cases) by asking open questions, having good eye contact and not interrupting our patients.

National Institute for Health and Clinical Excellence. *Depression: management of depression in primary and secondary care: NICE clinical guideline 23.* **London: NIHCE; 2007.** www.nice.org.uk/nicemedia/pdf/CG23NICEguidelineamended.pdf
This guidance uses the International Classification of Diseases – version 10 (ICD-10)

The recommendations are presented in a practical stepped care (Step 1 to 5), starting with recognition of depression and going through treatment options based on severity of symptoms.

The key priorities for implementation build upon the NSF for Mental Health.

This is a very useful guide to read alongside the NICE Anxiety 2004 publication.

The guidance was amended in May 2006 to take into account new guidance on venlafaxine.

NICE Guidelines for the management of depression

BMJ 2005; 330: 267-8
This editorial outlines the view that the guidelines are clear for moderate to severe depression, but less so for mild to moderate depression (partly because of lack of understanding about what happens when individuals seek help for emotional problems).

Screening questionnaires

These are useful to aid diagnosis and monitor progress. Although there is some data about reliability in certain age groups, less is known about the sensitivity and specificity cross culturally.

+ *Patient Health Questionnaire (PHQ-9):* not ideal for older patients.
+ *Hamilton Depression Rating Scale:* not ideal for older people as it includes a number of somatic items that may be positive in older people who are not depressed.
+ *Geriatric Depression Scale (see below):* designed for elderly people, it avoids somatic items.
+ *Beck Depression Inventory:* designed for patients with more severe depression, it tackles suicidal thinking.
+ *Edinburgh Postnatal Depression Scale:* more sensitive than other scales in use with postnatal women.
+ *Abbreviated Mental Test Score:* can be used as a guide to dementia.

Geriatric Depression Scale

1	Are you basically satisfied with your life?	Yes/ **No**
2	Have you dropped many of your activities or interests?	**Yes**/ No
3	Do you feel that your life is empty?	**Yes**/ No
4	Do you often get bored?	**Yes**/ No
5	Are you in good spirits most of the time?	Yes/**No**
6	Are you afraid that something bad is going to happen to you?	**Yes**/ No
7	Do you feel happy most of the time?	Yes/ **No**
8	Do you feel helpless?	**Yes**/ No
9	Do you prefer to stay at home rather than going out and doing new things?	**Yes**/ No
10	Do you feel you have more problems with memory than most?	**Yes**/ No
11	Do you think it is wonderful to be alive now?	Yes/ **No**
12	Do you feel pretty worthless the way you are now?	**Yes**/ No
13	Do you feel full of energy?	Yes/ **No**
14	Do you feel your situation is hopeless?	**Yes**/ No
15	Do you think that most people are better off than you are?	**Yes**/ No

Scoring: Answers indicating depression are in bold type. Each scores 1 point. This scoring guidance should not be seen by the patient. A score greater than 5 indicates probable depression.

Psychometric comparison of PHQ-9 and HADS for measuring depression severity in primary care
Br J Gen Pract 2008; 58(546): 32–6
In satisfying QOF it is now important to record a depression scale score.

Both of these scales (advocated by the British Medical Association) were shown to be highly consistent and equally reliable. They differed in how they categorised severity (which may have an impact on treatment decisions), PHQ-9 categorising a greater severity than HADS.

Should we screen for depression?
BMJ 2006; 332:1027–30
Screening for depression would be in keeping with the National Screening Committee criteria. However, screening alone cannot improve management and outcome of depression and the cost would be significant (currently we see case finding as part of the chronic disease QOF criteria. *See* questions below). The literature suggests screening is unlikely to improve the wellbeing of the population.

Effect of the addition of a 'help' question in two screening questions on specificity for diagnosis of depression in general practice
BMJ 2005; 331: 884–6
The following questions were asked of 1025 consecutive patients receiving no psychotropic drugs and in whom substance misuse had been excluded.
+ During the past month, have you often been bothered by feeling down, depressed or feeling hopeless?
+ During the past month have you often been bothered by little interest or pleasure in doing things?
+ Is this something with which you would like help?

The questions had a sensitivity of 94% and specificity of 79%. The third question regarding help is what improved the specificity from 57% to 79%. The first two questions have been adopted as part of the QOF screening in chronic disease, asking if patients have experienced the symptoms over the last two months.

The Defeat Depression Campaign was run by the Royal College of Psychiatrists and the Royal College of General Practitioners from 1992 to 1996. It aimed to educate GPs in recognition and management of depression, as well as enhancing public awareness.

New research by the Mental Health Foundation showed that GPs would like greater access to treatments alternative to medication, but lack of service provision or long waiting lists preclude this. The Foundation has produced two excellent leaflets on depression (including the role of exercise) which can be ordered online at www.mentalhealth.org.uk.

Drug treatment in depression

You need to ask yourself what you are trying to achieve:
+ improvement in mood, social and occupational function, quality of life
+ reduction in morbidity and mortality
+ prevention of a recurrence
+ minimisation of adverse effects of treatment.

Antidepressants

Systematic reviews have shown that there is no clinically significant difference in effectiveness between different classes of drugs. All have an improvement of 50–60%. On average people on selective serotonin reuptake inhibitors (SSRIs) are less likely to stop treatment because of side effects. The SSRIs are now prescribed first line (NICE, 2004). It is important to be aware of potential drug interactions, and to use recognised side effects to benefit the patient, e.g. if the patient is suffering from insomnia use those drugs with sedative side effects.

If there are no side effects the drug should be used for six weeks before changing class or increasing dose. When stopping the drug, tail off over four weeks (depending upon the patient and symptoms).

SSRIs and gastrointestinal bleeding

BMJ 2005; 331: 529–30

This editorial explains the pathophysiological basis behind why SSRIs deplete platelet seretonin (so they are less likely to clot/more likely to bleed) and can cause gastrointestinal bleeding; and why some patients would benefit from gastroprotection.

St John's Wort (*Hypericum perforatum*)

This is a low-grade monoamine oxidase inhibitor that is widely dispensed over the counter for low mood and depression. A systematic review of 27 studies (Cochrane Library 1999) concluded that it was more effective than placebo. However various different preparations of *Hypericum* were used in each study.

Acute treatment of moderate to severe depression with St John's Wort: rct versus paroxetine

BMJ 2005; 330: 503–6

This study found that 90 mg/day of hypericum extract (WS5570) three times a day (increased if no response after six weeks) was at least as effective after 42 days (assessed with the Hamilton Depression Scale) as paroxetine 20 mg (or 40 mg if the dose had to be increased).

It is worth noting that *Hypericum* can induce liver enzymes and may interact with digoxin, theophylline, warfarin and COCP (consult the BNF). Also *Hypericum* products differ widely in composition.

Non-drug treatments

Cognitive behavioural therapy (CBT)

This is a structured treatment aimed at changing dysfunctional beliefs and negative automatic thoughts that contribute to a patient's problems. This form of treatment requires the therapist to have a high level of training.

The simple understanding is that CBT and problem solving are successful, whereas counselling is less so, although it does have high patient satisfaction. More recent studies looking at long-term outcomes have, on the whole, seen no difference between groups.

The case for psychological treatment centres

BMJ 2006; 332: 1030–2

This editorial on health policy considered the cost of expansion, given the recommendations by NICE that talking therapy should be offered to all but the mildest cases of depression and anxiety. It is estimated that some extra 10 000 therapists would be needed to meet demand and that this number could feasibly be trained over a seven-year period.

Cognitive therapy for prevention of suicidal attempts: rct

JAMA 2005; 294(5): 263–4

This is a randomised, controlled trial of 120 patients who had recently attempted to commit suicide (either 10 sessions CBT or enhanced usual service). CBT was effective at preventing further suicide attempts.

Chocolate craving when depressed: a personality marker

Br J Psychiatry 2007; 191: 351–2

We all know that chocolate isn't all bad, and we probably subscribe to the fact that it increases serotonin levels, albeit temporarily, in the brain. It has been shown to reduce blood pressure. This study looked at 2692 people over 18 and found 45% craved chocolate when depressed, a significant association between craving and severe depression.

The future

Urinary screening may allow neurochemical profiling of depression subtypes, enabling more rational prescribing of antidepressants.

Counselling in general practice

Around 51% of general practices have an on-site counsellor.

Counselling is designed to help people work on their problems and become more skilled in helping themselves. It is a disciplined psychological intervention, requiring specialist training in the different styles (e.g. directive, informative, confrontational, supportive). There is documented evidence that, if selected appropriately, it is effective. Counsellors have their own professional code of ethics and practice; and must hold a current membership of a professional body, the British Association of Counselling.

Appropriate referral and assessment is essential for cost-effective intervention. Most counselling consists of 6–12 sessions.

Suitable candidates for brief focal counselling include those who:
+ are able to express feelings and thoughts
+ are able to trust the counsellor
+ have mild to moderate difficulties, e.g. depression, relationship problems, anxiety, bereavement, emotional or psychological difficulties
+ are able to bear disturbing or conflicting feelings.

Unsuitable candidates include those who:
+ have moderate to severe difficulties, e.g. schizophrenia, dementia, substance abuse, personality disorders, risk of suicide
+ are silent or withdrawn
+ are prone to over-intellectualisation
+ have no close relationships
+ lack ability to think about self.

The Royal College of Psychiatry (www.rcpsych.ac.uk) has a useful site with access to information on cognitive behavioural therapy and psychotherapy in the Mental Health Information section.

Schizophrenia

www.rcpsych.ac.uk/mentalhealthinformation.aspx

The first description of schizophrenia appeared in the eighteenth century. There is a 1% lifetime prevalence (mainly seen in 20- to 30-year-olds), with 25% of patients being cared for by their GP. The diagnosis is made on the basis of the WHO International Classification of Disease (ICD-10), which looks for clear evidence of past or present psychosis, absence of prominent affective symptoms and a minimum duration of illness. We also need to look for negative symptoms such as blunted affect or poor motivation.

Schneider's first-rank symptoms are summarised below:
+ auditory hallucinations

- thought withdrawal or insertion
- thought broadcasting
- somatic passivity
- feelings or actions perceived as being under external control
- delusional perceptions.

National Institute for Health and Clinical Excellence. *Schizophrenia 2002: Core interventions in the treatment and management of schizophrenia in primary and secondary care: NICE clinical guideline 1.* **London: NIHCE; 2002.**
www.nice.org.uk/nicemedia/pdf/CG1NICEguideline.pdf
The guidelines are relevant to adults older than 18 years of age and to those diagnosed with schizophrenia below the age of 60 years. There are three phases.

1 *Initiation of treatment (first episode):*
   - early referral to secondary care and involvement of other services
   - early treatment – suggests discussion with psychiatrist and urgent referral Consider atypicals first line, e.g. olanzepine.

2 *Treatment of acute episode:*
   - single drug – administer in BNF dose range for minimum six weeks, and monitor response
   - may need rapid tranquillisation
   - be aware of side effects, e.g. risk of diabetes and weight gain with some atypicals
   - address other needs: psychological, social, occupational and others.
   - there is a high risk of relapse: if treating a relapse you need to continue treatment for one to two years and slowly withdraw treatment thereafter, monitoring for two years after the last acute episode.

3 *Promoting recovery (primary care):*
   - care register (essential)
   - monitor mental health and treatment alongside secondary care
   - consider referral in the following circumstances
     - problem with compliance
     - poor response to treatment
     - suspected co-morbid substance misuse
     - increased risk to self or others
     - new to practice list (for assessment and care programme)
     - where service users prefer not to receive care from GP.

Document everything clearly.
The following are essential across all phases:
- optimism
- get help early

+ assessment
+ working in partnership
+ consent and accurate information
+ addressing language and culture
+ addressing the issue of advance directives (although limited in schizophrenia).

Schizophrenia
BMJ 2007; 335: 91-5

This clinical review article, written by Picchioni and Murray, takes a broad overview of the illness. It details the following causes.

+ *Genes:* although schizophrenia is multifactorial, it seems likely (given that the incidence is 40% in monozygotic twins) that many risk genes exist.
+ *Environmental factors:* people with schizophrenia are more likely to have experienced obstetric complications, premature birth, low birth weight and perinatal hypoxia; and in adult life stressors such as social isolation, migrant status and urban life.
+ *Drug use:* stimulants such as cocaine and amphetamines can induce a similar picture; recent reports have also implicated cannabis.

Early recognition, treatment and long-term management are discussed as is the prognosis – 80% of people with a first episode will recover although fewer than 20% will never have another episode. There is little published on prevention of schizophrenia. This article is no exception.

Antipsychotics in schizophrenia: a message from CATIE
MeReC Extra July 2006; Issue 23

The Clinical Antipsychotic Trials of Intervention Effectiveness (CATIE) has provided useful insight into the effectiveness of antipsychotics. This study randomised 1492 people with chronic schizophrenia and found (although only 26% of patients completed the trial) that there was little to choose in effectiveness between antipsychotics (olanzapine, quetiapine, risperidone, perphenazine and one other not licensed in the UK – ziprasidone). Clozapine was excluded from the trial as it needed careful monitoring (as it reduces the white cell count). The study advocated individualised antipsychotic treatments.

The new antipsychotics should be considered as first line in newly diagnosed cases, where there has been no response to first line therapy, or where extrapyramidal side effects have been a problem. Non-compliance is a complex issue, the new dissolve-in-the-mouth tablet goes some way to addressing this.

Eating disorders
www.rcpsych.ac.uk

Anorexia nervosa
BMJ 2007; 334: 894–8

The prevalence for anorexia is 0.3% (there is an even distribution across all social classes). Between 80% and 90% of patients are young females, with the average age of onset being 15 years. It is the most common cause of weight loss in women. Up to 20% will die as a result of their illness, death being more likely if weight fluctuates rapidly.

Many people do not ask for help, so as GPs we can play a vital role in detection of these illnesses. Look for presenting features such as depression, obsessive behavior, infertility and amenorrhoea. All five IDC-10 criteria must be met before a diagnosis is made (the American Psychiatric Association (1994) stated that if the diagnostic criteria for both bulimia and anorexia are met, the diagnosis of anorexia takes precedence).

Recognised risk factors include: genetic factors (we don't know what is inherited, possibly a vulnerable personality type), cultural values, childhood obesity, early onset of puberty, adverse life experiences, extreme shyness, bullying, family functional style and low self-esteem.

Early diagnosis and intervention gives better outcome. Cognitive behavioural therapy and SSRIs have both been shown to improve short-term outcome compared to placebo. It is not clear if remission rates are reduced, as yet (Cochrane Library).

Standards 2 and 3 of the Mental Health NSF outline the need to improve health care for patients with anorexia nervosa and bulimia nervosa.

SCOFF Questionnaire
BMJ 1999; 319: 1467–8

This was designed at St George's Hospital, London, by Dr J Morgan and colleagues to give specialists a simple screening tool with which to identify eating disorders. It consists of five questions, and 1 point is scored for each 'Yes' answer. A score greater than 2 indicates a probable problem.

- Do you make yourself **S**ick because you feel uncomfortably full?
- Do you worry you have lost **C**ontrol over how much you eat?
- Have you recently lost more than **O**ne stone in a three-month period?
- Do you believe yourself to be **F**at when others say you are too thin?
- Would you say that **F**ood dominates your life?

The researchers compared this tool with more lengthy questionnaires and had excellent results of 100% sensitivity and 87.5% specificity (12.5% false-positive rate).

Chronic fatigue syndrome/myalgic encephalomyelitis

National Institute for Health and Clinical Excellence. *Chronic fatigue syndrome/myalgic encephalomyelitis (or encephalopathy): diagnosis and management of CFS/ME in adults and children: NICE clinical guideline 53.* London: NIHCE; 2007
www.nice.org.uk/nicemedia/pdf/CG53NICEGuideline.pdf

Chronic Fatigue Syndrome (CFS), also known as myalgic encephalomyelitis or myalgic encephalitis (ME) is defined as disabling fatigue associated with other symptoms, e.g. musculoskeletal pain, sleep disturbance, impaired concentration and headaches. The cause is not understood. A polypeptide involved in the antiviral response was more common in CFS but this has no clinical application.

+ Overall population prevalence is 0.2–0.4%.
+ In a practice of 10 000 patients, around 40 will have CFS.
+ It is classified as a neurological condition by the WHO.
+ Communication is the key to good management providing
  - acceptance and understanding
  - information about the illness
  - assistance with occupational and social care issues.

Treatment of CFS/ME

+ Function and quality of life management:
  - sleep management to avoid napping
  - rest periods
  - exercise, encourage pacing and not overdoing things on a good day
  - healthy diet
  - consider cognitive behavioural therapy.
+ Pharmacological intervention:
  - low dose tricyclic for pain, e.g. amitriptyline
  - melatonin may be considered in young people who have sleep difficulties.
+ Setbacks and relapse:
  - management is about understanding the experience and going back to the basics set out above.
+ Ongoing review, as with any chronic disease.

Chronic fatigue syndromes or myalgic encephalomyelitis

BMJ 2007; 335: 411-12

The guidelines have been criticised for not being sufficiently evidence-based, but this editorial is somewhat more optimistic. It highlights the message that this is a recognised condition (interestingly a significant number of doctors still do not believe it exists), with positive treatment options. Rehabilitation trials for CFS by the UK Medical Research Council are under way.

Medically unexplained symptoms

Drug Ther Bull 2001; 39(1): 5

Around one in five new consultations by adults (and one in ten children) are by patients with physical symptoms for which there is no organic cause. In a third of cases the symptoms persist and can cause distress and disability.

General practice is about dealing with symptoms that don't fit the disease model. Do not make the mistake of labelling symptoms MUS until a thorough clinical assessment and appropriate investigations have been carried out. If no physical explanation can be found, the psychological and emotional issues need to be considered. Malingering is rare.

It is thought that, although by definition the cause is unknown, these symptoms are due to a complex interaction of biological, psychological, social and cultural factors. Although seen in all specialties, this is addressed mainly in psychiatry, probably due to the links with anxious personality types and the tendency to develop psychological symptoms (www.rcpsych.ac.uk).

Understanding the narratives of people who live with medically unexplained illness
Patient Educ Couns 2005; 56(2): 205–10

This paper identified three features of patients' narrative: a chaotic history of the illness narrative; concerns that their symptoms were all in their mind; and their status as medical orphans. There was genuine concern to secure some form of ongoing medical and social support.

Management

It is important to acknowledge the symptoms and distress, as well as to provide continuity of care.

Management of medically unexplained symptoms (Editorial)
BMJ 2005; 330: 4–5

This is a discussion of some of the issues and options available. It highlights that some of the essential elements in medical models are to make the patient feel understood, then to broaden the agenda and finally to negotiate a new understanding of the symptoms, including psychosocial factors.

Antidepressants

These can be useful, especially if the patient is experiencing pain or difficulty in sleeping, whether or not they are depressed. Benefit is usually seen in one to seven days (i.e. quickly!). The number needed to treat is three.

Reattribution

This involves demonstrating understanding of the patient's complaints by taking a history of related physical, mood and social factors. Make the patient feel understood and make the link between symptoms and psychological problems.

Cognitive behavioural therapy

This has been shown in systematic review to be beneficial, particularly in reducing physical symptoms.

Recent developments in the understanding and management of functional somatic symptoms in primary care
Curr Opin Psychiatry 2008; 21(2): 181–8

The authors consider the training in primary care and recent stepped care approaches. The latter, they explain, need further evaluation. They feel names that 'presuppose a mind-body dualism (such as somatisation, medically unexplained)' should not be used and that treatment offered must be professional as in any other condition.

Frequent attenders

This is usually a different group of people to those with unexplained symptoms.

The average GP attendance per patient is three to four times per year.

Part of the problem can include lack of reassurance, loss of confidence with the doctor, fear and concern.

Characteristics of high attenders include the following:

◆ multiple health problems
◆ lower social class
◆ medically unexplained symptoms
◆ belief that reattendance is necessary to get the right treatment.

Is frequent attendance in primary care disease-specific?
Fam Pract 2006; 23(4): 444–52

This study looked at a random sample of 1000 adults in North Staffordshire, in nine general practices, who had attended at least once in the last 12 months.

It then categorised them as either frequent (high or very high), moderate- or low-frequency consulters. It found that frequent attenders were not statistically limited to specific diseases, although certain pathologies did consult more frequently.

Paediatrics

Paediatrics is concerned with patients from 0 to 18 years. Guidance for all doctors can be found at www.gmc-uk.org/. This is the first publication from the GMC issuing guidance on children. It outlines roles and expectations and may help in making decisions that are in the best interest of the child/young person, assess capacity and consider consent issues.

Child health surveillance

There have been four editions of the Hall Report, *Health for all Children.*
+ The first set out a programme of routine reviews for all pre-school children.
+ The second suggested how this may be delivered.
+ The third is a response to evolving professional perceptions of preventative healthcare coupled with rapid changes in the political context in which that care is provided (1996).
+ The fourth report adds to the emphasis of health promotion and moves away from a medicalised model of screening.

In September 2003 the Green Paper *Every Child Matters* was published, highlighting the need to maximise opportunity, minimise risk and support children to be healthy, safe, make a positive contribution and achieve economic wellbeing. It sets out the strategy for child health promotion. This report was followed in March 2004 by *Every Child Matters: the next steps*, which started to set out the plan for delivery. In September 2004 the National Service Framework for Children, Young People and Maternity Services was launched (www.dh.gov.uk). It consists of 11 standards. The first five apply to all children, Standards 6 to 10 apply to children in special circumstances and Standard 11 is for maternity services.

Standard 1   Promoting health and well being, identifying needs and intervening early
Standard 2   Supporting parenting
Standard 3   Child, young person and family-centred services
Standard 4   Growing up into adulthood
Standard 5   Safeguarding and promoting the welfare of children and young people

Standard 6   Children and young people who are ill
Standard 7   Children and young people in hospital
Standard 8   Disabled children, young people and those with complex health needs
Standard 9   The mental health and psychological wellbeing of children and young people
Standard 10 Medicines for children and young people
Standard 11 Maternity services

The Child Health Promotion Programme replaced the Child Health Surveillance Programme and includes:

- the assessment of the child and the family's needs
- health promotion
- childhood screening
- immunisations
- early interventions to address identified needs.

The table below sets out an overview of health promotion services that will be offered.

Age	Intervention
Soon after birth	General physical examination with emphasis on heart, eyes and hips. Administration of vitamin K, BCG and hepatitis B vaccinations in high-risk babies.
5–6 days old	Blood spot test for hypothyroidism and phenylketonuria. Sickle cell and cystic fibrosis screening are also being implemented.
New birth visit	This is usually around 12 days and done by the health visitor or midwife. As well as assessing the family's needs, the family is also given the personal child health record and the 'Birth to Five' guide.
6–8 weeks	Physical examination and administration of first set of immunisations: polio, diphtheria, tetanus, whooping cough, Hib and meningitis C.
3 months	Second set of immunisations.
4 months	Third set of immunisations.
By 12 months	Further developmental assessment.
Around 13 months	Immunisation against measles, mumps and rubella.
2–3 years	Health visitor performs further developmental assessment.
3–5 years	Further immunisation against MMR, polio, diphtheria, tetanus and whooping cough.

cont.

Age	Intervention
4–5 years	A review at school entry (usually school nurse). The foundation stage profile assessment by the child's teacher to look at development of physical, emotional, social and creative development as well as communication, language and literacy.
10–14 years	BCG vaccination given to those who require it.
	Tetanus, diphtheria and polio boosters (age 13–18 years).

From 2009, screening for medium-chain acyl-coenzyme A dehydrogenase deficiency (MCADD) will be offered to babies in England. This is a rare, life-threatening autosomal recessive condition in which it is difficult for the body to change fat into energy. It is a known cause of sudden infant death and is treatable.

Assessment framework

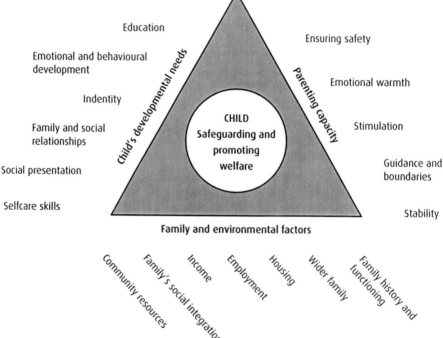

FIGURE 1.2 NSF for Children, Young People and Maternity Services 2004.

Screening
www.nsc.nhs.uk/ch_screen/child_ind.htm
It is important to make parents aware that screening tests are just that: screening

tests. If they have any worries or concerns they need to seek advice from their GP or health visitor.

Developmental dysplasia of the hip

This is a spectrum of conditions where the head of the femur is partly or completely displaced from the acetabulum. If this is not treated it can lead to a significantly abnormal gait and disability. Risk factors include family history, breech presentation, oligohydramnios, postural deformities of the feet, first born, caesarean delivery and female. It affects around five in 1000 babies at birth, one in 1000 at three weeks.

Early detection and conservative treatment are often successful, avoiding the need for surgery. Routine screening with Ortolani and Barlow (valid up to three months) misses up to 70% of cases. This is a falsely reassuring screening test for both parents and doctors. Some European countries now have a universal ultrasound screening programme. The UK targets babies with risk factors or with a positive Ortolani or Barlow, aiming for an ultrasound scan by eight weeks. A later sign would include asymmetrical leg creases.

Ultrasonography in screening for developmental dysplasia of the hip in newborns: systematic review
BMJ 2005; 330: 1413-5

A total of 188 studies were selected for full assessment, of which 10 met the inclusion criteria for analysis. There were three important findings. Firstly, there is insufficient evidence for the use of ultrasound as a screening tool. Secondly, ultrasound is likely to increase treatment rates, possibly unnecessarily; and finally, the duration of intervention was likely to be lowered by ultrasound screening.

Screening for hearing defects
http://hearing.screening.nhs.uk/

+ Around 840 children are born with permanent hearing impairment each year.
+ This equates to around two babies in every 1000 born.
+ Around 50% are not diagnosed until they are 18 months old.
+ Around 25% are not diagnosed until they are three years old (i.e. the distraction test did not pick up some children early enough).

Permanent hearing impairment affects communication skills, educational attainment and quality of life. If there is intervention by six months the outcome for all of the above, as well as the cost to society, is improved.

The Government announced the National Newborn Hearing Programme to screen all babies within 48 hours of birth. This is done by *otoacoustic emissions testing*. It has been known since the 1970s that for each sound heard by the ear, the ear produces a tiny corresponding sound ('echo') known as otoacoustic emission. This can now be measured by a computer and used clinically. Absence of, or a barely audible, echo indicates the child has a hearing problem. Sensitivity is in the range of 80–90% and costs are less than the distraction tests previously performed at eight months.

Early hearing: what is the best strategy?
Int J Pediatr Otorhinolaryngol 2007; 71(7): 1055-60
Although a number of factors increase the risk of hearing impairment (low birth weight, prematurity, perinatal hypoxia, jaundice and others), it can occur without any of these.

This French study looked at screening after birth (before discharge) compared with at two months in 5790 infants. Screening before discharge led to fewer false-positive results, which in turn had the effect of less maternal anxiety because of fewer false positives. It concluded that early neonatal screening was the better option.

Vaccination programme
www.immunisation.nhs.uk
The immunisation schedule has saved more lives than any other public health measure (apart from the publication of the Sanitary Act in 1866, requiring provision of clean water and effective sewage disposal). The success of a vaccine is not the number of primary cases of the disease, but the number of secondary cases generated from the one primary source. *See* table for ages recommended for each vaccination.

Childhood immunisation

Routine childhood immunisation programme		
When to immunise	What vaccine is given	How it is given
2 months old	Diphtheria, tetanus, pertussis (whooping cough), polio and *Haemophilus influenzae* type b (Hib) (DTaP/IPV/Hib)	One injection
	Pneumococcal infection (Pneumococcal conjugate vaccine, PCV)	One injection
3 months old	Diphtheria, tetanus, pertussis, polio and *Haemophilus influenzae* type b (Hib) (DTaP/IPV/Hib)	One injection
	Meningitis C (meningococcal group C) (MenC)	One injection

cont.

Routine childhood immunisation programme

When to immunise	What vaccine is given	How it is given
4 months old	Diphtheria, tetanus, pertussis, polio and *Haemophilus influenzae* type b (Hib) (DTaP/IPV/Hib)	One injection
	Meningitis C (meningococcal group C) (MenC)	One injection
	Pneumococcal infection (Pneumococcal conjugate vaccine, PCV)	One injection
Around 12 months old	*Haemophilus influenza* type b (Hib) and meningitis C (Hib/MenC)	One injection
Around 13 months old	Measles, mumps and rubella (German measles) (MMR)	One injection
	Pneumococcal infection (PCV)	One injection
Three years four months to five years old	Diphtheria, tetanus, pertussis (whooping cough) and polio (DTaP/IPV or DTaP/IPV)	One injection
	Measles, mumps and rubella (MMR)	One injection
13 to 18 years old	Diphtheria, tetanus, polio (Td/IPV)	One injection

Measles, mumps and rubella

A recent report from the WHO includes England and Wales in the seven European countries that can expect a measles epidemic in the near future. Their objectives and advice include:

- aim to maintain a high vaccine uptake
- strengthen routine vaccination programmes
- target catch-up campaigns at susceptible age groups
- stress the safety of the vaccine
- aim for eradication of measles by 2010.

Although the ongoing surveillance has discredited the link with autism and Crohn's disease, this is an emotive topic for all parents. The single vaccines are not licensed for use in the UK (other than rubella). If a single vaccine is requested it must be done on a named patient basis and be approved by the Medicines Control Agency. The website www.mmrthefacts.nhs.uk is an excellent reference site and gives direct links to other sites and evidence.

The MMR scare from 1998 resulted in a 4% drop in uptake reducing immunisation to 85%. To eliminate measles there needs to be an uptake of 94–96%. Figures from the NHS Information Centre show a small increase, with current uptake running nationally at 85% for the first vaccine (still only around 75% for the booster), which is 9% lower than seen for other vaccines (94%).

Measles in the United Kingdom: can we eradicate it by 2010?
BMJ 2006; 333: 890–5

This clinical review article looked at smallpox and polio for comparison. Following the late 1990 controversy over the safety of the vaccine, there was a decline in vaccine uptake, increasing the risk of epidemic (particularly in London). This led to the 2004–5 Capital Catch-up Campaign. There is also advice on postexposure prophylaxis (giving the MMR within 72 hours of exposure if older than nine months of age, or using immunoglobulin within five days of exposure in immunocompromised patients, pregnant women and infants under nine months). The article concludes that we will reach the 2010 goal for eradication only if we maintain high levels of vaccination.

MMR litigation

The High Court has said that 'no positive link has ever been established' with autism and the Medical Research Council has confirmed this. Judges have gone on to say that 'unsubstantiated health scares endanger children and enrich lawyers'.

The Joint Committee on Vaccination and Immunisation is an independent group that was first set up in 1963 to advise the Government on matters relating to communicable disease preventable through immunisation. Its role continues.

Chickenpox vaccine

The Joint Committee on Vaccination and Immunisation is considering whether to include varicella in the childhood immunisation schedule because of the severity and sequelae in some children and patient groups.

Hepatitis B vaccination
BMJ 2007; 335: 950

This editorial by Andrew Pollard considers that 55% of the world's children are being vaccinated against Hep B following a call from the World Health Organisation. To date this is not offered in the UK. The vaccine could be combined safely with the diphtheria, tetanus, pertussis, Haemophilus influenza b and polio as a hexavalent vaccine and included in the primary immunisation schedule. It is also considered that it could be combined with the HPV vaccine programme.

Thiomersal in vaccines

Thiomersal is a mercury-based antimicrobial preservative that is found in some DTP preparations (and some Hib vaccines outside the UK). This caught media attention because of suspected links with autism. It has never been part of live vaccines (MMR and BCG). The theoretical concerns are that, in combination, the cumulative mercury dose could exceed recommended safety levels. The US and Europe regulatory bodies have recommended that it is phased out. This has been endorsed by the WHO, which has also stressed that if thiomersal-free vaccines are not available, vaccination programmes should not be compromised (i.e. children should still be vaccinated).

Three DTP vaccinations with or without Hib would give a maximum cumulative dose of 75 mcg ethylmercury – less than half the 187 mcg dose that causes concern. This is cleared quickly and is not known to be cumulative. A thiomersal and vaccine fact sheet can be found at www.dh.gov.uk.

Feverish illness in children
National Institute for Health and Clinical Excellence. *Feverish illness in children: NICE clinical guideline 47.* London: NIHCE; 2007
www.nice.org.uk/nicemedia/pdf/CG47NICEGuideline.pdf
BMJ 2007; 334: 1163–4

This problem-focused guidance was published for use in the assessment and initial management of children younger than 5 years with a feverish illness. There are no targets, just advice based on evidence and consensus opinions. It recommends that the guidelines are followed until a diagnosis is made. At that point the child should be treated according to guidelines for that condition.

Assessing the severity of fever uses a traffic light system taking into account colour, respiratory symptoms, hydration and miscellaneous factors. It also highlights that even if a child is apyrexial when you see him/her, it is important to take all reports of fever seriously.

Measure and record	Assess for signs of dehydration
• Temperature	• Prolonged capillary refill time
• Heart rate	• Abnormal skin turgor
• Respiratory rate	• Abnormal respiratory pattern
• Capillary refill time	• Weak pulse
	• Cool extremities

The above findings should be recorded.

The guidelines look at criteria for admission, antipyretic interventions and care at home, including advice about when to seek further advice.

Autism
Autism is a lifelong developmental disability affecting social and communication skills with varying degrees of severity on a somatic pragmatic scale. Onset is usually by the age of three years, but can go undiagnosed. Early diagnosis enables behavioural therapy, facilitated communication and educational techniques to be introduced, hopefully improving long-term outcome.

SIGN, following the National Autism Plan for Children in England and Wales, produced evidence-based guidelines for autistic spectrum disorders (a group of developmental disorders that include autism, Asperger syndrome and atypical autism) in 2007. NICE is in the process of developing guidelines.

CHAT, the check list given below, is frequently used. These guidelines consider various warning signs in both pre-school and school-age children. Communication and social impairments are most easily recognisable, but impairment in interest with lack of flexibility and recognition of other odd behaviour is also important in coming to a diagnosis.

Early identification of autism by the Checklist for Autism in Toddlers (CHAT)
J R Soc Med 2000; 93: 521–5
This is a screening tool that can be used at the 18-month check by GPs or health visitors.

Section A

1	Does your child enjoy being swung, bounced on your knee, etc?	Yes/No
2	Does your child take an interest in other children?	Yes/No
3	Does your child like climbing on things, e.g. stairs?	Yes/No
4	Does your child enjoy playing peek-a-boo/hide and seek?	Yes/No
5	**Does your child ever pretend, for example, to make a cup of tea, using a toy cup and teapot, or pretend other things?**	**Yes/No**
6	Does your child ever use his/her index finger to point to *ask* for something?	Yes/No
7	**Does your child ever use his/her finger to point to indicate interest in something?**	**Yes/No**
8	Can your child play properly with small toys, e.g. bricks, cars without just mouthing or fiddling with them?	Yes/No
9	Does your child ever bring objects over to show you something?	Yes/No

Section B

1	During the appointment has the child made eye contact with you?	Yes/No
2	**Get child's attention and then point across the room at an interesting object and say, 'Oh look! There's a – (name the toy)'.**	
	Does the child look across and see what you are pointing at?	**Yes/No**
3	**Get the child's attention, then give the child a toy cup and teapot and say 'Can you make a cup of tea?' Does the child pretend to make or drink the tea?**	**Yes/No**
4	**Say to the child 'Where is the light?' Does the child point?**	**Yes/No**
5	Can the child build a tower of bricks (how many?)	Yes/No

If the items in bold print are absent at 18 months then the child is at high risk for a social communication disorder. If 'No' is the response to all five questions in bold, then the child is at high risk

A 12-point autism check list is in the process of being validated. It is not dissimilar to the questionnaire above but is based on a scoring system.

Attention-deficit hyperactivity disorder

Hyperactivity affects 1–2% of children. There are both ICD-10 and DSM-IV classifications in use. The consequences can be far reaching, affecting education and causing behavioural problems and social isolation. Benefits can be obtained with medication, behavioural therapy and educational support. Dietary supplements such as flax oil, vitamin C and omega-3 are receiving a lot of attention and there is anecdotal evidence for excluding some colourings and preservatives.

Access to treatment is influenced by both the parents and the GP. It can lead to conflict, misunderstanding and dissatisfaction if a parent's concerns are not taken seriously.

Current research is focusing on cognitive processing, genetic factors, brain function abnormalities and the significance of co-morbidity factors.

Attention-deficit hyperactivity disorder
Lancet 2005; 366(9481): 237-48
This review estimates that this disorder of inattention and impulsivity and hyperactivity can affect up to 12% of children worldwide, and that at least half of the children affected will have impairing symptoms into adulthood. It also considers treatment with methylphenidate and amphetamine effective as well as targeted psychosocial treatments.

Methylphenidate, atomoxetine and dexamfetamine for ADHD in children and adolescents (NICE 2006)

Prescribing in ADHD has gradually increased over the last few years and currently costs the NHS around £5 milllion a year. Although these treatments are licensed, it is recommended that they are prescribed only following specialist input.

- Methylphenidate is a sympathomimetic amine that works on dopamine receptors.
- It is used as part of the comprehensive treatment programme (paediatric and psychiatric).
- It is not licensed for children under six years, or in cases of thyrotoxicosis or tics.
- Continued prescribing and monitoring may be performed by GPs under a shared care agreement.

NICE is developing guidance on ADHD: pharmacological and psychological interventions in children.

Sudden infant death syndrome

www.fsid.org.uk/coni.html

The interim report of the confidential enquiry into maternal and child health dated October 2007 is available to view at www.cemach.org.uk.

Risk factors in the infant include the following:
+ low birth weight
+ prematurity
+ sex (60% of cases are boys)
+ multiple births
+ high birth order (parity).

Risk factors in parents for sudden infant death of their child include the following:
+ young maternal age
+ unmarried mothers
+ maternal smoking in pregnancy
+ *smoking after birth* – this increases the risk five-fold, and is the biggest risk.

Environmental risk factors include:
+ low socioeconomic class
+ sleeping prone (the Back to Sleep campaign was launched in 1994)
+ winter
+ over heating
+ used cot mattresses (this factor is being considered in more detail).

Recent data suggest that babies sleeping with a dummy have a reduced risk of cot death.

CONI (Care of the Next Infant) and the Foundation for the Study of Infant Deaths have been established to support parents. They provide counselling and apnoea alarms as well as many other resources.

Uncertainty in classification of repeat sudden unexpected infant deaths in Care of the Next Infant Programme

BMJ 2007; 335: 129–32

It is rare for a family to experience SID, and even more so to experience two such deaths.

This article states that a recent study of families with two sudden infant deaths concluded that 13% of second deaths were homicide. A review of published material shows this to be a minimum estimate, as the cause of many second deaths could not be ascertained (cf. screening for MCADD).

Child protection

In 2007 there were 27 900 children under a Child Protection Plan (CPP). These children are on a child protection register because they are at risk of ongoing abuse. Such abuse could be physical, sexual (this includes contact and non-contact), neglect and emotional ill-treatment.

Following the Victoria Climbié trial there has been renewed effort to keep us all informed on child protection issues and *Working to Safeguard Children* was published. As GPs we are not expected to be trained in forensics, but we should remain vigilant, keep good records, be prepared to set investigations in motion through the child protection agency and maintain close contact with other health professionals and the family. This is often tricky in that, although the welfare of the child must be placed above all other considerations, usually all members of the family are under our care and often at the start of an investigative process you may be reporting only suspicions.

The NSPCC (www.nspcc.org.uk) is a very good site to help you understand more about child protection issues.

The Royal College has also published a toolkit that has been developed with the NSPCC. This can be downloaded from: www.rcgp.org.uk/continuing_the_ gp_journey/circ/ safeguarding_children_toolkit.aspx.

Women's health

Hormone replacement therapy

Hormone replacement therapy (HRT) is a collective term to encompass a variety of sex steroids, oestrogens and progesterones given in various forms. Treatment with HRT is a curious ethical problem and is always topical.

Menopause in the UK is around 51 years of age. The target population of women who should be given the opportunity to make an informed decision on whether to take HRT or not includes the following:

- women with menopausal symptoms affecting quality of life (usually short-term use)
- women who have had a premature menopause (under the age of 45 years)
- women who have had a surgical menopause (hysterectomy and oophorectomy) under 40 years of age. Use of HRT in this group is usually until the age menopause would have occurred.

Managing the menopause
BMJ 2007; 334: 736–41
Helen Roberts wrote this clinical review. It discussed most issues and provided

the type of simple table I find most helpful when explaining risk to patients, i.e. a table of absolute risk. The table shows the number of extra women (aged 50–79) who would suffer an event if they took HRT for one year. A negative number means there is a risk reduction.

Difference in absolute event rates for hormone replacement therapies compared with placebo/10000 women/year		
Event	Oestrogen and progestogen vs. placebo	Oestrogen only vs. placebo
Breast disease	8	-7
Heart disease	7	-5
Pulmonary embolus	8	7
Stroke	8	12
Hip fracture	-5	-6
Colorectal cancer	-6	1

Managing the menopause – British Menopause Society Council Consensus Statement on HRT, 10 June 2005

This concludes that results from recent papers have thus far given no reason to make any changes in current clinical practice. Below is a brief summary of the statement.

Benefits
1 *Vasomotor symptoms* – there is good evidence from randomised controlled trials (RCT) with improvement usually noted within four weeks.
2 *Urogenital symptoms and sexuality symptoms* – respond well to oestrogens (topically or systemically), long-term treatment is often needed.
3 *Osteoporosis* – there is evidence from RCTs (including the Women's Health Initiative and the Million Women Study) that HRT reduces hip as well as other osteoporotic fractures. It is not advised that HRT be used as first line treatment for prevention of osteoporosis. Benefit wears off rapidly after cessation of use.
4 *Colorectal cancer* – results from the oestrogen progestogen arm (WHI) show only that HRT reduces the risk of colorectal cancer. It is not advised that HRT be used for prevention.

Risks
1 *Breast cancer* – mammographic density is increased in about 25% of women. HRT appears to confer a similar degree of risk as that associated with a late natural menopause (2.3% compared with 2.8% per year respectively).

The lifetime risk is significantly increased with current long-term use when started over 50 years (relative risk of 1.35, 95% confidence interval 1.2–1.49). Such effect is not seen in women who start HRT for a premature menopause, indicating that it is the duration of lifetime hormone exposure that is relevant. Progesterone addition increases the risk of breast cancer and has to be balanced against the fact that if not used, the risk of endometrial cancer will increase. Breast cancer risk falls after cessation of use, and by five years is no greater than if never exposed to HRT.

2 *Endometrial cancer* – unopposed oestrogen increases endometrial cancer, sequential progesterone does not eliminate this risk.
3 *Venous thromboembolism* – HRT increases the risk two-fold, the highest risk being in the first year of use. Absolute risk is small at 1.7 per 1000 in women over 50 years of age.
4 *Gallbladder disease* – HRT increases the risk (confirmed in WHI).

Uncertainties
1 *Cardiovascular disease* – the role of HRT for primary and secondary prevention remains uncertain. WHI showed a transient increase in coronary heart disease; absolute risk at 50–59 years was 5, and at 60–69 years was 1.
2 *Dementia and cognition* – while oestrogen may delay or reduce the risk of Alzheimer's, it does not seem to improve established disease.
3 *Ovarian cancer* – in oestrogen-only, after more than 10 years of use there seems to be an increase in the risk. In continuous combined therapy this does not seem to be the case.
4 *Quality of life* – this is difficult to evaluate, and there is no conclusion as yet.

Women's Health Initiative (WHI)
This was two separate, parallel, multicentre, randomised, double blind, placebo-controlled studies evaluating the risk and benefit of conjugated equine oestrogen both alone and in combination with medroxyprogesterone acetate in healthy postmenopausal women.

It looked at 16 608 postmenopausal women with an intact uterus (there was a further arm of 10 739 patients who had previously undergone a hysterectomy), aged 50–79 years. Participants were randomly assigned to either placebo or conjugated equine oestrogens (0.625 mg per day) plus medroxyprogesterone acetate (2.5 mg per day). The women were followed up for a mean of 5.2 years.

Results were published over several papers (mainly in *JAMA*) and the main findings were as follows:
◆ HRT does not confer cardiovascular or cognitive protection   *ie in combined oe + Pr*
◆ HRT increases breast cancer in women with a uterus
◆ HRT increases the risk of venothromboembolism
◆ HRT does not improve overall quality of life

◆ HRT reduces fracture rates
◆ HRT reduces vasomotor symptoms.

There are many facets to this trial (for example breast cancer risk is further broken down into association with obesity, exercise and use of non-steroidal anti-inflammatories – all in separate articles). The latest article (*JAMA* 2005; 293: 935–48) shows that HRT worsens urinary incontinence where it had previously been thought to improve it.

Criticism related to the WHI Study
This is a general collection of thoughts from many authors across many publications and is by no means exhaustive.
◆ A high dose of conjugated equine oestrogens was the choice for HRT.
◆ Women were on average 63 years at the start of treatment (most women use HRT from 45–55 years and are symptomatic).
◆ It looked at postmenopausal women so cannot be extrapolated to women with an early menopause.
◆ Women taking HRT in the UK are a self-selecting group, usually educated and in a higher socioeconomic class, with a better diet, and are less likely to come from ethnic minority backgrounds (the trial included all women).
◆ There is a danger that trials that are stopped early are at a random high, so it is important to be cautious about fast tracking results into practice.

WHI clinical trial revisit: imprecise scientific methodology disqualifies the study's outcomes
Am J Obstet Gynaecol 2005; 193(5): 1599–604
This is a discussion paper about the lack of independent, nonbiased analysis of the quality of methodology. The authors feel that the questions over validity make it difficult to apply the WHI results to healthy postmenopausal women, different ethnic groups or as general postmenopausal prevention.

Postmenopausal hormone therapy and risk of cardiovascular disease by age and years since menopause
JAMA 2007; 297(13): 1465–77
Until WHI contradicted findings, the general belief from data and trials was that cardiovascular events were lower in women who took HRT by up to 33%. This study was a secondary analysis of the data from the WHI. The authors found a slightly increased risk of stroke but no increase in the risk of coronary heart disease or mortality in women taking HRT from around the time of the menopause.

The Million Women Study
Breast cancer and HRT in the Million Women Study
Lancet 2003; 362(9382): 419-27

This is an observational study that was set up to investigate the effects of specific types of HRT on incident and fatal breast cancer. A total of 1 084 110 UK women aged 50–64 years were recruited between 1996 and 2001. They provided information about their use of HRT and other personal details and were followed up for cancer incidence and death.

The study found that current users of HRT were more likely than never-users to develop breast cancer (relative risk 1.66, 95% CI 1.58–1.75), $p < 0.0001$) and die from it (RR 1.22, 95% CI 1.00–1.48, $p = 0.05$). Past users were not at increased risk. The associated risk was greater for oestrogen-progestogen than other forms of HRT ($p < 0.0001$). The risk varied little between the strength and type of HRT.

Cancer incidence and mortality in relation to body mass index in the Million Women Study: cohort study
BMJ 2007; 335: 1134-9

A total 45 037 incident cancers and 17 203 deaths from cancer were examined. Having adjusted for various lifestyle factors, age and use of HRT, increasing BMI was associated with increasing risk for incident cancers for 10 out of 17 cancer types considered: endometrial, oesophageal adenocarcinoma, kidney, leukaemia, postmenopausal breast cancer, multiple myeloma, pancreatic cancer, non-Hodgkin's lymphoma and ovarian cancers. An inverse relationship was seen for squamous cell carcinoma of the oesophagus and lung cancer. Premenopausal breast cancer, stomach, malignant melanoma, colorectal, brain, cervical and bladder cancers showed no relationship with BMI of statistical significance.

Main morbidities recorded in the women's international study of long duration oestrogen after menopause (WISDOM): a randomised controlled trial of hormone replacement therapy in postmenopausal women
BMJ 2007; 335: 239-44

Contrary to the WHI, this study was designed to look at oestrogen use after the menopause in women aged 45–60 years (this was later changed to 50–69 years), that would be a slightly more representative group of women. Recruitment began in 1999 and included women from the UK, Australia and New Zealand. The paper presents the initial results of 6498 women followed for 11.9 months. This was of short duration as the study was closed following publication of the WHI. At this point cardiovascular risk and thromboembolic risk were both seen to increase when HRT was started after the menopause.

HRT and stroke: clinical trials review

Stroke 2004; 35(11 Suppl 1): 2644–7

Observational data suggest that postmenopausal HRT is associated with a 25–50% lower cardiovascular disease incidence. However, observational data for HRT is associated with the potential for bias.

Of the three major trials on stroke and postmenopausal women, two focus on secondary prevention:

+ the heart and estrogen/progestin replacement study (HERS)
+ women's estrogen for stroke trial (WEST).

And one examined primary prevention:

+ The Women's Health Initiative (WHI).

All indicate that postmenopausal hormone therapy is not effective at reducing stroke either in established vascular disease or as primary prevention.

Association between HRT and subsequent stroke: a meta-analysis

BMJ 2005; 330: 342–5

This analysis looked at 28 trials with 39 769 subjects. It found that HRT was associated with increasing stroke, particularly of ischaemic type. Of the people who had a stroke, those taking HRT seemed to have a worse outcome.

Alternatives to HRT

The research base for these products is limited. Undoubtedly some women get very real relief from these products. Some of these may contain oestrogenic properties and women need to be aware of the implications of this if they have a history of oestrogen-sensitive tumours.

For hot flushes:

+ phyto-oestrogens – chick peas, lentils, soya products, red clover

There have been several small RCTs comparing, for example, soy flour to wheat flour. They have found no significant reduction in hot flushes

+ black cohosh – a recent study (*Maturitas* 2005; 16: 134–46) found that it offered no significant benefit
+ dong quai (*Angelica sinensis*)
+ evening primrose oil (*Oenothera biennis*)
+ *Ginkgo biloba*
+ *Agnus castus* (also suggested for premenstrual tension)
+ clonidine (an alpha adrenoceptor agonist available on prescription)
+ selective serotonin reuptake inhibitors
+ acupuncture (usually a small tack left in at the ankle that can be massaged).

For osteoporosis:
- bisphosphonates, e.g. alendronate, etidronate, residronate
- strontium ranelate.

For mood disturbances:
- St John's Wort
- antidepressant medication.

Cervical cancer
www.cancerresearchuk.org
- The incidence of cervical cancer in the UK is 9.6 per 100 000.
- The mortality rate is 5 per 100 000.
- The incidence of disease peaks at 30–35 and 70–75 years of age.
- Around 95% of cervical cancers are squamous cell, 5% are adenocarcinomas.
- The most important risk factor is human papillomavirus (HPV); at least 50% of sexually active people will get HPV (type 16, 18, 31, 33 or 35). Smoking and the age at first intercourse are also important factors.

Cervical screening
- Around 80% of women aged 25–64 years have been screened (3.8 million women).
- Cervical screening prevents around 5000 deaths per year in the UK. The incidence of cervical cancer fell by 42% between 1988–96 (in England and Wales) as a direct consequence of the cervical screening programme.
- The screening programme currently costs around £157 million per year.

Protocol for cervical screening

Age group	Frequency
25	First invitation
25–49	3-yearly invitation
50–64	5-yearly invitation
Over 65	Only if the last 3 tests include an abnormal result or if not been screened since the age of 50

Liquid based cytology
This is now being implemented across the UK. In conventional smear taking (with a wooden spatula or brush with cells being fixed on a slide) up to 80% of cervical cells are not transferred to the slide. In 2003 it was announced that liquid based cytology (LBC) would become the test of choice in the UK.
- LBC reduces inadequate smears from 9% to 2%.

- LBC is currently a more expensive option, but a cost saving would be made by a reduced need for repeats.
- Cells from the sample brush are washed off in the vial. The fluid is then spun down and the cells are filtered out under pressure onto a slide to be read (the reading is not yet automated). Please note there are differing LBC kits on the market.

Accuracy of liquid based versus conventional cytology: overall results of new technologies for cervical cancer screening: randomised controlled trial
BMJ 2007; 335: 28–31

This Italian study looked at women aged 25–60. A total of 22 466 had conventional screening and 22 708 had the experimental LBC arm. The study found that there was no statistical difference in sensitivity for detection of cervical intraepithelial neoplasia (CIN) grade 2 or more. LBC detected more grade 1 CIN (p = 0.0006). There was a reduction in inadequate smears as there was no obscuring inflammation.

Human papillomavirus vaccine

Around 95% of all cervical cancer is attributed to HPV and development of a vaccine that prevents this is one of the most exciting occurrences in modern medicine. The Joint Committee for Vaccination and Immunisation and Department of Health have published guidance for the start of the vaccination programme in 2008/9 (Year 8 girls) with a catch up to include women up to 18. Gardasil (quadrivalent HPV 6, 11, 16 and 18 recombinant vaccine) has been found to prevent 100% of cases of high-grade pre-cancerous lesions as well as non-invasive cancers (CIN II and III or AIS) associated with HPV 16 and 18. This was seen after a two-year follow-up following a three-dose regime. Cervarix (bivalent: HPV types 16 and 18) is also licensed in the UK and this is the vaccine that has been chosen for the immunisation campaign. Women outside of this cohort are being advised to discuss vaccination with their GP.

The need for booster vaccines, questions around administering the vaccine in women already infected with HPV, changes to the cervical screening programme, the therapeutic role of vaccines and cost effectiveness (as well as whether men should be included in the vaccination programme) are all areas that will need clarification.

Human papillomavirus vaccination programmes
BMJ 2007; 335: 357–8

This editorial on the analysis reported in the same issue of the *Journal* (*BMJ* 2007; 335: 375–7) brings to our attention that focusing on vaccine uptake alone will not be adequate but should be part of a comprehensive, integrated system of cervical cancer prevention. Such a strategy should tackle adolescent sexuality, and parental control and protection of children. It advocates giving the vaccine before exposure and developing public policies that have a broader perspective.

Ovarian cancer

◆ Ovarian cancer is the fourth most common female cancer in the UK.
◆ The incidence in the UK is 20 per 100 000 (and it appears to be increasing).
◆ Each year there are 6900 new cases.
◆ Women with BRCA1 gene have a 50% lifetime risk and those with BRCA2 have a 30% lifetime risk (the same risk as if two first-degree relatives have ovarian cancer).

Ovarian screening

There is no proven role for screening, but methods would include Ca125 and transvaginal ultrasound scanning. In some areas women with one or more first-degree relatives with ovarian cancer may be offered a yearly Ca125 and ultrasound scan. They should be made aware of the limitations and the lack of evidence for this approach. Trials looking at the success of screening for ovarian cancer have not been encouraging.

The Medical Research Council launched a 10-year trial (UK Collaborative Trial of Ovarian Cancer Screening) of 200 000 postmenopausal women looking at transvaginal ultrasound scan vs. Ca125 on a yearly basis to try to establish effectiveness of each method in terms of their impact on mortality, morbidity and cost.

Researchers at Yale University have isolated 35 proteins that are significantly higher in women with ovarian cancer; and are currently validating the use of four (leptin, prolactin, osteopontin and insulin-like growth factor-2).

The Prostate, Lung, Colorectal and Ovarian (PLCO) American trial is enrolling 143 000 individuals aged 55–74 years into a screening trial, the follow-up of which will last for 13 years, having started in 1993. At the time of printing, the results for this had not been published – but watch out for them.

Ovarian cancer and oral contraceptives: collaborative reanalysis of data from 45 epidemiological studies including 23 257 women with ovarian cancer and 87 303 controls

Lancet 2008; 371: 303-14

This analysis, using data from 41 studies over 21 countries, was trying to ascertain how long the protective effects of the oral contraceptive pill lasted after discontinuing use. It found that the risk reduction (31% of cases and 37% of controls had used contraceptive pills) lasted for 30 years, although it became attenuated over time.

Population risk reduction after five years of use was 29% (95% CI 23–34%).

For use that had ceased 20–29 years previously the risk reduction was 15% (CI 9–21%).

Although the contraceptive pill is not yet advocated in the prevention of ovarian cancers, this paper certainly makes one wonder how much this positive spin off should be promoted.

Breast cancer

Breast cancer accounted for 27% of all female cancers in 1995. It is the most common female cancer and it is the cause of 18% of all female deaths.

- Around 5% of all breast cancers are linked to specific single gene defects.
- Some 50–80% are due to BRCA (breast cancer genes) 1 or 2.
- BRCA1 and 2 are linked with colon cancer and possibly prostate cancer.
- Women with dense breasts on mammography are more likely to develop breast cancer (*NEJM* 2007; 356: 227–36).

Breast screening

www.cancerscreening.nhs.uk/breastscreen/index.html

The NHS breast screening programme was introduced in England and Wales in 1988 on the recommendation of the Forrest Committee. In one year 1.3 million women were screened and 8345 cancers were diagnosed with mammography. Mammography is currently the best tool for screening for breast cancer and it is offered to all women aged 50–70 years of age every three years (women over 70 years may request ongoing three-yearly screening).

It is estimated that the NHS screening programme saves 1400 lives per year in England. (It is worth noting that a 2007 Cochrane Review did not feel there was enough evidence to determine whether screening did more harm than good.)

Scientists are developing salivary tests that measure genetic markers of cancer. Although these will not replace mammography for many years, the tests so far predict breast (and oral) cancers with 95% accuracy.

The Leningrad and Shanghai studies are large randomised controlled trials that have both failed to demonstrate a reduction in mortality from breast cancer or increased detection by teaching self-examination.

Mammography has been shown in a Swedish RCT to reduce mortality by up to 40%, the benefit being greatest in 50–70-year-olds. Compared with symptomatic breast cancers, screen-detected cancers are smaller and more likely to be non-invasive. If they are invasive they are more likely to be better differentiated and node negative.

It has been calculated that for every two million women screened, one extra cancer after 10 years may be caused by the radiation delivered to the breast from mammography.

No increase in anxiety has been found in women invited to attend for screening unless there is a need for recall.

HRT reduces the sensitivity of mammography (from 77% to 65%) and is associated with more false-positives.

Participation in mammography screening
BMJ 2007; 335: 731-2
Although this editorial was written because USA guidance changed to offer women aged 40–49 inclusion in screening, it discusses the real pros and cons of screening and the importance of encouraging women to decide what is right for them, rather than being told what to do. The main benefit of screening is to avoid death from breast cancer.

The relative risk of death from breast cancer for women who are screened is 0.85 for women in their 40s and 0.78 for those 50 or older. The main drawbacks of screening are false-positives and over diagnosis, creating the impact of increased anxiety and unnecessary further investigation including biopsies.

Model outcome of screening mammography: information to support informed choices
BMJ 2005; 330: 936-8
This argues that risk and benefit should be set out in a more straightforward way for patients, using decision-making models. The paper presents age-specific estimates of benefits and harms of screening mammography:
+ for every 1000 women screened over 10 years, 167–251 (depending upon age) receive an abnormal result and are recalled
+ from 56 to 64 of these have at least one biopsy
+ from nine to 26 have an invasive cancer detected by screening
+ about 0.5, 2, 3 and 2 fewer deaths from breast cancer occur every 10 years per 1000 women aged 40, 50, 60 and 70 years respectively, who choose to be screened compared to those who do not.

Maximising benefit and minimising harm of screening
BMJ 2008; 336: 480-3
The opening sentence of this article states: 'all screening programmes do harm; some do good as well, and, of those, some do more harm than good at a reasonable cost'. It suggests successful screening has a total quality approach from the outset; clear objectives and standards; single national protocols to help compare results and identify trends, as well as a dataset with well understood definitions; complete data of good quality; and there should be a clear reference point, such as a randomised controlled trial.

Breast cancer risk assessment tool
This is a tool to calculate 10-year risk of breast cancer, including age, age at first menstruation, age of first live birth, number of first-degree relatives with breast cancer, number of previous biopsies (positive or negative) and one biopsy with

atypical hyperplasia. There are ongoing studies to look at validity and whether the statistical model can be improved. This can be viewed online at www.cancer.gov/bcrisktool/breast-cancer-risk.aspx.

Heavy menstrual bleeding

National Institute for Health and Clinical Excellence. *Heavy menstrual bleeding: NICE clinical guideline 44.* London: NIHCE; 2007

www.nice.org.uk/nicemedia/pdf/CG44NICEGuideline.pdf

Heavy menstrual bleeding (menorrhagia) is a loss of more than 80 mls of blood per cycle (with either regular or irregular cycles). It is important to assess the condition properly for primary and secondary causes.

♦ Around 28% of women feel menstruation is excessive and 5% consult their GP.
♦ One in 20 women aged 30–49 years consult their GP each year with menorrhagia.
♦ One in five women will have a hysterectomy before the age of 60 years.
♦ Quality of life issues should be focused on by GPs.

The NICE guidelines consider important factors in the history, and necessary initial investigations (full blood count is the only routine test advocated). Further investigations should be directed, depending upon the history. For example high vaginal and *Chlamydia* swabs if there is a suspicion of infection; clotting studies should be considered if there is a significant family history. Ultrasound scan should be considered where there is a pelvic mass or the uterus is palpable abdominally, or where there is treatment failure.

Referral for endometrial biopsy should be considered:
♦ in women over 45 years
♦ where there is persistent intermenstrual bleeding
♦ where treatment has failed.

Premenstrual syndrome

This is a distinct disorder (with emotional and physical symptoms) that occurs in the luteal phase of the cycle, due to release of progesterone triggered by ovulation, and continuing until menstruation. There is no evidence of a specific hormonal imbalance. Meta-analyses have confirmed that treatment with progesterone products is no more effective than placebo. There is no diagnostic test. The best way to diagnose premenstrual syndrome (PMS) is by asking the patient to keep a three-month diary which should show cyclical premenstrual deterioration with postmenstrual cure.

Premenstrual dysphoric disorder (PMDD) symptoms (DSM-IV 1994)

♦ Depressed mood and interest.

◆ Marked anxiety, tension, difficulty concentrating.
◆ Marked affective lability, lethargy with either hypersomnia or insomnia.
◆ Marked anger, irritability or increased interpersonal conflicts.
   This is an extreme part of the PMS spectrum.

Treatment

Patients can be treated in two broad ways.

Suppressing ovulation:
◆ combined oral contraceptive pill has a variable response
◆ danazol (several randomised controlled trials prove benefit, although long-term use is limited due to masculinising effects)
◆ oestrogen patches or implants – progestogenic endometrial protection (e.g. Mirena) is needed as well as assessment of the endometrium at the outset of treatment so as not to risk falsely reassuring women that bleeding is normal when they may have endometrial cancer
◆ gonadotrophin-releasing hormones (pharmacological menopause – time-limited unless add-back HRT or tibolone is used)
◆ oophorectomy and hysterectomy (rarely justified).

Changing serotonin status:
◆ vitamin B_6 (50–100 mg maximum as there is risk of peripheral neuropathy) has been shown to give some improvement; vitamin E may be of benefit in breast tenderness
◆ selective serotonin reuptake inhibitors (SSRIs) appear to be seven times more effective than placebo, but must not be prescribed with St John's Wort.

Luteal phase dosing with paroxetine controlled release in the treatment of premenstrual dysphoric disorder
Am J Obstet Gynaecol 2005; 193(2): 352–60
This multicentre randomised double-blind placebo-controlled trial looks at either 12.5 mg or 25 mg of paroxetine daily in the luteal phase versus placebo (in a total of 373 patients). Both doses were found to be effective, well tolerated and significantly better than placebo.

Other treatment options

Agnus castus fruit extract, the fruit from the Chaste tree, has been a traditional remedy for PMS.

Treatment for PMS with *Agnus castus* fruit extract: prospective, randomised, placebo-controlled trial

BMJ 2001; 322(7279): 134-7

A total of 178 German women were randomised for three cycles. *Agnus castus* fruit was found to be significantly more effective than placebo, and it appears to be safe.

Additional options include:

* *St John's Wort* – initial studies have shown a possible benefit; it does help depressive features irrespective of other symptoms
* *dietary changes* – for example, increasing soy isoflavins has been seen to give some improvement
* *complementary therapies*
  * acupuncture has been shown to help features of dysmenorrhoea
  * homeopathy has been found in a pilot study of 20 women to have a 90% improvement compared to placebo
  * Qi therapy, aromatherapy, reflexology, photic stimulation and magnetic therapy all have some supporting anecdotal evidence.

Contraception

The global population is estimated to reach 8.9 billion by 2050, creating significant risks of overpopulation. The goals of contraception are, ultimately, to reduce the number of unplanned and unwanted pregnancies by safe, well-tolerated and reversible methods.

Hormonal methods of contraception have been slow to change over the last four decades due to social, political and legal reasons, as well as medical complications encountered.

Combined oral contraception

In the UK 25% of women aged 16–49 years and 50% of women in their twenties are on the pill. Currently all pharmacological methods of contraception are reversible and made from synthetic steroids, containing no natural oestrogens or progesterones.

There are three generations of combined pill:

1 First generation (e.g. Norinyl-1, Ovran)
  * first produced in 1960s, no longer used
  * high dose of oestrogen (increased risk of venothromboembolism (VTE))
2 Second generation
  * lower oestrogen
  * similar progestogen to first generation pills
3 Third generation
  * produced 1980s
  * lower dose of oestrogen

- new form of progestogen (less androgenic than second generation products)
- 1995 pill scare – Committee on Safety of Medicines stated that VTE risk was doubled in users of pills that contained gestodene or desogestrel. This was based on unpublished trials with no confidence intervals. It was the first time progestogens had been implicated.

Risk assessment

www.ffprhc.org.uk

The UK Medical Eligibility Criteria (UKMEC) for the combined contraceptive pill is printed in summary in the Faculty of Family Planning's guidance on prescribing the combined contraceptive pill.

It is important to assess risk before initiating treatment and at each review.

- VTE risk increases with increasing age.
- BMI greater than 35 kg/m² quadruples the risk of VTE; there are other alternatives so use them if you possibly can.
- Smoking doubles the risk of VTE.
- Family history – if patients have a first-degree relative younger than 45 years of age with VTE/primary thrombotic tendency, combined pills should not be used.
- Ask about migraines (focal), breast cancer, pregnancy, undiagnosed vaginal bleed and diabetes.
- Measure blood pressure.

Venothromboembolism

In one year:

- a total of 5 in 100 000 women will develop VTE
- the number is 15 in 100 000 if taking second generation pill (levonorgestrel/norethisterone)
- the number is 25 in 100 000 if taking third generation pill (gestodene/desogestrel)
- and it is 60 in 100 000 in pregnancy.

The absolute risk, as opposed to the relative risk, is small.

If after one year of pill use a woman has not experienced a clot, it is thought that the subsequent risk will then be much lower.

Since the 1980s, the accepted risk for VTE due to combined oral contraceptives has been 30 in 100 000. Therefore, studies did not necessarily suggest an increased risk in third generation pills but a reduced risk, and a greater risk with second-generation pills than originally thought.

In 1999 the Department of Health announced an end to the 1995 restrictions on prescribing third generation pills.

UK studies

Cancer risk among users of oral contraceptives: cohort data from the Royal College of General Practitioners' oral contraception study
BMJ 2007; 335: 651–4

It is thought that use of the combined contraceptive pill increases the risk of breast, cervical and liver cancers and reduces the risk of endometrial, ovarian and possibly colorectal carcinomas. This study began in 1968. A total of 23 000 women using the pill and 23 000 women who were not, were recruited by 1400 GPs in the UK. In this cohort there was no increased risk in cancer; if anything, there was a 3–12% reduction in cancer (depending upon which dataset was used), with significant reduction in ovarian, uterine body, large bowel and rectal cancers. The absolute risk reduction is estimated at 10 or 45 per 100 000 women years of use.

Combined oral contraceptives and cervical cancer
Curr Opin Obstet Gynaecol 2004; 16(1): 27–9

This was a literature review that included eight studies conducted by the International Agency for Research on Cancer. The epidemiological links suggest an increased risk of cervical cancer (up to two-fold), but only of women who are long-term users (five years or more) and who had persistent human papilloma-virus infections of the cervix.

Long Acting Reversible Contraceptives (LARCs)
NICE October 2005

NICE recommends the profession take into account women's individual needs and preferences. The following recommendations have been identified as priorities:

Contraceptive provision:
+ information and choice of all methods of contraception should be offered
+ contraceptive service providers should be aware that all currently available LARC methods (IUD, IUS, injectables and implants) are more cost effective than the pill at one year. IUDs, IUS and implants are more cost effective than injectables, and increasing the use of LARCs will reduce the risk of pregnancy.

Counselling and provision of information:
+ these should be both written and verbal and include efficacy of method, duration of use, risk and possible side effects, non-contraceptive benefits, procedure for initiation and discontinuation, and when to seek help whilst using the method
+ they should include advice on safer sex.

Implanon

This was launched in September 1999 (following withdrawal of Norplant, relating to the insertion and removal of six rods insertion). It consists of a single semi-rigid rod with dimensions of 40 mm × 2 mm, and insertion should be subdermal. It releases 30–40 µg etonogestrel/day, the device lasting for a total of three years. It has a Pearl Index of 0.

Amenorrhoea is reported in around 21% of women and irregular bleeding can be problematic (as expected with progesterone methods) in around 17% of women, although by six months this has often settled.

Enzyme inducers such as antiretrovirals and probably St John's Wort can reduce effectiveness (antibiotics are still thought to be safe). There is no need to replace the rod early in obesity, although you may do so if there is an early return of bleeding.

Coils

- Copper coils (380 mm copper) are relatively easy to insert, even in nulliparous women. The licence is usually from 8–10 years, depending upon the type of coil and the time of insertion related to the menopause. The failure rate at two years is around 1.6 per 100 women (60% were due to expulsion). At least 300 mm of copper is needed for contraception to be effective.
- Mirena is licensed for five years (seven years if fitted over the age of 45 years) for contraception and four years for endometrial protection in HRT. The NICE guidelines state that if the woman is amenorrhoeic the IUS can be kept *in situ* until it is no longer needed for contraception. (This is not as straightforward as it might seem, given the need for contraception is usually based on having stopped menses with no hormonal influence.)
- Gynaefix is a frameless IUD consisting of six copper tubes on a nylon thread, knotted at one end, which anchors into the uterine fundus. The failure rate is less than 1% in up to five years of use and the expulsion rate is low.

Current contraceptive issues

- *Depomedroxyprogesterone* – there has been a drive to limit the use of this drug in younger women and to limit the duration of use to two years following a better understanding that it affects the bone mineral density.
- *Evra patch* (norelgestromin and ethinyloestradiol) was licensed in the UK in 2003. It is worn for three weeks out of a four-week cycle and the patch needs to be changed weekly.

New product review (Sep 2003) Norelgestromin/ethinyloestradiol transdermal contraceptive patch (EVRA)
J Fam Plann Reprod Health Care 2004; 30(1): 43–5

The overall Pearl Index was 1.24 (95% CI 0.19–2.33), similar to triphasic contraceptive pills. Self-reported compliance was 10% better with the patch (88.2%) compared to the pill (77.7%). This is an additional choice for women wanting combined hormonal contraception.

◆ *YAZ* – a new combined pill not yet licensed in the UK with ethinyloestradiol and drosperidone. It has 24 active pills with a four-day pill-free interval.

◆ *Immunocontraception* – a novel approach that is receiving a considerable degree of attention. Sperm have unique proteins, and targeting antibodies to these gamete-specific antigens could be successful. Currently vaccines targeting the HCG molecule are undergoing phase I and phase II trials on humans.

◆ *Folic acid supplemented contraception* – is being given consideration as there are still some preventable foetal abnormalities occurring. This would help, for example, in women who stop the pill to conceive but forget to take folic acid. A recent trial has found in favour of a woman who claimed she did not receive folic acid advice from her GP.

Emergency contraception

A MORI survey has indicated that 43% of 15–24-year-olds reported having casual sex in the last 10 years, of whom 40% had failed to use a condom. Around 12% of patients who require emergency contraception are under 16 years of age. Emergency contraception is available free of charge on prescription from GPs, family planning clinics, youth clinics, walk-in centres, genito-urinary clinics, some Accident and Emergency departments and pharmacists. In 1983 the Attorney General ruled that emergency contraception is not a form of abortion as there is no pregnancy to terminate. This was further supported in 2002. Life legally begins at implantation (in England).

Levonelle is now first line, although PC4 is still available, and has been shown to be effective with a stat dose of 1.5 mg. Levonelle has been available from pharmacists since January 2001 following pilot studies that showed a high demand, and also showed that patients were using the drug appropriately and that it was safe.

The demand through pharmacists is increasing (especially following the new pharmacy contract) and the Office of National Statistics has published data showing that demand through pharmacists has increased from 27% (2003/4) to 50% (2004/5); and demand through GPs has fallen from 41% to 33%.

If a patient weighs over 70 kg the Oxford Family Planning Association study has confirmed a higher failure rate of progesterone-only pills. Advice for Levonelle is that patients take one 1.5 mg tablet as soon as possible after unprotected sexual intercourse and that the dose is repeated after 12 hours (a 100% increase in the dose). This also follows for women on enzyme-inducing drugs. Women should be warned of the greater risk of ectopic pregnancy following emergency contraception.

Advance provision of emergency contraception for pregnancy prevention: a meta-analysis
Obstet Gynecol 2007; 110(6): 1379–88

The logic behind these studies is to enable timely use of emergency contraception and, hopefully, to reduce pregnancy rates. This meta-analysis looked at eight randomised trials and concluded that advanced provision did not reduce pregnancy rates.

Awareness of emergency contraception
J Fam Plann Reprod Health Care 2005; 32(2): 113–4

This was a study of 78 women who attended for termination. Sixty per cent of the women felt that emergency contraception was easily available; only 37% of them had ever used it.

It concluded that there are many reasons why emergency contraception is underused.

Community pharmacy supply of emergency hormonal contraception (EHC): a structured literature review of international evidence
Hum Reprod 2006; 21(1): 272–84

This systematic review (January 1990 – January 2005) included 24 peer-reviewed papers: one randomised controlled trial (RCT) and 23 qualitative or observational studies.

The pharmacy supply of EHC enables most women to receive it within 24 hours of unprotected intercourse, which is a feature rated highly by women. The RCT showed it did not reduce the use of other contraceptive methods; neither did it lead to an increase in risky sexual behaviour or infection.

One study found that pharmacy supply has led to a reduction in their Accident and Emergency attendance. This data was further supported by an article in *BMJ* 2005; 331: 271–3.

Other options for emergency contraception

The copper coil can be used up to five days after unprotected intercourse (i.e. up to day 19 of a regular 28-day cycle, but should be based on the shortest cycle if periods are irregular). Medico-legally this is not procuring an abortion (having been tested in the courts).

Improving teenagers' knowledge of contraception: cluster RCT of teacher-led intervention
BMJ 2002; 324: 1179–83

This study found that teachers giving a single lesson on emergency contraception to year 10 pupils improved the number of boys and girls who knew the correct time limits for both types of emergency contraception. It did not change sexual activity or use of emergency contraception.

Young people: sex, contraception, consent and the law

The age of consent for heterosexual sex is 16 for both men and women. In England, Scotland and Wales the age of consent for sex between men is also 16. The Sexual Offences Act 2003 updated offences. A significant attempt was made to protect children under the age of 13. The Act does not prevent a GP providing confidential sexual health advice, information and treatment.

Working to Safeguard Children is a document written as part of the new child protection guidelines. There is a duty under the Children Act 2004 to report any concerns of abuse or exploitation against anyone under 18, using the Child Protection Procedures.

Working Together (2006) gives a checklist, which includes:
+ whether the young person is competent to understand and consent to the sexual activity in which they are involved
+ the nature of the relationship – consider age and power imbalances
+ whether aggression, coercion or bribery was involved (including drug or alcohol use)
+ whether a young person's behaviour places them at risk
+ whether there have been any attempts to secure secrecy by the sexual partner.

Action to be taken where under-13s have disclosed sexual activity:
+ consult the child protection lead
+ always refer, except in exceptional circumstances (keep full records of the reasons not referred).

Gillick Test and Fraser competence

Judging whether a child under 16 is mature enough to understand what treatment involves, including the risks, is the Gillick test. It determines whether a child is competent to consent to treatment (such as contraception and vaccinations). In issues such as contraception, where an adult with parental responsibility is not necessarily involved, the Fraser guidelines on competence can be applied:
+ the young person understands the doctor's advice
+ the doctor cannot persuade the young person to inform his/her parents that contraceptive advice is being sought

- the young person is likely to begin or continue having sex whether or not you prescribe contraception
- physical or mental health is likely to suffer unless the young person receives contraception.

Gillick or Fraser? A plea for consistency over competence in children
BMJ 2006; 332: 807

This is an excellent editorial by Robert Wheeler. He explains the original case brought by Victoria Gillick, who challenged the health service guidance that would have allowed her daughters, aged under 16, to receive confidential contraceptive advice without her knowledge; and then explains Lord Fraser's concern over the dilemma of providing contraceptive advice to girls where their welfare may depend on it. Gillick competence provides an objective test of competence, whereas Fraser guidelines are more narrow, relating only to contraception.

Teenage pregnancy
www.bpas.org

Teenage sexual health, pregnancy and termination is always topical. The age of consent (from a legal perspective) to any form of sexual activity is 16 for both men and women. There is a series of laws to help protect children aged 13 to 16 years from abuse; there is a maximum provision for life imprisonment for rape of children under 13 years old, and there is no defence of mistaken belief about age as there is in 13–15-year-olds.

Teenage Pregnancy Unit statistics have found:
- in England there are 39 600 conceptions per year to teenagers
- the teenage (under 18) conception rate is 42–48 per 1000 conceptions per year, and almost half lead to termination
- nationally the rate is starting to fall (London remained stable from 1998–2003), but the UK still has the highest teenage pregnancy rate in Western Europe
- in England a total of 174 000 terminations are performed each year, and 12.4% of these are to women under 18 years, following either a previous birth (5%) or previous termination (7.4%)
- one in every ten babies in the UK is born to a teenage mother.

It is well recognised that teenage pregnancies:
- are seen at higher rates in deprived areas
- mean that teenage mothers are less likely to finish their education or find a job
- mean teenage mothers are more likely to bring their children up in poverty
- generally lead to poorer antenatal health and low birth-weight babies

◆ when resulting in a birth, mean the infants have twice the mortality rate seen in the population.

Health of the Nation 1990

This initiative increased priorities to under-16s and aimed to halve the rate of teenage pregnancies by 2000. This goal was not met for a number of reasons, including the fact that GPs have little influence on risk-taking behaviour.

Modernising Health and Social Services 2000/01–2002/03

This highlights the tackling of teenage pregnancies in the light of the Health of the Nation findings, especially in preventing conception and supporting teenage parents.

National Teenage Pregnancy Strategy

www.dfes.gov.uk/teenagepregnancy/dsp

This strategy is set out in the *Social Exclusion Unit Report on Teenage Pregnancy Issues* and was launched in 1999 with the following aims:
◆ to halve under-18 conception rates in England by 2010
◆ to increase the participation of teenage mothers in education, training or work by 60% by 2010, in order to reduce the risk of long-term social exclusion.

Progress so far:
◆ a decline of 11.8% in the conception rate among under-18-year-olds (the lowest rate for 20 years)
◆ a decline of 12.1% in the conception rate among under-16-year-olds (lowest rate for 20 years)
◆ forty-six per cent of conceptions still end in abortion (this has been static since 1998).

Issues relating to teenage pregnancies

1 *Provision of health and sex education:* teenagers are often unaware how to obtain contraceptive advice and believe they have to be over 16 years of age to obtain treatment. However, since the Gillick ruling of October 1985 (the Fraser guidelines), this is no longer the case. Teenagers are often willing to run the risk of sexually transmitted infections and pregnancy because they think their parents will find out if they see their GP (confidentiality is needed at all levels).
2 *Contraceptive services need to be accessible:* this includes GPs/family planning services/school nurses/youth clinics, etc.
3 *Role of schools:* this includes sex education/behavioural interventions as well as the need to develop communication skills and sustain the truth that virginity is still in the majority (apparently).

Sexual health in adolescents
BMJ 2007; 334: 103-4

This *BMJ* editorial discusses whether, rather than improving sexual health, sex behaviour interventions make it worse. Delay in first intercourse and parental involvement are both key factors in improving outcomes and reducing risk behaviour (and, maybe, teenage pregnancy).

What impact has England's Teenage Pregnancy Strategy had on young people's knowledge of and access to contraceptive services?
J Adolesc Health 2007; 41(6): 594-601

This paper looked at a random selection of 8879 adolescents aged 13 to 21 years. It found that young women had increasingly used the availability of school services to obtain contraceptive supplies (increased from 15.4% to 24% over a four-year period). There was no increase in overall service use.

Impact of a theoretical-based sex education programme (SHARE) delivered by teachers on NHS registered conceptions and terminations: final results of cluster randomised trial
BMJ 2007; 334: 133-6

This work looked at 4196 women in 25 secondary schools in Scotland and found no difference between the control group and the intervention group. The lack of effectiveness was not due to lack of quality of delivery.

Positive experiences of teenage motherhood: a qualitative study
Br J Gen Pract 2004; 54: 813-18

This was a small study of nine teenage mothers. They had recognised that they were all still young enough to further their education and were realistic about their futures, making plans about their careers. A nice twist, showing it doesn't have to be all doom and gloom.

National Strategy for Sexual Health and HIV (2001)

www.dh.gov.uk

In July 2001 a consultation document was published that outlined the Government's proposed strategy for sexual health and HIV. The main aim of the strategy is to prevent sexual causes of premature deaths and ill health, as well as to ensure that services are available for those patients who need them.

Local networks of providers will be based on three service levels.

Level 1: to be provided by GPs

+ Sexual history and risk assessment.
+ Contraceptive information and services.
+ Pregnancy testing and referral.
+ Cervical cytology screening and referral.
+ Sexually transmitted disease testing for women.
+ Assessment and referral for men.
+ HIV testing and counselling.
+ Hepatitis B immunisation.

Level 2: intermediate care to be provided by primary care teams with a special interest (e.g. an enhanced service), genito-urinary medicine or family planning clinics

+ IUD and contraceptive implants.
+ Testing and treatment of STDs.
+ Invasive STD testing for men.
+ Partner notification and contact tracing.
+ Vasectomy.

Level 3: specialist clinical teams across more than one primary care group

+ Outreach contraceptive services.
+ Outreach STD prevention.
+ Specialised infection management, including contact tracing.
+ Specialised HIV treatment and care.

A large proportion of GPs already provide level 1 services (the exception being HIV testing). The Additional Services of the current GP contract covers contraceptive services, whilst the enhanced service would allow a greater role of sexual health provision, as per the strategy.

Primary care and the national Strategy for Sexual Health and HIV: an evaluation of one primary care trust.
Int J STD AIDS 2006; 17(3): 189–92
This study from Windsor, Ascot and Maidenhead PCT looked at the level of sexual health service provision. It found that the main gaps in the system were for male and asymptomatic female screening and sexual health promotion.

Sexual health care training needs of general practitioner trainers: a regional survey
J Fam Plann Reprod Health Care 2005; 31(3): 213–18
Following the aims of the sexual health strategy to improve access to sexual health care, primarily in general practice, this study surveyed 374 GPs (295 (79%)

of these questionnaires were returned). The main drawback to implementation (from GPs at ground level) was the training needed; 82% of respondents felt considerably more training was needed to support the strategy.

Chlamydia

Sexually Transmitted Infections in Primary Care 2006 is available for download from www.rcgp.org.uk/PDF/clinspec_STI_in_primary_care_NLazaro.pdf.

- Reported rates of *Chlamydia* are 1339 in 100 000 in 16–19-year-olds, rising steadily (9%) from 2002 to 2003.
- Around 70% of women and 50% of men are asymptomatic. There may be non-specific symptoms.
- It may affect 3–5% of sexually active women in the UK.
- It is the most common curable sexually transmitted disease in Europe.
- It can cause ectopic pregnancy, pelvic inflammatory disease (in 10–30% of cases), infertility, perihepatitis (Fitz-Hugh–Curtis Syndrome) and there can be neonatal transmission.

High-risk groups are 16–25-year-olds and women undergoing a termination of pregnancy. Behavioural risk factors include teenagers leaving school at a young age, women with multiple partners, being single, and people from ethnic minorities.

Evaluation of nucleic acid amplification tests (NAATs) in the absence of a perfect gold standard test: a review of the statistical and epidemiological issues
Epidemiology 2005; 16(5): 604-12

This is an interesting insight into the limitations of NAATs, polymerase chain reaction, ligase chain reaction and transcription-mediated amplification tests and their limitations in diagnostic testing for sexually transmitted diseases. The study found that NAATs (currently used as the test of choice in the UK) had a sensitivity of around 97.6% and a specificity of 95.3%.

Screening for *Chlamydia*
www.chlamydiascreening.nhs.uk/

It is important not to confuse opportunistic screening of asymptomatic men and women with the need for a full complement of swabs and blood tests in high-risk individuals where it is important to consider all sexually transmitted infections.

In 1996 the Chief Medical Officer's Advisory Group called for a national screening programme and, following pilot studies, the chlamydia screening programme was outlined in the National Strategy for Sexual Health and HIV. The aim is to implement this for men and women under 25 years of age by 2008.

National Chlamydia Screening Programme

This was launched in 2003 with the following aims:

◆ to control chlamydia through early detection and treatment of asymptomatic infection
◆ to reduce onward transmission
◆ to prevent the consequences of untreated infection.

Opportunistic genital chlamydia screening will be offered to sexually active individuals:

◆ under 25 years
◆ under 16 who are deemed Fraser competent
◆ whenever there is a change in sexual partner.

In men, a first-pass urine has 75–100% sensitivity and in women a self-taken vulvo-vaginal swab has over 80% sensitivity with 99% specificity (urine in women has been shown to be less sensitive). Endocervical swabs at the time of a cervical smear may also be used.

Although the screening is initiated in primary care (general practice, antenatal clinics, family planning, colposcopy clinics, etc), the chlamydia screening office then co-ordinates the result notification, treatment if needed (azithromycin 1 gm stat is first line, taking one week to work), and contact tracing. The person undergoing the test has the option of receiving the results by phone (text messaging is offered in some regions) or in person.

Further pilots are in place with Boots the Chemist looking at its role in offering screening.

Screening implications for general practitioners

1 Extra time is needed by clinical staff:
   • for taking samples from at-risk patients or explaining how to do a self-test
   • for training practice staff
   • for taking a sexual history from all patients under 25 years
   • for pre-test counselling
   • for counselling patients who test positive. Although the office will co-ordinate things, it is inevitable that there will be some fall out
   • for partner notification and treatment
   • to ensure compliance and follow-up to treatment.
2 Extra resources are needed
   • for staff training
   • for laboratory tests.
3 Issues:
   • compliance requires sexual abstinence for one week
   • contact tracing (six-month history from patients)

- consider a test of cure
- genito-urinary referral confidentiality issue/ insurance forms, etc.

New point of care Chlamydia Rapid Test – bridging the gap between diagnosis and treatment: performance evaluation study
BMJ 2007; 335(7631): 1190–4

This study was looking at sensitivity and specificity of a Chlamydia Rapid Test (which identifies *Chlamydia lipopolysaccharides*) for vaginal swabs in 1349 women, as compared to polymerase chain reaction (chosen as the gold standard). For self-collected vaginal swabs the Chlamydia Rapid Test had a sensitivity of 82.7% and specificity of 98.8%. The instructions were found easy to understand by 99.4% of women (mean age of 18.5 years). The test would allow same-day results (the test takes 30 minutes), which would allow immediate treatment of infected patients.

With appropriate incentives, general practice can improve the coverage of the National Chlamydia Screening Programme
Br J Gen Pract 2006; 532(56): 892–3

This essay gives a brief summary and outlines plans for coverage of all PCTs by April 2007. In reality, although this is possible, rolling out the measures and underpinning them with the necessary resources is going to take some time (even excluding the complication of the enhanced service and the fact you may be paid twice for the same work). There has to be high coverage for the screening to be successful and, as some areas are not implementing or are withdrawing screening, the effectiveness of the programme is at risk.

Antenatal care
www.nice.org.uk/nicemedia/pdf/CG062NICEguideline.pdf

In March 2008 NICE published its updated guidance *Antenatal Care: routine care for healthy pregnant women*. The NSF for Children, Young People and Maternity Services was published in 2004. This looks at all areas from pre-conception, pre-birth, birth and postnatal community care.

Down's syndrome screening
Down's syndrome is the most common chromosomal abnormality at birth. The incidence is related to maternal age and the Down's syndrome screening programme is part of antenatal modernisation. All hospitals have a Down's syndrome co-ordinator who co-ordinates the development of services and offers support to pregnant women, GPs and midwives.

NICE indicates that by 2007 pregnant women should be offered the following tests (which would provide detection rates above 75%).

- From 11 to 14 weeks

- the combined test (nuchal translucency (NT), hCG and PAPP-A).
- From 14 to 20 weeks
  - the quadruple test (hCG, AFP, uE3, inhibin A).
- From 11 to 14 weeks and 14 to 20 weeks
  - the integrated test (NT, PAPP-A + hCG, AFP, uE3, inhibin A)
  - the serum integrated test (PAPP-A + hCG, AFP, uE3, inhibin A).

A non-invasive test for prenatal diagnosis based on fetal DNA present in maternal blood: a preliminary study
Lancet 2007; 369: 474–81

This study compared alleles on chromosome 21 (children with Down's carry three rather than two copies) and chromosome 13 (which served as a reference as it is not associated with Down's). Using a polymerase chain reaction it allowed the ratio of the single-nucleotide polymorphisms to be calculated. These were then compared to amniocentesis reports (or findings at birth). The test correctly predicted 58 out of 60 samples.

Although it was recognised that the test needed further refinement this may, in the future, replace amniocentesis and chorionic villus sampling.

HIV testing
- If an HIV infected woman is unaware of her infection status her baby has around a one in four chance of being infected.
- Around 300 babies per year are born with HIV (mainly in London).
- Up to 80% of infections of babies by vertical transmission could be prevented with the use of antivirals (antenatally, during delivery and for the infant), lower segment caesarean section and avoidance of breast feeding.

Women are now being offered HIV screening at booking to reduce the risk of transmission (national targets were adopted in 1999). Although screening is offered there is not always counselling to fully explain the implications of not having the test or of a positive test. HIV testing antenatally is becoming a more acceptable, routine test, given the scope of treatment for the neonate and the mother.

Social and ethical inequalities in the offer and uptake of prenatal screening and diagnosis in the UK: a systematic review
Public Health 2004; 118(3): 177–89

This systematic review identified 20 relevant papers. None found any significant social inequalities in testing, although some suggested that women of South Asian origin might be up to 70% less likely to receive prenatal testing for haemoglobin disorders and Down's syndrome than white women. The review concluded that there may be some evidence of ethnic inequalities to prenatal testing but there is little understanding behind why.

Group-B *Streptococcus*

USA, Canada and Australia encourage routine screening for Group-B *Streptococcus* (GBS) antenatally (vaginal and rectal swabs at 35–37 weeks), as it is known to cause severe early onset of infection in neonates. The incidence of early onset GBS disease in the UK is 0.5/1000 births. Screening is not advocated in the UK as it is still not clear whether screening may cause more problems that it would solve. The Royal College of Obstetrics has printed Green-top guidelines on the topic, discussing the data from studies available.

Pre-eclampsia

Green-top guidelines www.rcog.org.uk

This condition complicates 2–8% of pregnancies. Six per cent of maternal deaths are due to eclampsia (as reported in the *Confidential Enquiry into Maternal Deaths*). There are many theories on reasons for development of pre-eclampsia: genetics (maternal, paternal and foetal); raised homocysteine levels in initially normotensive women; and factor V Leiden gene are all being given consideration in current journals. As yet there are no useful screening tests. UK research is recruiting 1000 women in order to look into a saliva test to detect raised urate levels. The Green-top guidelines consider severe pre-eclampsia and eclampsia in more detail.

The *Confidential Enquiry into Maternal Deaths* (2003–05) reported 18 deaths from eclampsia, and detailed the incidence as 26.8 cases per 100 000 pregnancies (95% CI 23.3–30.7), which was a significant decrease from 1992.

Risk factors for pre-eclampsia at antenatal booking: systematic review of controlled trials

BMJ 2005; 330: 565-7

The authors looked at trials published from 1966 to 2002 and found an increased risk in the following cohorts:

- a previous history of pre-eclampsia (Relative Risk 7.19, 95% CI 5.85–8.83)
- the presence of antiphospholipid antibodies (RR 9.72, 95% CI 4.34–21.75)
- pre-existing diabetes (RR 3.56, 95% CI 2.54–4.99)
- twin pregnancies (RR 2.93, 95% CI 2.04–4.21)
- nulliparity (RR 2.91, 95% CI 1.28–6.61).

Family history, raised blood pressure (greater than 80 mmHg diastolic) at booking, maternal age over 40 years, raised BMI before pregnancy, and multiparous women were also shown to increase the risk.

The pre-eclampsia community guideline (PRECOG): how to screen for and detect onset of pre-eclampsia in the community
BMJ 2005; 330: 576–80

This is a simple comprehensive guideline giving a structured approach to the risk assessments we make for our antenatal patients. It was developed because 46% of maternal deaths and 65% of foetal deaths due to pre-eclampsia could have had a different outcome if they had been managed differently. The guideline looks at assessment in early pregnancy, referral criteria to specialist units and community monitoring. Important signs and symptoms to identify are: new hypertension; new proteinuria; headaches and/or visual disturbance; epigastric pain and/or vomiting; reduced foetal movements; and babies that are small for their gestational age.

The only weakness identified is the lack of evidence to support recommendations of more frequent assessment. Although criteria for screening have not been met, that is not a concern that will limit the implementation of this commonsense, workable guide.

Aspirin and pre-eclampsia

There is a theoretical belief that antiplatelets may have a role in prophylaxis but there is a lot of conflicting evidence. The CLASP trial and subsequent meta-analyses showed no benefit.

Antiplatelet agents for prevention of pre-eclampsia: a meta-analysis of individual patient data
Lancet 2007; 369(9575): 1791–8

This meta-analysis of 31 randomised trials looked at data from 32 217 women and 32 819 babies to assess whether the use of antiplatelets was of use in primary prevention of pre-eclampsia. Women in the antiplatelet arms of the trials had a relative risk of developing pre-eclampsia of 0.9 (95% CI 0.84–0.97, NNT 114) and of a serious adverse outcome of 0.90 (0.85–0.96). There was no significant risk of death to the foetus. This did not seem to favour a particular group of women.

Low dose aspirin in pregnancy and early childhood development: follow-up of the collaborative low dose aspirin study in pregnancy. CLASP Collaborative group
Br J Obstet Gynaecol 1995; 102 (11): 861–8

This was the 12- and 18-month follow-up of children born to women who had been at high risk of complications from pre-eclampsia. The findings were reassuring about the safety of aspirin, but it showed no clear evidence of benefit.

Pre-eclampsia and risk of cardiovascular disease and cancer in later life: systemic review and meta-analysis
BMJ 2007; 335: 974-7

This study looked at a data set of 3 488 160 women, of whom 198 252 had been affected by pre-eclampsia. Although there was no association with cancers, there were cardiovascular links identified (95% confidence intervals):

- hypertension 3.70 (2.7–5.05)
- ischaemic heart disease 2.16 (1.86–2.52)
- stroke 1.81 (1.45–2.27)
- venous thromboembolism 1.79 (1.37–2.33).

Overall mortality was increased 1.49 (1.05–2.14).

Postnatal depression
DTB 2000; 38(5): 33-7

- One in 10 women become depressed after childbirth (70 000 women/year).
- Around 50% are still having problems six months postnatally.
- This is different from 'baby blues', which are common from day 3 to 5 (up to day 10) and which do not require treatment; and it is less severe than puerperal psychosis.
- Postnatal depression tends to start around four to six weeks after delivery.
- It is important to diagnose and treat early to minimise problems with bonding within the family.

National Institute for Health and Clinical Excellence. *Antenatal and postnatal mental health: clinical management and service guidance: NICE clinical guideline 45.* London: NIHCE; 2007
www.nice.org.uk/CG45

The guidance considers the role of GPs in detecting problems, referring to psychiatric services and prescribing based on a risk-benefit assessment.

Edinburgh PN Depression Scale
Br J Psychiatry. 1987; 150: 782-876

This scale was developed in primary care to improve detection through screening. It is used at six to eight weeks postnatally and is scored by a health professional (GP, Health visitor or midwife).

1 I have been able to laugh and see the funny side of things	
As much as I always could	0
Not quite so much now	1
Definitely not so much now	2
Not at all	3

2 I have looked forward with enjoyment to things

As much as I ever did	0
Rather less than I used to	1
Definitely less than I used to	2
Hardly at all	3

3 I have blamed myself unnecessarily when things went wrong

Yes, most of the time	3
Yes, some of the time	2
Not very often	1
No, never	0

4 I have been anxious or worried for no good reason

No, not at all	0
Hardly ever	1
Yes, sometimes	2
Yes, very often	3

5 I have felt scared or panicky for no good reason

Yes, quite a lot	3
Yes, sometimes	2
No, not much	1
No, not at all	0

6 Things have been getting on top of me

Yes, most of the time I haven't been able to cope at all	3
Yes, sometimes I haven't been coping as well as usual	2
No, most of the time I have coped quite well	1
No, I have been coping as well as ever	0

7 I have been so unhappy that I have had difficulty sleeping

Yes, most of the time	3
Yes, sometimes	2
Not very often	1
No, not at all	0

8 I have felt sad or miserable

Yes, most of the time	3
Yes, quite often	2
Not very often	1
No, not at all	0

9 I have been so unhappy that I have been crying

Yes, most of the time	3
Yes, quite often	2
Only occasionally	1
No, never	0

10 The thought of harming myself has occurred to me

Yes, quite often	3

Sometimes	2
Hardly ever	1
Never	0

If the calculated total score is greater than 13 there is a 92.3% chance that the woman is suffering from a depressive illness. The score should not override clinical judgement.

Treatment of postnatal depression

Treatment of proven benefit includes cognitive behavioural therapy and counselling by a health visitor. SSRIs and tricyclic antidepressants appear to be safe in pregnant and breast feeding women. Guidance is to use the lowest effective dose and drugs in the group with the most data (fluoxetine, amitriptyline and imipramine).

Psychosocial and psychological interventions for prevention of postnatal depression: systematic review
BMJ 2005; 331: 15-18
This study took into account results of different trials (7697 women) and found that diverse psychosocial or psychological interventions do not significantly reduce the number of women who develop postnatal depression. The most promising intervention was the provision of individual, intensive, professionally based post partum care (RR 0.76, 95% CI 0.59–1.0)

Confidential Enquiry into Maternal Deaths 2003-05
www.cemach.org.uk/
The leading cause of death postnatally was suicide. The report detailed 37 women who had committed suicide from 2003–05. Twelve had occurred whilst pregnant or in the first postnatal year.

Men's health

Several studies have shown that men seek help for a given illness later than women. Although they do care about health issues, men find it more difficult to express their fears.

Prostate cancer screening
www.cancerbackup.org.uk/Cancertype/Prostate
◈ Prostate cancer is the most common cancer in men.

- Around 32 000 new cases are diagnosed each year.
- Around 25% of men with a PSA of 4–10 ng/mL will be found to have cancer.
- Around 20% of men with prostate cancer do not have a raised PSA.
- Around 60% of cases have metastatic disease at the time of diagnosis.

PSA is the current tumour marker that is being used when investigating for prostate cancer. The use of PSA for a population-based screening programme is being evaluated. Digital rectal examination (DRE) has had a lot of text time and, although still included in some ongoing trials, it is unlikely that this would form a significant part of a screening test. Although there is no screening programme, any man can have a PSA test if requested. Hence screening may creep in, although PSA does not satisfy the criteria for a screening programme. Evidence is lacking that screening for prostate cancer would be beneficial, but early detection and treatment may improve morbidity and mortality. In the UK a Prostate testing for cancer and Treatment (ProtecT) study is under way. The American PLCO (Prostate, lung, colorectal and ovary) screening trial results are awaited and should soon be published. In the USA the advice is that all men with a life expectancy of more than 10 years should be offered PSA testing.

Arguments against screening with PSA include the following:
- there is a lack of consensus on treatment for early disease and a risk of harm with diagnostic biopsy
- despite the widespread use of PSA testing there is lack of evidence that it reduces mortality
- for every 100 men with a raised PSA only 30 will have a prostate cancer
- only a minority of cancers spread to shorten life expectancy
- the PSA is unable to distinguish between indolent and aggressive tumours
- PSA is not tumour specific; it can also be raised in prostatitis, benign prostatic hypertrophy, urinary retention, instrumentation and ejaculation
- there is no specific cut-off below which the risk of prostate cancer is zero
- the values we currently use would be unreliable in obesity, where PSA levels are often lower
- recent advances in genetics could mean a screening programme may be possible with no PSA.

Active surveillance for prostate cancer detected in three subsequent rounds of a screening trial: characteristics, PSA doubling time and outcome
Urol Oncol 2007; 25(6): 527–8

Although the European Randomised Study for Screening of Prostate Cancer (ERSPC) is ongoing, this study looked at the Rotterdam arm, where 278 patients and their physicians had made decisions together (not governed by protocol). This preliminary outcome showed beneficial features of being under active surveillance: median age at diagnosis was 69.8 years; tumour type was T1c in

79% and T2 in 20.9% of cases. It is impractical to try to extrapolate, given this is an interim report and not randomised; but it puts forward more of a case for screening.

Screening decreases prostate cancer mortality: 11 year follow-up of the 1988 Quebec prospective randomised controlled trial
Prostate May 2004; 59(3): 311-18

Two studies have now found that yearly screening reduces mortality by as much as 8%. This particular study looked at 46 486 men in Quebec aged from 45 to 80 years, and found 74 deaths due to prostate cancer occurred in the unscreened group compared to 10 deaths in the screened group (mean follow-up of 7.93 years). The statistics used were a Cox proportional hazards model of the age at death from prostate cancer, which showed a 62% reduction ($p < 0.002$) in screened men.

Individualised screening interval for prostate cancer based on PSA level: results of a prospective, randomised population based study
Arch Intern Med 2005; 165(16): 1857-61

The study included 5855 men aged 50 to 66 years who had accepted the invitation to take part in the study. Men with a PSA greater than 3.0 ng/mL were offered biopsy. After a mean follow-up of 7.6 years, 539 cases (9.2%) of cancer were detected. If the PSA was found to be less than 1 ng/mL, then not a single case developed prostate cancer within three years. The researchers concluded that the resting interval should be individualised, based on PSA level at the time of testing.

It's a maybe test: men's experiences of PSA testing in primary care
Br J Gen Pract 2007; 57(537): 303-10

This study was undertaken because little was known about the views of men regarding PSA testing. It found that men were uncertain about the test, the results and further interventions offered, all of which caused anxiety. The decision to have the test was based on social and media factors rather than being patient-led.

Prostate cancer prevention
The influence of finasteride on the development of prostate cancer
NEJM 2003; 349(3): 215-24

This was a study of 18 882 men aged 55 years and older who had a normal DRE and a PSA of less than 3 ng/mL. They were randomised either to treatment with finasteride or placebo for seven years. Finasteride was found to have a reduction of 24.8% of prostate cancer, although tumours of Gleason grading 7–10 were more common in this group, as were sexual side effects.

Prostate cancer vaccine

Prostate-specific membrane antigen (PSMA) has been a target for vaccines, as has radioactively labelled monoclonal antibodies against PSMA. Although certain vaccines are in the clinical trial phase, as yet there are no conclusive results on efficacy.

Benign prostatic hypertrophy/lower urinary tract symptoms

www.gpnotebook.co.uk

+ There is benign prostatic hypertrophy (BPH) in 3.3 million men in the UK.
+ One in three men over 50 years of age will have symptoms.
+ The prime concern in management, besides symptom control, is to ensure that those men with outflow obstruction do not go on to develop renal failure.

The International Prostate Symptom Score (IPSS)

www.gp-training.net/protocol/docs/ipss.doc

This is a way of assessing symptoms over time with treatment. The BPH Impact Index is a way of assessing how troublesome symptoms are.

Management

1 *Alpha-blockers* (e.g. prazosin, indoramin). These relax the smooth muscle of the prostate and in randomised controlled trials have proved more effective than placebo. They usually show an improvement within two to three weeks. If there is no improvement within three to four months, an alternative should be tried.

2 *5-alpha-reductase inhibitors* (e.g. finasteride). These inhibit 5-alpha-reductase, which converts testosterone to dihydroxytestosterone (DHT), and is known to influence prostate growth. Randomised controlled trials have confirmed that they are more effective than placebo. They cause hyperplasia to regress over three to six months (allow 12 months for maximum effect), so are especially suitable if the prostate is enlarged. These may reduce the PSA by up to 50%.

Impact of baseline symptom severity on future risk of benign prostatic hyperplasia-related outcomes and long-term response to finasteride. The PLESS study group

Urology 2000; 56(4): 610–16

The Proscar long-term efficacy and safety study has published several outcome studies.

A total of 3040 men with BPH were treated for four years with either finasteride or placebo. Finasteride reduced the risk of surgery and acute urinary retention in all groups ($p < 0.001$).

3 *Dutasteride* has been shown to reduce symptom scores, reduce retention, reduce prostate volume, improve flow rates and reduce the need for surgery.

4 *Plant extracts*
  - Saw palmetto (*Serona repens*) (Permixon). This is an extract from a cactus-like plant. It has had some success (although the trial did not use a placebo arm) and is thought to work in a similar way to finasteride.
  - β-sitosterol. Trials have shown that this is more effective than placebo in the short term. The side-effects include gastrointestinal symptoms and impotence.
  - Rye grass pollen extract. It has been suggested that this is beneficial but trials as yet are inconclusive.

5 *Botulinum A toxin.* When this is injected into the prostate it has been shown to improve symptoms of BPH.

Erectile dysfunction
www.bssm.org.uk/downloads/BSSM_ED_Management_Guidelines_2007.pdf
- Around 50% of men aged 40–70 years experience some degree of erectile dysfunction (ED).
- ED is frequently a manifestation of underlying vascular disease and men should be screened for risk factors and signs of vascular disease as part of the assessment.
- The incidence is doubled in hypertensives, tripled in diabetics and quadrupled in men with coronary heart disease.
- Cigarette smoking increases the prevalence of all of the above, two-fold.
- Lipids and glucose should be measured in all patients.

If there is a normal libido and secondary sexual characteristics, it is unusual to find a low testosterone (if measuring, the sample should be taken between 8.00am and 11.00am). If sex hormone binding globulin (SHBG) and testosterone are requested, a ratio can then be determined (i.e. the availability of testosterone), which may help management. Also consider whether testing for thyroid hormone and prolactin are needed.

Treatment
Involve the partner as well as the patient where possible.

Patients who received an NHS prescription before 14 September 1998 can continue to receive erectile dysfunction treatment (not just the first method they were prescribed) on the NHS (the script should be endorsed 'SLS'). Otherwise treatment is available on the NHS only for patients with certain medical problems, e.g. prostate cancer, diabetes, spinal cord injury, Parkinson's disease, multiple sclerosis (there are 12 in total). Private scripts can be written for those not eligible for NHS treatment.

Lifestyle – reduce alcohol, if excessive, stop smoking and lose weight if overweight.

These factors should also help reduce cardiovascular risks and treatment of cardiovascular risk should be as per guidelines.

Phosphodiesterase type 5 (PDE) inhibitors (sildenafil, tadalafil and vardenafil)
These are selective inhibitors of phosphodiesterase type 5 and are currently the favoured option, but are contra-indicated in patients taking nitrates. The best responders are those with psychogenic causes. They are mainly effective in arousal because they prolong the production of nitric oxide (a vasodilator). The response may be less marked after around two years of use. There is an understanding that if the treatment is used regularly the response is better than if used infrequently. A study recently found that in men with a history of ischaemic heart disease and hypertension, using sildenafil and tadalafil increased the risk of non-arteritic anterior ischaemic optic neuropathy (NAION) blindness (*Br J Ophthalmol* 2006; 90(2): 154–7). Use is not contra-indicated but it would be prudent to warn patients.

An open-label, multicentre, randomised cross-over study comparing sildenafil citrate and tadalafil for treating erectile dysfunction in men naïve to phosphodiesterase 5 inhibitor therapy
BJU 2005; 96(9): 1323–32
Following a four-week baseline assessment, 367 men with ED (average age of 54 years) were randomised to receive sildenafil for 12 weeks followed by tadalafil for 12 weeks, or vice-versa.

Both treatments were seen to be effective. After treatment 29% of men chose sildenafil and 71% chose tadalafil for an eight-week extension. Tadalafil is known to have a 24-hour duration of action and to work within 30 minutes, so although it is more expensive you usually get more 'bang for your buck'.

Apomorphine (Uprima) (dopamine receptor agonist)
This drug has been licensed for ED. Currently there are no prescribing restrictions. There is a 1 in 500 risk of syncope due to vasovagal response, so care is needed with the first dose and when increasing from 2 mg to 3 mg.

Intracavernosal prostaglandin E1 (Alprostadil)
Around 80% of men have a satisfactory erection with this method. There is a greater need for education on how to self inject.

Intraurethral prostaglandin E1
The MUSE system of pellets gives around 30% of men some discomfort after use, which causes discontinued use of treatment. One randomised controlled trial showed a satisfactory effect in 40% of men.

Yohimbine (alpha-blocker)
This drug is not yet licensed. It has been found to be effective in some placebo-controlled trials but its effectiveness is probably inadequate for treatment of most.

Ophthalmology

Age-related macular degeneration (ARMD)
This is the most common cause of blind registration in industrialised countries. It impairs central vision and progresses slowly over a period of years. There is no cure. There are around 300 000 cases in the UK.

Legal blindness is vision less than 20/200 (6/60). This means a person can see 20 feet (six metres) when a normally sighted person could see 200 feet (60 metres).

Dry ARMD is the most common form (85–90% of cases). It is gradual in onset and caused by drusen (thickening of Bruch's membrane between the retina and the choroid) and atrophy of retinal pigment epithelium. Around 15% of cases of dry ARMD will progress to the exudative form, wet ARMD.

Possible protective factors for prevention of ARMD
Although you can't modify age, sex (men are seen to be at greater risk) or genetics (yet) the following lifestyle changes have been found to be of importance:
* wearing sunglasses and brimmed hats in bright light
* stopping smoking (smoking reduces antioxidants which can more than double the ARMD risk)
* nutrition – carotenoid-rich vegetables (green leafy vegetables). Lutein and zeaxanthin are the carotenoids found in the macula and are thought to be of most importance. A low-fat diet and a healthy approach to food underpin the general principles.

Dietary antioxidants and primary prevention of age related macular degeneration: systemic review and meta-analysis
BMJ 2007; 335: 755–9
This analysis included 12 studies and 149 203 people with 1878 cases of early ARMD. It found that a range of dietary antioxidants (including vitamin A, C and E, zinc, lutein, lycopene and β-carotene had little or no effect).
* statins have been largely discounted, but it was thought that they may help by reducing cholesterol (preventing deposition in Bruch's membrane), through antioxidant properties and by inhibiting endothelial cell apoptosis.

Cholesterol lowering drugs and risk of age related maculopathy: prospective cohort study with cumulative exposure measurements
BMJ 2003; 324: 255–6

This Dutch study with 26 781 person-years follow-up found no association between cholesterol-lowering drugs and age-related maculopathy. The authors discussed the fact that previous studies had low statistical powers.

⚬ regular eye tests would identify eye problems (two-yearly; this is free to people over 60 years of age).

Wet ARMD accounts for 10% of cases but up to 90% of sight loss in ARMD. It occurs as growth of new blood vessels (stimulated by secretion of vascular endothelial growth factor, VEGF) behind the retina leak blood and fluid, causing damage and more rapid loss of vision. This form is amenable to treatment with photodynamic therapy or Argon laser. In photodynamic therapy with verteporfin dye, a non-thermal laser activates the dye once injected to close the new choroidal vessels (in exudative/wet AMD). This treatment looks promising. There is no real evidence for radiotherapy or submacular surgery.

A view on new drugs for macular degeneration
DTB 2007; 45(7): 49–52

This review looks at two new drugs (pegaptanib sodium and ranibizumab) that block the effects of VEGF and that are now licensed in the UK for neovascular age-related macular degeneration. They are administered by intravitreal injection. Both have been found to prevent further deterioration (34% were seen to have improved) in vision but lack robust safety evidence.

ENT

ENT is one of the largest components of primary care. We manage acute problems, but recurrent and chronic problems are often referred. Although there is now a good evidence base for the more common ailments it isn't quite as straightforward as it may seem.

Sore throat

This is the most common, overtreated, controversial and mundane (or is it?) symptom in general practice. Symptoms last for up to 10 days and may be associated with systemic features such as fever, malaise and vomiting.

A Cochrane Review looked at antibiotics and complications with sore throats and concluded that antibiotics offered a small clinical benefit. They were found to reduce the risk of rheumatic fever by up to 30%, but this would be barely significant in the Western world. The incidence of acute otitis media was reduced by 25%.

National Institute for Health and Clinical Excellence. *Referral advice.* London: NIHCE; 2001
www.nice.org.uk/nicemedia/pdf/Referraladvice.pdf
In recurrent episodes of acute sore throat in children aged up to 15 years the following should be considered:
- outcomes are likely to be improved if the parent, child and health professional decide on a treatment in partnership. Communication is key
- agree on analgesia that can be used (ibuprofen and/or paracetamol)
- avoid prescribing antibiotics if acceptable (children issued antibiotics may be at increased risk of further infection and attend more frequently)
- issue antibiotics if there are
  - features of systemic upset
  - peritonsillar cellulitis
  - a history of rheumatic fever
  - increased risk from infection (e.g. a child with immunodeficiencies or diabetes mellitus)
- a specialist referral should be considered:
  - acutely if there is suspicion of a quinsy, airway obstruction or swelling causing dehydration
  - routinely if there is a history of sleep apnoea, failure to thrive, five or more episodes of infection in the last 12 months for the previous two years (Paradise criteria) or the child has guttate psoriasis caused by recurrent tonsillitis.

A quinsy might be more common in unwell patients with three out of four Centor criteria (fever greater than 38°C, purulent tonsils, tender anterior cervical nodes and no cough). The incidence has been seen at 1 in 60 if these criteria are met, compared to 1 in 400 when not systemically unwell. It is worth offering antibiotics to patients who have been unwell for 48 hours and fit the Centor criteria.

Public beliefs on antibiotics and respiratory tract infections: an internet-based questionnaire study
Br J Gen Pract 2007; 57(545): 942–7
Patient expectations are one of the strongest predictors of antibiotic prescribing decisions. This study was based in the Netherlands and 20 questions were given to an Internet panel. Only 44.6% identified that antibiotics were effective against bacteria, not viruses. The study identified misconception of the effectiveness

of antibiotics for treatment of viral infections and highlighted the fact that by prescribing we positively reinforce the misconception.

Lemierre's syndrome: a forgotten complication of oropharyngeal infection
J Ayub Med Coll Abbottabad 2005; 17(1): 30–33

Apparently *Fusobacterium necrophorum* is the usual aetiological agent which may rarely complicate oropharyngeal infection as septicaemia, septic thrombo-phlebitis of the internal jugular vein and metastatic lesions (usually in the lungs). In this study of 156 patients admitted with oropharyngeal infection, two (1.28%) patients had features suggestive of Lemierre's syndrome. This will be, undoubtedly, even more rare in the UK but the authors conclude that the wide-spread use of antibiotics significantly reduced incidence. Lemierre's is potentially fatal. Recognition, early diagnosis and prolonged treatment with appropriate antibiotics are usually curative.

Acute otitis media

♦ Around 66% of cases are due to *Haemophilus influenzae* and *Streptococcus pneumoniae.*
♦ Around 25% of cases are sterile (no organism can be isolated).
♦ Some 10–20% are due to mycoplasma and anaerobes.
♦ About 4% are viral (although titres are raised in 25%, possibly preceding bacterial infection).

Use of antibiotics for otitis media

Several meta-analyses have shown that the effectiveness of antibiotics is limited in terms of clinical improvement. The advantages of antibiotics include the following:
♦ there is a bacterial aetiology
♦ antibiotics are cheap and relatively safe
♦ there is a reduction in complications (e.g. mastoiditis)
♦ use can reduce symptoms more quickly.

The disadvantages include:
♦ the cost escalates when you consider prescribing in mass numbers
♦ it may discourage natural immunity
♦ it may promote drug resistance
♦ it may promote dependence on doctors by prescribing.

A randomised, double-blind, placebo-controlled non-inferiority trial of amoxicillin for clinically diagnosed otitis media in children 6 months to 5 years of age
CMAJ 2005; 172(3): 335–41

This study randomly assigned 512 children aged six months to five years, with otitis media, to receive either amoxicillin (60 mg/kg daily) or placebo for 10 days. Follow-up was on days 1, 2 and 3 and for a final time between day 10 and 14.

At 14 days 84.2% of children receiving placebo and 92.8% of children receiving amoxicillin had clinical resolution of symptoms. More pain and fever was seen in the placebo group in the first two days. There was no difference in recurrence rates by three months. The cure rates were not substantially worse in the placebo groups than the treatment group.

One of the questions we need to ask is whether we are justified in withholding antibiotics when we know that they improve symptoms in children, especially in those who have systemic symptoms and those who are too young to express their symptoms, especially symptoms of pain.

Otitis media with effusion (glue ear)

This is the most common cause of conductive hearing loss in children aged two to five years. Up to 80% of children, by the age of four years, will have been affected with it at some time. Hearing loss has knock-on effects to speech development, school performance in writing and spelling and behaviour (which may be over-boisterous or clingy).

Around 50% of cases resolve spontaneously within three months and 95% within 12 months.

Risk factors for developing OME include:
+ passive smoking (environmental tobacco smoke)
+ children attending day care (due to transmission rates of infection)
+ bottle feeding (breast feeding may offer some preventative benefits)
+ rhinitis, asthma and reflux.

Does passive smoking affect the outcome of grommet insertion in children
J Laryngol Otol 2005; 119(6): 448–54

In this study 606 children (with 1174 ears) who underwent grommet insertion were followed up until the grommets were extruded. The median survival rate for grommets was 59 weeks in children who were exposed to passive smoking and 86 weeks for non-exposed children. The extrusion rate was 36% higher at the end of one year if both parents smoked compared to the non-smoking group. Post-operative infection rates, attic retraction, post-extrusion myringosclerosis and permanent perforations were more common in children exposed to passive smoking.

Grommets (ventilation tubes) for hearing loss associated with otitis media with effusion in children
Cochrane Database 2005; (1): CD001801

This review was to assess the effectiveness of grommet insertion compared to myringotomy or non-surgical treatment in children with OME. The outcomes studied were hearing level, duration of middle ear effusion, wellbeing and prevention of sequelae attributable to hearing loss. The authors conclude that an initial period of watchful waiting is appropriate. No evidence is available for subgroups of children with speech and language delays or learning problems. The dramatic improvements following grommet insertion are usually seen only in the short term.

Gastric reflux in children can mean that gastric juices reflux, via the Eustachian tube, into the middle ear. This can cause inflammation and ideal conditions for secondary infection.

Osteoporosis

This is defined by the NHS Consensus Development Conference as a 'progressive skeletal disorder characterised by low bone mass and microarchitectural deterioration of bone tissue with a consequent increase in bone fragility and susceptibility to fracture.'

The WHO Definition is as follows:

+ osteoporosis: bone density greater than 2.5 SD below the mean (femoral neck)
+ osteopenia: bone density greater than 1 SD below the mean

Note that one definition is a pathological process and the other is an arbitrary point on a scale. The T-score criteria were proposed for epidemiological studies to compare populations and for defining thresholds in clinical trials. Unless stated otherwise the measurements will be from the femoral neck. They were not intended for diagnosis or management decisions in individual cases.

+ It is estimated that up to 3 million women in the UK have osteoporosis.
+ The prevalence (in women) increases from 2% at 50 years to 25% at 80 years.
+ Osteoporosis causes over 180 000 fractures per year (mainly wrist, vertebral and hip fractures) in England and Wales.
+ It costs the Government £1.5 billion per year (87% of this is due to hip fractures).
+ One in five hip fracture patients dies within one year, 50% have severely impaired mobility.
+ A third of vertebral fractures cause chronic pain (i.e. there is a huge impact on morbidity and mortality).

Risk factors include:

+ postmenopausal women

- early menopause (before 45 years of age, e.g. following a hysterectomy or oophorectomy)
- immobility
- long-term steroid use (it is suggested that this group receive preventative treatment)
- previous fragility fracture
- high systolic BP (higher rate of bone loss)
- secondary causes will affect up to 50% of men and 10% of women with osteoporosis
  - alcoholism
  - thyroid problem (hypothyroidism and hyperthyroidism)
  - liver disease
  - malabsorption
  - hypogonadism in men
  - connective tissue disorders (e.g. rheumatoid and SLE)

Treatments

Monitoring the effect of treatment has usually been done with repeat DEXA scans, after at least 18 months of treatment. However bone turnover markers (such as P1NP) may be of more use in the short term and are currently being evaluated.

Prevention/lifestyle changes
- Stop smoking, avoid excess alcohol and take regular weight-bearing exercise.
- Fall prevention – assessment of safety in the home can be provided in primary care.
- Protection of sites of high impact – hip protectors are of proven benefit, with up to 50% reduction in some studies (residential care based).

Calcium supplements
- The recommended daily dose is 1 gram for people over 50 years of age.
- There is no evidence that calcium reduces fractures unless it is taken with vitamin D.

Vitamin D
- The recommended daily dose is 400 iU, too low for fracture prevention. More usually, 800 iU would be used.
- Two trials have shown that vitamin D and calcium reduced risk of fracture by up to 50% over five years. The best results are seen in institutionalised frail elderly.

Bisphosphonates
These are now first choice in management of osteoporosis. A once-monthly

preparation, ibandronate, has recently been released. Bisphosphonates have been identified as a cause of osteonecrosis of the jaw (one to three years after starting treatment)

Strontium ranelate
This is a dual agent (like teriparatide) that improves bone mineral density by increasing bone formation and reducing bone resorption.

Hormone replacement therapy
A meta-analysis suggests that this yields a relative risk reduction of 40% (for fractures). However, the benefits are lost within five years of stopping HRT. This is a treatment option that is no longer recommended for prevention because of the risk factor profile.

Tibolone (bleed-free preparation of HRT)
This has been shown to increase bone mass density in the spine over two years.

Selective oestrogen receptor modulators (e.g. Raloxifene)
These decrease the fracture rate by 30% over three years at best.

Osteoporosis – secondary prevention
National Institute for Health and Clinical Excellence. *Osteoporosis – secondary prevention: NICE technology appraisal 87.* **London: NIHCE; 2005**
www.nice.org.uk/TA087
Although guidance for primary prevention is almost complete (it is in an appeal process at present), the guidance for use of bisphosphonates, raloxifene and teriparatide in secondary prevention is already drawing a degree of criticism because of how restrictive it is.

   NICE standards are:
* all women over 75 years who have fractured should be treated for presumed osteoporosis without the need for a DEXA scan
* all women between 65 and 74 years of age should be treated if osteoporosis is confirmed by DEXA scan
* women younger than 65 years should be treated:
  * if they have a bone mineral density less than -3 SD
  * if they have a bone mineral density of -2.5 SD with one or more additional risk factors (BMI less than $19\,\mathrm{kg/m^2}$, a family history of maternal hip fracture if less than 75 years of age, untreated premature menopause, medical disorders associated with bone loss or conditions associated with prolonged immobility).

For treatment, NICE's preference is the bisphosphonates with raloxifene as an alternative. Teriparatide should be restricted for use in more severe cases.

Several articles have been published which raise concerns about the guidelines. Below are a number of issues that are often discussed:

- the guidelines are too restrictive and will exclude a lot of people who would benefit from treatment
- the research omitted a number of European articles, casting doubt on the cost-effectiveness calculations
- the T-score weighting means that under the guidelines patients need to be at a higher risk to qualify for treatment
- it does not take into account the Royal College of Physicians' guidance (2002), that patients on long-term corticosteroids should receive treatment at a T-score of −1.5 SD (−2.5 SD in NICE)
- NICE has now agreed that, due to the long delays, treatment can be given whilst awaiting a DEXA scan. How this would then affect treatment if, after scanning, a patient was found to be just outside the treatment criteria is not clear.

Screening

Fractures occur late and there are no symptoms prior to this. All women over 65 years of age in the USA are screened (it has been recognised that men are missing out on potential preventative advice). However there is no universal policy in the UK. When the NICE document *Osteoporosis – primary prevention* is published, this matter should be addressed at some level.

Shifting the focus in fracture prevention from osteoporosis to falls
BMJ 2008; 336: 124-6

This edition of the *BMJ* looks at several issues around falls and osteoporosis. No study to date has ever looked at whether preventing falls also prevents fractures with any sufficient power. Some randomised trials have reported a 50% reduction. The falls assessment looking at history, medical risk factors, movement, strength and gait are all part of how a GP should be assessing the risk of falling.

Royal College of Physicians Guidelines 1999

These guidelines suggest DEXA scanning should be offered to individuals with risk factors, as well as those with a low bone mass density (less than 19kg/m^2) and those with a strong family history (despite the Finnish study concluding that genetics were not thought to be important).

Useful information can be obtained from the National Osteoporosis Society www.nos.org.uk.

Back pain

+ Around 60–80% of the population will have back pain at some point in their life.
+ Up to 85% of acute episodes resolve in six weeks. If it persists for 12 weeks or more it is a chronic problem.
+ Around 7% of people consult their GP each year with back pain.
+ A total of 120 million work days per year are lost as a result of back pain.

These figures are based on 1998 data from the Office of National Statistics and ARC data 2007.

Diagnosis and management

Red Flags are symptoms and conditions that require urgent imaging, blood tests and referral. They include the following.
+ A past medical history of carcinoma, TB, drug abuse and HIV (cause of immunosuppression and infection).
+ Previous prescription drug use (e.g. steroids).
+ Symptoms of night sweats, fever and loss of weight.
+ A new structural deformity (e.g. kyphosis) suggestive of fracture.
+ Widespread neurology:
  • cauda equina symptoms – these need immediate referral as there is a risk of permanent damage and incontinence. These symptoms include:
    – loss of sphincter control
    – bilateral neurological leg pain
    – saddle loss of sensation.

Patients with simple back pain or isolated nerve root irritation can be managed conservatively. Multilevel or progressive neurological problems require urgent referral.

Clinical Evidence gives a comprehensive outline of current trials for each modality of treatment (www.clinicalevidence.com). Advice includes:
+ simple analgesia regularly
+ take regular exercise as soon as the pain allows.

Randomised controlled trial of exercise for low back pain: clinical outcomes, costs and preferences
BMJ 1999; 319: 279-83
This study showed that early access to a doctor (within three days) and physiotherapist (within one week) for exercise for new-onset back pain was associated with good outcome. Early mobilisation increases the speed of recovery, reduces

the length of time off work and reduces the number of recurrences.
+ Muscle relaxants may help if there is a degree of spasm unresponsive to
  analgesia.
+ Physiotherapy.
+ Complementary therapy: chiropractor, osteopath and acupuncture may all
  be beneficial, although there are no randomised trials confirming this.

Use of complementary and alternative therapies by patients with self-reported chronic back pain: a nationwide survey in Canada
Joint Bone Spine 2005; 72(6): 571-7
Complementary and alternative medicine (CAM) use was associated with younger age, being married, having a higher level of education and earning a higher income. Overall CAM users were more active, healthier and had a more involved social life.

Osteoarthritis

Around 20–25% of visits to GPs relate to the musculoskeletal system. Most of these cases are secondary to osteoarthritis. Osteoarthritis, by definition, cannot be cured, but the previously held belief that it would inevitably progress is being challenged as the understanding of the metabolic process develops. Risk factors for development of osteoarthritis include being female, older age, obesity, nutrition, bone density and muscle strength.

Management
Diet
Other than weight loss, specific diets have no role to play in the management of osteoarthritis and rheumatic conditions. There are reports of vitamin C reducing rates of progression and improvements with certain seeds and cod liver oil.

Exercise and physiotherapy
Exercise improves muscular tone and joint function, so should not be avoided. Physiotherapy reduces pain, improves joint range and muscle strength as well as improving mobility and independence.

Investigation of clinical effects of high- and low-resistance training for patients with knee osteoarthritis: a randomised controlled trial
Phys Ther 2008; 88(4): 427-36
This is a recent paper from Asia comparing the effects of high- and low-resistance strength training in elderly subjects with knee osteoarthritis. A total

of 102 patients were assigned for eight weeks either of treatment or of none (the control group). Pain, function, walking time, and muscle torque were examined before and after intervention. Improvement for all measures was observed in both exercise groups, with no significant difference between intensity.

Glucosamine

Glucosamine sulphate is a natural substance that forms proteoglycans (part of the articular cartilage). It is thought to be chondroprotective, although the jury is still out on how clinically effective it is for pain relief. This is available as a dietary supplement, which is expensive. There is an option to prescribe on an FP10 (a dose of 1500 mg/day), although availability will depend on the individual PCT.

Effect of glucosamine sulphate on hip osteoarthritis: a randomised trial
Ann Intern Med 2008; 148(4): 315–16

This study looked at whether glucosamine sulphate had an effect on the symptoms and progression of hip osteoarthritis during two years of treatment. It examined 222 patients with hip osteoarthritis who were recruited by their general practitioner and randomised to two years of treatment with 1500 mg of oral glucosamine sulphate or placebo once daily. Glucosamine sulphate was no better than placebo in reducing symptoms and progression of hip osteoarthritis.

Local injections

Intra-articular hyaluronic acid gives symptomatic benefit. This has been confirmed in several randomised controlled trials. The lasting effect is uncertain, as is the benefit compared to steroid injection.

Intra-articular hyaluronic acid for treatment of osteoarthritis of the knee: systematic review and meta-analysis
CMAJ 2005; 172(8): 1039–43

This study included 22 trials published up to April 2004. It concluded that intra-articular hyaluronic acid injection has not been proven to be clinically effective and may be associated with greater risk of adverse events.

Rubefacients

Topical creams and gels are often used by patients, especially when they are unable to tolerate systemic treatments. This is often an area targeted in prescribing budgets because of relative lack of evidence and associated costs.

Systematic review of topical rubefacients containing salicylates for the treatment of acute and chronic pain
BMJ 2004; 328: 995–8

This study looked at randomised double-blind trials comparing rubifacients to placebo, all of which were fairly small in number. The conclusion was cautious but probably indicates that topically applied rubefacients containing salicylates are effective in treating acute pain. At best the NNT is 5.3 (Relative Benefit 1.5, 95% CI 1.3–1.9)

Complementary therapies

These are all used regularly in subgroups of the population with good effect. Specific randomised trials are lacking.

COX-2 inhibitors

+ Around 15% of people on long-term NSAIDs get ulcers, accounting for 2000 deaths per year.
+ In 1999 more than £170 million was spent on NSAIDs, not including the co-prescribing of gastroprotective agents.
+ COX-2 inhibitors are as effective as other NSAIDs in reducing inflammation and pain.

NICE Guidelines on cyclo-oxygenase inhibitors (2001)

+ These drugs are indicated for pain and stiffness in inflammatory arthritis and short-term pain relief in osteoarthritis.
+ They are not recommended for routine use.
+ They are recommended for those over 65 years of age who are taking other drugs that could cause gastrointestinal side effects (e.g. steroids and anti-coagulants), and those patients who have existing gastrointestinal problems.

NICE's holding statement (February 2005) advises that it will be reviewing its advice, and at time of print this is still under full review.

Rofecoxib (Vioxx) has been withdrawn from the market (September 2004) following an increased incidence of stroke and heart disease in patients using these drugs. Current advice on cyclo-oxygenase-2 (COX-2) drugs from the European Medicines Agency is that:
+ they are contra-indicated in patients with established ischaemic heart disease
+ caution should be exercised in patients with cardiovascular risk factors
+ we should use the lowest dose for the shortest time necessary.

Risk of adverse gastrointestinal outcomes in patients taking cyclo-oxygenase-2 inhibitors or conventional non-steroidal anti-inflammatory drugs: population based nested case-control analysis
BMJ 2005; 331(7528): 1310–16

Cases were taken from 367 general practices contributing to the UK RESEARCH database. There were 9407 incident cases identified and 88 867 matched controls. Increased risk of adverse gastrointestinal events was associated with COX-2 and NSAIDs. After adjustment for confounders the risk remained significantly higher for naproxen (OR 2.12, 95% CI 1.73–2.58), diclofenac (1.96, 1.78–2.15) and rofecoxib (1.56, 1.30–1.87) but not for current use of celecoxib (1.11, 0.87–1.41). The research found that use of ulcer healing drugs removed the risk for adverse gastric events in all groups of NSAIDs except diclofenac, which still had an increased odds ratio (1.49, 1.26–1.76).

Meta-analysis of cyclo-oxygenase-2 inhibitors and their effects on blood pressure
Arch Intern Med 2005; 165(5): 490–6

The review looked at 19 studies (totalling 45 457 people). Although COX-2 and NSAIDs raised systolic and diastolic blood pressure (by 3.8 mmHg and 2.83 mmHg respectively), this was not significantly more than placebo. A further meta-analysis published showed that there was no significant increase in cardiovascular risk with celecoxib.

Obesity

Obesity is defined as a Body Mass Index (BMI) greater than 30 kg/m².
* Over 20% of men and women in the UK are obese. It is a huge medical, public health and economic problem, with genetic and environmental determinants.
* Six per cent of all deaths can be attributed to obesity (National Audit Office 2001).

Reducing obesity is one of the six priorities of the *Choosing Health* White Paper. The strategies go beyond the recommendations of the House of Commons Select Committee's Report of May 2005. The Government's response to the report lays out 52 recommendations. These include the recognition that further data collection is needed; the approach schools should take; the role of OFSTED in assessing these directives; a national walking strategy; the roles of healthcare professionals (pharmacological, surgical, psychological and behavioural aspects); and the need for a dedicated framework for obesity, building on the current

National Service Frameworks. One specific recommendation is that there should be a wide-ranging programme of solutions:

+ health promotion
+ education about food
+ restriction of promotion of unhealthy foods for children
+ a comprehensive care pathway on obesity.

Obesity Care Pathway 2005

www.nationalobesityforum.org.uk

This publication offers a toolkit for healthcare professionals and considers the following:

+ the need for baseline patient data and investigations
+ patient motivation
+ healthy eating
+ physical activity
+ integrated weight management programmes
+ the role of pharmaceuticals.

It highlights the use of waist circumference alongside BMI as an aid to stratifying risk and monitoring success.

National Institute for Health and Clinical Excellence. *Obesity: guidance on the prevention, identification, assessment and management of overweight and obesity in adults and children: NICE clinical guideline 43.* **London: NIHCE; 2006**

www.nice.org.uk/nicemedia/pdf/CG43NICEGuideline.pdf

Staying a healthy weight improves health and reduces risk of diseases associated with being overweight or obese. These recommendations focus on health promotion (in schools and in a health context) and management of lifestyle depending on co-morbidities and a willingness to change. They also grade obesity based on BMI.

Multicomponent interventions should encourage:

+ increased physical activity
+ improved eating behaviour (stimulus control, self monitoring, goal setting)
+ healthy eating.

Medication options look at orlistat and sibutramine (not rimonabant/Acomplia) with the following guidelines for adults:

+ prescribe if BMI is $28.0 \, kg/m^2$ (27 for sibutramine) with risk factors or BMI $30.0 \, kg/m^2$ without
+ continue at three months if there has been 5% weight loss (less strict for NIDDM)

◆ continue at 12 months after discussion, depending on progress (for orlistat, sibutramine is not recommended for longer than 12 months).

The *Drugs and Therapeutic Bulletin* (2007; 45(6): 41) article compared drug treatments (including rimonabant) based on the evidence available and concluded that orlistat had the better efficacy and safety profile. Medication for children was not recommended under 12 years, and for over 12 only if there are co-morbidities (prescribing should be started by a multidisciplinary team).

Comparison of the Atkins, Ornish, Weight Watchers and Zone diets for weight loss and heart disease risk reduction. A randomised trial
JAMA 2005; 293: 43–53

The investigators enrolled and randomised 160 adults (mean BMI 35) with known dyslipidaemia, hypertension or fasting hyperglycaemia, to look at which diet worked best. The dropout rate was 42% by 12 months, the most common reason being that the diet was too hard to follow. In each group, 25% sustained a 5% weight loss, and 10% a loss of 10% of initial body weight at one year. Improvement in cardiac risk factors was directly proportional to the amount of weight loss and was similar among the diet groups. The study concluded that all diets were successful – the key is patient motivation and self-selection of the diet that suits them best.

Prognosis in obesity (we all need to move a little more and eat a little less)
BMJ 2005; 330: 1339–40 (Editorial)

A fantastic title that, no matter how many guidelines are produced, says it all.

This discussion touches on lots of points, most topically the 2004 White Paper *Choosing Health* and the subsequent action plan *Choosing a Better Diet*, which have both set tough targets to reduce childhood obesity. Both sides of the energy balance equation must be tackled and are well within the range of day-to-day variability in activity and diet.

Obesity and cancer
BMJ 2007; 335: 1107–8

This editorial discusses the work commissioned by the International Agency for Research on Cancer (IARC) to look at epidemiological, clinical and experimental data to evaluate the risk between weight and cancer. As previously discussed, there was an association with postmenopausal breast cancer, endometrial cancer, kidney cancer and adenocarcinoma of the oesophagus. Higher BMI was also significantly related to leukaemia, multiple myeloma, non-Hodgkin's lymphoma, and pancreatic and ovarian cancers.

Metabolic syndrome

Metabolic syndrome is known to be associated with cardiovascular disease and type 2 diabetes. There is a school of thought that all we are doing by labelling someone as having metabolic syndrome is medicalising obesity, when what we should be doing is tackling obesity to prevent impaired glucose tolerance and diabetes. Many feel that the term is imprecise and, indeed, there are a number of definitions.

The International Diabetes Federation (2005) diagnostic criteria

Essential requirements:
* central obesity, waist measurement
  * males, greater than 94 cm
  * females, greater than 80 cm
* plus any two of
  * raised fasting glucose greater than 5.6 mmol/L (or previously diagnosed type 2 diabetes)
  * raised triglycerides greater than 1.7 mmol/L (or on treatment)
  * reduced HDL-cholesterol (less than 1.03 mmol/L in men; less than 1.29 mmol/L in women; or on treatment)
  * raised blood pressure (greater than 130/85 mmHg; or on treatment for previously diagnosed hypertension).

Exercise

Active adults live longer!

Obesity in the UK, both in children and adults, is increasing. This has numerous implications for health (non-insulin dependent diabetes, coronary heart disease, osteoarthritis, etc). Exercise is effective for long-term weight reduction/regulation, although it is difficult to perform blinded trials. The White Paper *Choosing Health*, National Service Frameworks and care pathways are some of the documents that touch on the importance of exercise. Practice Based Commissioning schemes are expected to incentivise reductions in lifestyle risks by 2008/9.

The current advice (from the British Heart Foundation) is to take 30 minutes of moderate exercise every day (in a healthy adult), although shorter bouts of more physical exercise can give similar benefits.

Exercise on prescription is something to be wary of as 'prescription' implies a full understanding of the possible side-effects and complications. The defence unions have advised against prescribing exercise if you do not have the skill to evaluate the patient. However, you could recommend it.

Effects on cardiovascular disease

+ Exercise reduces primary and secondary cardiovascular disease.
+ Coronary heart disease can be reduced by 20–30% in men.
+ Stroke could be reduced by 30–40%.
+ Blood pressure can be reduced by up to 10 mmHg systolic and 8 mmHg diastolic.
+ Exercise increases HDL-cholesterol levels.

Musculoskeletal effects

+ Exercise has been shown to increase mobility and reduce falls in the elderly.
+ It can reduce the rate of hip fracture by up to 50%.
+ If weightbearing, it can increase bone density.

Psychiatric effects

+ Exercise reduces and relieves anxiety.
+ It appears to have an anti-depressant effect.

Other effects

+ Exercise can prevent non-insulin dependent diabetes in 25% of cases.
+ It improves glucose tolerance in NIDDM.
+ People who exercise live longer.
+ Graded aerobic exercise improves fatigue, functional capacity and fitness in patients with chronic fatigue syndrome.

Four commonly used methods to increase physical activity: brief interventions in primary care, exercise referral schemes, pedometers and community based exercise programmes for walking and cycling
www.nice.org.uk/nicemedia/pdf/PHYSICAL-ALS2_FINAL.pdf
This guidance looks at how effective these four methods are at encouraging people to be more active. It recommends that we opportunistically encourage people to be more active (30 minutes exercise, five days a week or more), using their judgement as to when this would be appropriate. It is suggested we could use the General Practitioners' Physical Activity Questionnaire to identify inactive individuals. In giving advice we should take into account their individual needs, preferences and circumstances and supply written advice.

Physical activity and health (Editorial)
BMJ 2007; 334: 1173
This editorial walks quickly through the evidence on exercise and health, from the American Attorney General ruling (1997) to the Cochrane Review (2007). An identified weakness in many of the trials is the lack of assessment on health gains, although the nurses' health study did show a reduced risk of cardiovascular disease, type 2 diabetes and all causes of mortality.

Alcohol misuse

The Office of National Statistics is reporting a steady increase in the number of alcohol-related deaths.
+ 13.4 per 100 000 deaths per year were alcohol related in 2006.
+ Around 7% of the UK population have features of mild alcohol dependence.
+ Around 21% of 11–15-year-olds drink twice a week (an increase of 4% since 1994).

In men, alcohol consumption greater than 300 g/week is associated with an increased blood pressure and stroke. Drinking one to four units/day in men and one to two units/day in women on five to six days of the week appears to be protective against CHD and possibly stroke. Tackling those patients who misuse alcohol and getting them to recognise they are drinking too much is probably where we as GPs could make the biggest impact. Brief intervention by a GP can be effective, depending upon where your patient is in the cycle of change. A recent editorial in the *BMJ* (*BMJ* 2008; 336: 455) highlights the need for higher taxes and restricted availability.

The first alcohol needs assessment for England was conducted in 2004 and published by the Department of Health in 2005.

The key findings were the following.
+ 38% of men, and 16% of women (aged 16 to 64 years) have an alcohol use disorder (equivalent to 8.2 million people).
+ More than 50% of these are binge drinkers.
+ Around 1.1 million people are dependent on alcohol.
+ The general practice research database study found low levels of formal identification, treatment and referral of patients with alcohol use problems. GPs identify 1 in 67 males and 1 in 82 females who are harmful drinkers.
+ There is a large gap between the need for alcohol treatment and access to alcohol treatment (only 5.6% of individuals needing help are receiving it).

The Alcohol Harm Reduction Strategy for England
BMJ 2004; 328: 905–6 (Editorial)

This editorial discusses the strategy and the differences between the interim and final reports. It finds it disappointing that a strategy to reduce any increase in alcohol-related harms doesn't adequately focus on reducing alcohol consumption. The author states that 'the complex relation people have with alcohol and how deeply embedded the use of alcohol is in our culture is not sufficiently acknowledged in the report'.

The strategy will tackle the following areas:
- alcohol-related disorder in towns and city centres (crime and disorder)
- improved treatment and support for people with alcohol problems (identification and treatment)
- clamping down on irresponsible promotions by the industry (supply and industrial responsibility)
- providing better information about the dangers of alcohol (education and communication).

Screening tools

CAGE and AUDIT are the most widely validated methods of screening for alcohol-use disorders. CAGE seems to be more popular in the UK.

CAGE questionnaire
- Have you ever felt you should **C**ut down?
- Have you ever been **A**nnoyed by someone criticising your drinking?
- Have you ever felt **G**uilty about your drinking?
- Have you ever had an **E**ye opener (early morning drink) to steady your nerves/get rid of your hang over?

A score of 2 or more has a high correlation with alcoholism, but this screening tool has a low sensitivity and specificity.

AUDIT (Alcohol Use Disorders Identification Test)
This WHO screening tool is thought to be a more suitable screening test for excessive drinking at the less severe end of the spectrum. It has been found to have a higher sensitivity and specificity than the CAGE questionnaire.

FAST
This is another quick screening test. Here the focus is on the frequency of risky levels of consumption of alcohol. Patients are asked to rate the following:
- how often they drink
- to what extent they drink

◆ whether a friend or health professional has ever been concerned about the amount they drink.

Drug misuse

Illicit drugs are used for their mind-altering effects and the highs achieved. The harmful effects from long-term use, both medically and socially, are well recognised and the driving force behind the current initiatives. NICE has published guidance on opioid withdrawal (methadone or buprenorphine first line) and psychosocial support.

◆ It is estimated that 250 000 people in the UK suffer from problems related to drug misuse.
◆ It is estimated that 20 000 young people become adult problem drug users every year.
◆ One in 65 intravenous drug users has HIV (1 in 25 in London).
◆ More than two in five intravenous drug users have been infected with hepatitis C.

Modernising the Health Service looks at drug issues in part and aims to provide targeted prevention activity for at least 30% of young people most vulnerable to drug misuse.

Guidelines on Clinical Management is a booklet containing guidance on drug use and treatment first published in 1984 and is regularly updated (most recently in 1999).

The Home Office recognises the problems caused by drug use, from the health implications through to crime and underachievement in education by young people, and has many initiatives under way.

◆ Blueprint – this is a five-year research programme looking at the effectiveness of drug prevention initiatives in school and community settings.
◆ The Drug Intervention Programme has screened 15 860 young offenders.
◆ Talk to Frank is a website and helpline for young people (www.talktofrank. com) to find out more information.
◆ Positive Futures aims to divert young people from drug misuse through sports and art.

There are many other plans through, for example, the National Service Framework for Young People.

The GP's role is primarily to identify patients who have problems and need specialist help. Although there has been an increase in the number of GPs providing specialist care (as part of enhanced services and as GPs with special interests), most would still refer patients on. Of equal importance is the recognition of problems such as mental health complications, infections (e.g. HIV and hepatitis) and thrombosis.

Although addicts want GPs to be involved in their treatment, doctors should not be pressurised into accepting responsibilities beyond their level of skill. This has been brought to our attention again most recently where a GP was charged with manslaughter when a teenage patient of his died of a methadone overdose.

Comparison of pharmacological treatments for opioid-dependent adolescents: a randomised controlled trial
Arch Gen Psychiatry 2005; 62(10): 1157–64

This study looked at treatment with either buprenorphine or clonidine for opioid dependence. After 28 days 72% of adolescents receiving buprenorphine compared to 39% on clonidine were retained in treatment ($p < 0.05$). The study concluded that buprenorphine with behavioural intervention was significantly more efficacious.

Air travel

When booking our holidays and long-haul flights few of us will give much thought to our health, but increasingly as GPs we will be asked questions on risk and recommendations for prevention of, for example, deep vein thrombosis. Deep vein thromboses (DVTs) in association with air travel have been reported since the 1950s; and in response to the House of Lords' report on health and air travel (Nov 2000), the Department of Health has published advice for passengers (this is available at www.dh.gov.uk).

The absolute risk of thrombosis is small. The longer the duration of travel the higher the apparent risk, although there is no lower limit below which it is safe. As the risks for thrombosis are additive, short sequential flights probably increase the risk. Factors that put people at risk on long-haul flights include cramped conditions, varying air pressure and oxygen concentration, and dehydration with or without excess alcohol consumption. Certain other factors put some people at higher risk than others. These include obesity, heart disease, pregnancy, the pill, HRT, a family history of DVT, recent major leg surgery and increasing age.

Evidence of what constitutes sensible advice is lacking. The general consensus is:

- move around in the seat and in the cabin as much as possible
- rotate ankles and flex calf muscles regularly
- avoid alcohol and caffeine
- avoid dehydration (i.e. drink plenty of water).

Air travel and venous thromboembolism: a systematic review
J Gen Intern Med 2007; 22(1): 7–14

This systematic review was to determine the efficacy of preventative treatments from 25 trials over a 40-year period. It compared duration of travel (less than six hours, to six to eight hours). A total of 27 pulmonary emboli were diagnosed per million flights and there was a 0.05% risk of venothromboembolism, diagnosed through ultrasound.

Graduated pressure stockings helped prevent VTE in four out of the six studies ($p < 0.05$), aspirin did not. The study concluded that all travellers should avoid dehydration and should exercise leg muscles. If a flight is less than six hours long and there are no known risk factors, no DVT prophylaxis is needed. Travellers with one or more risk factors should consider stockings for travel longer than six hours.

TED Stockings
Mediven travel stockings (which exert a pressure of 20 mmHg at the ankle) have been shown to reduce the incidence of DVT in travellers. There is no evidence for the use of lower-compression stockings.

Aspirin
The benefits of aspirin are arterial rather than venous. To my knowledge, no published study has shown any reduction in risk of thrombosis in travellers. It is important to be aware of the gastrointestinal haemorrhage risk, and that some clinics are advising taking 150 mg of aspirin the day before travel.

Subcutaneous heparin
This is indicated in high-risk patients and does reduce the risk of DVT. Usually one injection two to four hours before travelling is adequate. If the patient is on warfarin there is no additional benefit.

Airogym
This is an inflatable cushion placed under the feet that simulates walking when pressed. The results so far are encouraging, but as yet there are no published outcome trials.

Part 2

Non-clinical

Introduction

Now in its 60th year, general practice has never been more focused on the primary healthcare team and the necessity of team work as it is at present. There is increasing competition to offer general medical services, and general practice is always in a state of change.

This section is dedicated to non-clinical issues, the latest policies, and the more ambiguous topics that may be examined and are worth considering. These topics will become part of your everyday working knowledge. In exam terms, although you need to have an understanding of the issues (their application in formulating your answers shows a difference in the level of candidate being examined), you are most likely to have these topics assessed by your trainer, although around 10% of the applied knowledge test will include questions on health informatics and administrative issues.

A brief history of general practice

The first reference to general practice was around 200 years ago. Since then development has been slow, but has created an essentially stable primary healthcare system.

1815   General practice became a recognised profession

1841   Royal Pharmaceutical Society of Great Britain was established

1858   General Medical Council (GMC) established to control standards and conduct, educate doctors, and protect public and the profession from quacks

1911   David Lloyd George set up medical insurance

1942   Beveridge Report on the setting up of a welfare state

1946   NHS developed under Labour

1952   College of General Practitioners founded (Royal status granted in 1967)

1966   General Practice Charter – the main principles were better pay, seniority, group practices, designated area allowances, financial recognition of out-of-hours and reimbursement schemes for staff salaries

1968   Recommendation of a three-year vocational training scheme (VTS) by Royal College of General Practitioners; compulsory from 1982

1971   Direct access to laboratory facilities.

1990   Government paper *Working for Patients* (performance targets and related pay)

1991   Fundholding commenced

1995   General Medical Council's *Good Medical Practice*

1996   White Paper on *Primary Care: delivering the future*

1997   Summative assessment at completion of VTS became mandatory

1998   Primary care groups developed to replace fundholding

2000   NHS Plan
2002   New World Organisation of Family Doctors (WONCA) definition of general practice
2004   New General Medical Services (nGMS) contract
2005   Practice-based commissioning.
2007   White Paper: *Trust, Assurance and Safety*

GMC's *Duties of a Doctor*

www.gmc-uk.org

The GMC's guidance is slightly more modern than that of the Geneva Convention. It was developed because, in the job we undertake, patients must be able to trust us with their health and their life. The duties are as follows.

◆ Make the care of your patient your first concern.
◆ Protect and promote the health of patients and the public.
◆ Provide a good standard of practice and care:
  • keep your professional knowledge and skills up to date
  • recognise and work within the limits of your competence
  • work with colleagues in ways that best serve patients' interests.
◆ Treat patients as individuals and respect their dignity:
  • treat patients politely and considerately
  • respect patients' right to confidentiality.
◆ Work in partnership with patients:
  • listen to patients and respond to their concerns and preferences
  • give patients the information they want or need in a way they can understand
  • respect their right to reach decisions with you about their treatment and care
  • support patients in caring for themselves to improve and maintain health.
◆ Be honest and open and act with integrity:
  • act without delay if you have good reason to believe that you or a colleague may be putting patients at risk
  • never discriminate unfairly against patients or colleagues
  • never abuse your patients' trust in you or the public's trust in the profession.

You are personally accountable for your professional practice and must always be prepared to justify your decisions and actions.

WONCA European definition of general practice

WONCA is the World Organisation of Family Doctors. It published a new definition of family practice in 2002. An overview of this was published in *The New Generalist*, Spring 2003.

The discipline of general practice:
+ is normally the first point of medical contact in the healthcare system
+ makes efficient use of resources through co-ordination
+ develops a person-centred approach
+ has a unique consultation process that establishes a relationship over time
+ has a decision-making process based on prevalence and incidence of illness
+ manages acute and chronic problems
+ promotes health and well being
+ deals with health problems in their physical, psychological, social, cultural and existential dimensions.

The specialty of general practice was summarised as follows.
+ GPs are specialist physicians trained in the principles of discipline. They are primarily responsible for provision of comprehensive and continuing care.
+ They care for individuals in the context of their family, community, culture. They recognise they have a professional responsibility to their community.
+ They exercise their professional role by promoting health, preventing disease and providing cure or palliation.
+ They must take responsibility for maintaining their skills, personal balance and values.

The future of general practice

Parliament is responsible for the entire NHS. Prime Minister Gordon Brown's first major speech regarding the NHS emphasised its role not only in disease management but also in prevention and health promotion.

General practice is here to provide a primary care service to the whole population (i.e. it is the first point of contact with the NHS, together with Accident and Emergency, Family Planning, NHS Direct, GU Clinics and other primary care services). Everyone in the UK has the right of access to a GP.

Our role is demand led. It covers preventative healthcare, acute and chronic diseases, business and personnel management, research, audit, training and teaching, as well as co-ordination between services for patients and their families.

Over the past 10 years there have been some major changes:
+ in 2000, the NHS Plan was published
+ in 2004, the new GMS contract was introduced
+ in 2005, practice-based commissioning was introduced
+ in 2007, *The Future Direction of General Practice* was published.

The future direction of general practice: a roadmap
www.rcgp.org.uk/PDF/Roadmap_embargoed%2011am%2013%20Sept.pdf
The roadmap is a vision document mapping the way forward for general practice in a time of rapid change.

The focus is on three main points:
+ improving the quality of the doctor-patient relationship
+ developing general practices as learning organisations
+ encouraging collaboration between practices.

Interestingly, it cautions against the polyclinics that have received a great deal of recent media attention.

Our NHS, our future: NHS Next Stage Review
Darzi interim report October 2007: www.nhs.uk/ournhs
Lord Darzi's 10-year vision is that the NHS should be fair, personalised, effective and safe. There are eight specific areas targeted: maternity services, child health, mental health, planned care, staying healthy, long term conditions, acute care, and end-of-life care.

It considers there should be a central point for reporting adverse incidents: Patient Safety Direct. There would be implementation of new, innovative improvements, overseen by a new Health Innovation Council. It also recommends that the NHS would benefit from being a greater distance from the political process.

In 2002, as part of ongoing development, the discussion document *Shaping Tomorrow: Issues Facing General Practice in the New Millennium* was issued by Chris Mihill of the General Practitioners Committee (GPC) of the BMA. It collected views from the profession, politicians and patients, addressing topics such as what patients want and what model should replace the 'Dr Finlay icon of the all-purpose, 24-hour, home-visiting family doctor'. There are 12 chapters in the document, from which I have selected and summarised what I consider to be the most important issues.

My doctor or any doctor?
With regards to access directives, two main patient groups have emerged: the essentially well, who value easy access to healthcare with staff able to deal with their problems; and those with chronic diseases who prefer to see their own doctor. In countries where there is little continuity of care (or records) there are higher rates of investigation. Here lies an obvious argument for continuity of both care and records.

Should GPs let go and use the primary healthcare team?
This question really focuses on the purpose of the consultation. Although most patients are happy to see a nurse for triage or treatment of a minor illness, there

is the flip side of the coin that no consultation is trivial. Each is an opportunity for discovering hidden agendas and health promotion.

Independent contractor status vs. salaried service

Independent contractor status is deemed to allow GPs greater control over their working practice, hours, and staff, and to allow them to act as advocates on behalf of their patients. This is thought to encourage innovation, change and efficiency.

However, there is a widely held belief that independence is an illusion. Taking a salaried stance does not mean that you lose your autonomy, or that you can no longer be an advocate for your patient.

A job for life or a portfolio career?

Young doctors want flexible careers, to work part time, the chance to move between practices, or even to mix general practice with other careers.

Gatekeeper: is there still a role?

Will walk-in centres and NHS Direct change the game? It is anticipated that in the future this, or another form of triage, will be used in the first instance, with GPs further down the line.

Clinical autonomy: does it have a place any more?

This, in a way, goes back to the independent contractor status issue in that, whatever your opinion, we live in the world of NICE, National Service Frameworks, guidelines, protocols, evidence-based medicine and clinical governance.

Primary care groups: working together or professional straightjacket?

Primary care trusts mean increasing accountability and increasing pressure to deliver consistent care in an evidence-based way.

Promoting quality: what makes a good GP? Will revalidation stop bad doctors?

This chapter looks at issues such as quality (which in itself will not mean the same to all of us), consistency, and increasing the number of GP specialists (i.e. additional GP roles contracted by the primary care trust – patients would then be referred to secondary care from that point).

Future pressures

This looks at what patients want (not necessarily need), funding, and rationing. Pressure will come from all areas – the elderly, genetics, the Internet, consumerism and patient expectations – all of which will drive standards.

Shaping Tomorrow concluded that change is being imposed by the Government (like it or not) and the challenge is to retain those parts of general practice that hold value and satisfaction for patients and doctors. To do this we need to define what is special and central to what we do, and then fight to keep it. It is better to try and shape tomorrow rather than have it imposed on us.

It is not yet clear what the 'Millennium GP' should look like. (Yes, it actually says that.)

The 21st century GP: physician and priest
Br J Gen Pract 2007; 57 (543): 840–2

This discussion looks at what people expect from their GPs today, summarising that we need to play a variety of roles to different people, being able to address any condition that patients bring to us. Although we are capable doctors and quality can at times be measured, a significant part of what we do is not measurable. Patients use us for the skills that best suit their needs, but it is the significance of the immeasurable that creates our true worth.

NHS Plan

This is a 10-year reform plan/vision for the NHS that was published in July 2000. It outlines a new delivery system for the NHS with changes for social services and NHS staff groups. Whilst continuing to underpin the founding principles of the NHS (access to care for all on the basis of need, not ability to pay) it will bring about far-reaching changes across the NHS.

There are five main challenges that need to be addressed.
+ *Partnership* – across the NHS to ensure best possible care.
+ *Performance* – setting and delivering high standards within the NHS.
+ *Professions* – the wider NHS workforce must work together to deliver services for patients, breaking the traditional barriers.
+ *Patient care* – delivery should be fast and convenient, listening to need and letting patients know their rights.
+ *Prevention* – promoting healthy living across all societies, and tackling variations in care.

In January 2001, the Department of Health published *Primary Care, General Practice and the NHS Plan*, which covered much the same ground, but was aimed more specifically at primary care professionals. I have broken these down into digestible chunks with the initial timescale plans.

Planned investment

Chronic underfunding has been acknowledged and there is now a plan for sustained increases in funding.

By 2004:
+ 6500 more therapists

+ 2000 more GPs
+ 7500 more consultants
+ 20 000 more nurses
+ 1000 more medical student places
+ 7000 extra beds in hospital/intermediate care.

By 2010:
+ 100+ new hospitals
+ 500 one-stop primary care centres
+ 3000+ GP premises will be modernised.

In addition, child care support will be available for NHS staff, with 100 on-site nurseries.

Information technology/accessibility

By 2002 all GPs will have access to the NHS net.
  By 2004:
+ access to electronic personal medical patient records (EPR), 75% of hospitals and 50% PCT and primary healthcare teams will have implemented EPRs
+ electronic prescribing of medication
+ single call to NHS Direct will be a one-stop gateway to out-of-hours care.

By 2005:
+ electronic booking of appointments (Choose and Book)
+ local health services to have provision for telemedicine
+ maximum wait no longer than 48 hours for a routine GP appointment or 24 hours to see a practice nurse
+ maximum wait for any stage of treatment six months (three months by 2008).

General practice

+ By 2001 every primary care group (PCG) must have in place a system to monitor practice referral rates.
+ By 2002 a third of all GPs are expected to be working to Personal Medical Services (PMS) contracts.
+ By 2003 PCGs will have become PCTs. Occupational Health services to be extended to GPs and their staff.
+ By 2004 there will be extended nurse prescribing (over 50% will be able to prescribe). There will be deeper partnerships with the pharmaceutical industry.

Patient involvement
By 2002:
* patient advocates in every trust
* PALS (Patient Advocacy and Liaison Service).

There will also be:
* further overhaul of the complaints system; the NHS will act on concerns before they become complaints
* increased lay input at every level, including advising the National Institute of Health and Clinical Excellence (NICE)
* input of patients' views on local health services to help decide how much cash they receive
* copying of letters about patient care, to provide a copy for the patient
* if an operation is cancelled, the ability for the patient to choose the date within 28 days, or the hospital will pay for it to be done at another hospital of the patient's choosing.

Other points raised include:
* anti-ageism policy
* nursing care in nursing homes to be free
* better access to dental care
* better diet – fruit available in schools for four- to six-year-olds
* retirement health checks
* modern contracts for doctors
* new care trusts to commission health and social care in a single organisation.

The GMS contract: *Your Contract, Your Future*
www.gpcwm.co.uk/gms2/f_regulations.htm
The Red Book – our terms of service – was renegotiated and costs were estimated, looking at the workload, infrastructure, practice expenses and skill-mix changes that were necessary.

The contract is between the primary care trust and the practice (i.e. there will be no individual lists) and will be for essential and additional services. The contract will safeguard premises, allowing for improvement and development in the interest of quality patient care.

The final version was signed up to and launched in April 2004. The second round of 'renegotiation' is in April 2008.

Investing in general practice: the new GMS contract
The basis of the new GMS contract has been accepted and should:
* provide new mechanisms to allow practices greater flexibility to determine the range of services they wish to provide

+ reward practices for delivering clinical and organisational quality and for improving the patient experience
+ facilitate the modernisation of practice infrastructure, including premises and IT
+ provide for unprecedented and guaranteed levels of investment through a gross investment guarantee
+ support the delivery of a wider range of higher-quality services, and empower patients to make the best use of primary care services
+ simplify the regulatory regime.

UK expenditure on primary care should rise from £6.1 billion to £8 billion over three years (a 33% increase). One of the funding issues is that, as GPs, we have surprised politicians with our achievements in enhanced services, leading to anticipated shortfalls in budget allowances.

More flexible provision of services

All GMS practices will provide essential services and a range of enhanced services. Practices will have the opportunity to increase their income through opting to provide a wider range of enhanced services.

Primary care trusts are responsible for ensuring patient access is not compromised, and by 31 December 2004 should have taken full responsibility for out-of-hours services (6.30pm–8.00am weekdays, all weekends, bank holidays and public holidays). This will include GP co-operatives, NHS Direct/24, walk-in centres, paramedics, pharmacists, GP services in Accident and Emergency, commercial deputising services, and social work services.

How will the money flow?

+ *Protected global sum* will be paid directly to the practice from the PCT for essential and additional services. It includes a lot of the past Red Book payments.
+ *Enhanced services payments* will come from the PCTs and include development money.
+ *Wisdom and experience payments* are for more senior doctors and will come from the PCTs.
+ *Quality and outcome payments:*
  • infrastructure, e.g. premises, IT, staff
  • ten chronic disease frameworks and organisational achievements
  • aspirations – declared by the practice at the beginning of the year
  • reward – paid at the end of the year if aspirations are met.

Categorisation of services

Essential services

These are provided by every practice. The service is initiated by the patient.

They include the following:

- management of patients who are ill:
  - relevant health promotion
  - appropriate referral
- general management of patients who are terminally ill
- chronic disease management.

Additional services
Most practices would be expected to provide these but could opt out if necessary, e.g. because of staff shortages:

- cervical screening
- contraceptive services
- vaccinations and immunisations
- child health surveillance
- maternity services (intrapartum care would be an enhanced service)
- minor surgery.

Enhanced services
These are essential or additional services delivered to a higher specific standard, as well as innovative services. They will allow primary care trusts to invest in areas such as routine home visits, patient transport, and services for violent patients.

There will be:

- national direction with specifications and benchmark pricing, which all primary care trusts must commission
- national minimum specifications and benchmark pricing, which are not directed
- locally developed services.

Breadth of care will be rewarded through holistic care payments.

This categorisation would allow GPs to:

- control their workload
- receive guaranteed resources
- opt out of additional services if they were unable to provide them
- offer innovative services.

New services will only ever be introduced when the necessary additional resources have been provided.

Rewarding quality and outcomes (2007–08)
The quality framework has four main components focusing on four domains, each with key indicators.

1 *Clinical standards (18 areas):* coronary heart disease, heart failure, atrial fibrillation, stroke or transient ischaemic attack, hypertension, diabetes, chronic obstructive airways disease, epilepsy, cancer, palliative care, mental health, hypothyroidism, asthma, kidney disease, learning disabilities, obesity, dementia, depression, and smoking.
2 *Organisational standards (four areas):* records and information, information for patients, education and training, and medicines' management.
3 *Experience of patients (one area):* this will involve a satisfaction survey and the consultation length offered.
4 *Additional services (one area):* cervical screening.

At the beginning of the financial year the practice will receive a proportion of the quality payment for the standard aspired – the *aspiration payment* (payment per point is currently £124.60). Once the standard has been achieved the practice will receive the remainder – the *achievement payment.*

Exception reporting will be in place to ensure practices do not lose payments as a result of factors outside their control. Similarly, certain categories of patients will be excluded (e.g. those who are terminally ill, those on maximum medication, newly diagnosed patients).

As part of this original document, global sum payments were to be calculated on the Carr-Hill allocation formula. There were problems with the weighting of this, especially for practices with accurate practice lists. The allocation formula for the global sum will now be applied to the registered practice population from 1 April 2004. As a result of this, and concerns over income, a minimum practice income guarantee (MPIG) for the first few years has been confirmed.

A fresh new contract for GPs
BMJ 2002; 324: 1048-9
This is a firm critique of some of the philosophy behind the contract proposal.

'Currently, allocation of resources only poorly reflects patients' needs. It focuses on individual GPs and fails to recognise the role of the practice team. Quality measures are sparse and crudely applied and perverse incentives often serve to reward poor quality services'. National pricing of the new contract (announced 19 April 2002) will take into account changing demands on primary care, through an annual assessment of workload. If workload rises, new resources will be made available. In the future GPs will be better able to control their workload. Incentives for GPs will change; there will be greater focus on quality.

Effect of the new contract on GP's working lives and perceptions of quality of care: a longitudinal survey
Br J Gen Pract 2008; 58: 8-14
This longitudinal postal questionnaire survey in the UK was conducted over

19 months and looked at reported job satisfaction (7-point scale), hours worked, income, and impact of the contract. In 2004, 2105 doctors replied, and in 2005 there were replies from 1349. Mean overall job satisfaction increased from 4.58 (on the 7-point scale) in 2004, to 5.17 in 2005. The greatest improvements in satisfaction were with remuneration and hours of work. Mean reported hours worked fell from 44.5 to 40.8. Mean income increased from an estimated £73,400 in 2004 to £92,600 in 2005. Most GPs reported that the new contract had increased their income (88%), but decreased their professional autonomy (71%), and increased their administrative (94%) and clinical (86%) workloads.

Personal medical services

Personal medical services (PMS) are an alternative to GMS. The NHS Plan expected 30% of GPs to move to PMS by 2002 and all single-handers to move by 2004. This expectation was to change with the launch of the new General Medical Services contract (nGMS) which was to encompass some aspects of PMS. Recently, PMS practices are being offered minimum income guarantees to switch to GMS contracts.

PMS was introduced by the Conservatives in the Primary Care Act 1997, following the initial concept having been introduced in the *Choices and Opportunities*, a White Paper. It went live in April 1998 with a core contract that doctors had to fulfil. The contract was scrapped in favour of a broad framework with outcomes and targets to be agreed locally.

The intention of PMS was to address local service issues and pilot new ways of delivering and improving services by allowing local flexibility. The emphasis is on local funding for local issues, which will hopefully attract GPs into areas with recruitment problems.

PMS contracts have recently been renegotiated. The contract covers what people would normally expect from GMS, but delivery can be different. The focus is on competitive services; achieving targets; and a minimum of three audits per year. PMS providers will be accountable for delivery of NSFs and other key national clinical governance requirements (risk management, audits, work force planning and so on).

An introduction to PMS
An Introduction to PMS is a GPC publication that covers the original aims of PMS:
+ promoting persistently high-quality services
+ providing opportunities and incentives for primary care professionals to use their skills to the full

◆ providing more flexible employment opportunities
◆ addressing recruitment and retention problems
◆ reducing the bureaucracy involved in the management of primary care
   provision.

PMS has had a variable reception. As happens with all new developments, the initial money available (especially for growth) was quite substantial, but this is no longer the case. Also, interestingly, the PMS core contract for third-wavers is much more directive.

The King's Fund study, *Current thoughts on PMS so far*, was published in October 2001. It concluded that PMS had so far been 'disappointing'.

Personal Medical Services Pilots: modernising primary care? states: 'there is little strong or consistent evidence of a "PMS effect" on quality.'

A PMS contract is not enforceable by law but both parties are subject to binding arbitration by the Secretary of State for Health.

Benefits of PMS

◆ It is locally negotiated, and can reflect local circumstances.
◆ There was less management bureaucracy at the time it was launched.
◆ There are flexible employment opportunities, with opportunities and
   incentives to develop skills.
◆ There is improved integration of primary healthcare teams.
◆ More services are available for patients.
◆ It addresses some recruitment and retention problems in general practice.
◆ It promotes consistently high-quality services.
◆ It is practice based, not a contract with an individual doctor (i.e. illness,
   maternity leave and so on), much like the new GMS contract.

PMS practices have the right to alter the quality and outcome frameworks if agreed with the PCT.

Drawbacks of PMS

◆ It is local, not national, so is not aligned with national pay reviews.
◆ There is no agreement on pensions.
◆ There is annual renegotiation, and the contract is then fixed for a year, which
   may compromise income.
◆ The local medical committee statutory levy is not automatically taken.
◆ Funding for growth reduced with each new wave
◆ Discrepancies in earnings (where there is significantly more income than in
   GMS) are being looked into (i.e. to determine if there is provision of a better
   service for patients).

Continuity of care

Both swift access to care and continuity of care have long been identified as being important factors in patient care, the problem being that the faster the access, the harder it is to maintain continuity.

Continuity of care in GP surgeries: valued by many but hard to deliver
The New Generalist 2007; 5 (3): 53–5

George Freeman explains a programme he has been working on to determine patients' priorities. There is some criticism of Darzi's plans for polyclinics, and the lack of foresight as to the importance of and preference for continuity. Continuity can be segmented into information, management and relationship. The article is thoughtful and gives a robust overview of current thinking – definitely worth reading.

   The work is based on a qualitative paper (*BJGP* 2006; 56: 749–55) interviewing 31 patients to look at service use.

Out-of-hours care/24-hour responsibility

Patient demand for out-of-hours care has been steadily increasing over the last 40 years. It is reflected in the increase in night visits claimed, and the attendance in casualty departments. Deputising services and out-of-hours co-operatives have changed the way GPs fulfil their 24-hour responsibility to their patients. Following the new GMS contract, this is something for which we are no longer directly responsible.

   Raising Standards for Patients: new partnerships in out-of-hours care was published in October 2000, followed by the three-year guidance plan. It made various recommendations, including:

* triage through a single call to NHS Direct by 2004 (for all out-of-hours care)
* electronic records that out-of-hours staff can access
* quality assessments of medical staff, organisations and access through clinical governance.

NHS Direct

NHS Direct is a 24-hour telephone advice line staffed by specially trained nurses. It aims to empower patients by giving them 'easier and faster information about health, illness and the NHS' (i.e. going some way toward the Government's vision of a modernised healthcare system). It now allows single-call access to out-of-hours care (the Exemplar programme), offering a triage service, and has been gradually increasing in capacity since 1998. It also has a health website and the facility to ask for information if you are unable to locate it on the site (although it cannot answer specific health queries online). There is an NHS Direct digital TV service.

   Previously discussed points are summarised below.

Positive points include the following:
+ aimed at reducing NHS workload
+ easy access for patients
+ empowers patients
+ encourages self care
+ accompanying NHS Direct healthcare guide.

Concerns include the following:
+ may fuel workload/demand
+ issues surrounding continuity of care
+ missed diagnosis with telephone consultations
+ will there be adequate integration with out-of-hours cover? If not, this may cause confusion
+ not equally accessible to all, e.g. deaf, elderly, mentally ill, non-English speaking people.

The NHS Direct healthcare guide has been written by Dr Ian Banks (a GP in Northern Ireland) with the help of an editorial board. The literature is designed to be used in conjunction with NHS Direct. It gives basic information on health and illness using narratives and flow charts and gives a guide as to when patients should contact NHS Direct for further advice. It is available both as a printed book and on the Internet (www.nhsdirect.nhs.uk). Again, a large problem is promotion and accessibility to those most in need, e.g. the socially deprived or illiterate.

The National Audit Office's report, *NHS Direct in England*, found:
+ some co-operatives (in the North East) had an 18% drop in calls when callers were transferred to NHS Direct first
+ high customer satisfaction.

Impact of NHS Direct on general practice consultations during the winter 1999–2000: analysis of routinely collected data
BMJ 2002; 325: 1397–8
Introduction of NHS Direct had no effect on the number of consultations for influenza-like illness and other respiratory infections.

NHS direct was not introduced to increase or decrease the number of consultations but to make them more appropriate. This was not looked at in the study.

Effect of introduction of integrated out-of-hours care in England: observational study
BMJ 2005; 331: 81–4
This study aimed to quantify service integration achieved in the national Exemplar programme for single-call access to out-of-hours care through NHS

Direct and its effect on the wider healthcare system. Outcomes measured were extent of integration, impact on ambulance transport, attendance at Accident and Emergency, minor injury units, walk-in centres and emergency admissions to hospitals. It concluded that most patients made two calls to contact NHS Direct and then had to wait for nurse feedback (29% achieved single-call access). Emergency ambulance transports increased in three of the four exemplars. The overall concern was the lack of capacity within NHS Direct to support the National Implementation Strategy.

Walk-in centres

Walk-in centres have been developed to cover demand and integrate out-of-hours care, to off load some of the burden on Accident and Emergency departments; to improve access to healthcare professionals and to help reduce GP work load by providing treatment and information for minor conditions.

In the initial period, 40 centres were opened in England. The *King's Fund Report* released at the end of 2001 called for a halt in the expansion of the pilot programme and for more skills' training for nurses. It also suggested improved links with GPs and other healthcare providers.

When trying to determine the efficacy of walk-in centres it is worth bearing in mind that:

+ they direct funds from other areas of primary care
+ there can be a lack of continuity of care and delay in treatment
+ the service may generate a new demand.

The impact of co-located NHS walk-in centres on emergency departments
Emerg Med J 2007; 24(4): 265–9

This study looked at eight sites with co-located centres, and eight controls. As most hospitals had implemented the concept to a very limited extent, there was no evidence of any effect on attendance rates, process, costs or outcome of care.

Impact of NHS walk-in centres on primary care access times: ecological study
BMJ 2007; 334: 838

This study looked at 2059 practices in 56 primary care trusts, over a 21-month study period. It considered the number of people waiting for appointments over 48 hours and the distance from a walk-in centre. The waiting time of less than 48 hours increased from 67% to 87% over the study period. It was not related to proximity of a walk-in centre. The study was rerun to determine whether the improvement was artificial because of the Government target to improve access, but results were similar.

An observational study comparing quality of care in walk-in centres with GP and NHS Direct using standardised patients
BMJ 2002; 324: 1556–9

This looked at five clinical scenarios: postcoital contraception, chest pain, sinusitis, headache and asthma. Walk-in centres performed adequately and safely compared to GPs and NHS Direct for these conditions. The impact of referrals on the workload of other healthcare providers was deemed to need further research.

Intermediate care

Intermediate care is a new phrase for the old concept of bridging the gap between primary and secondary care. It is not just about providing social care for elderly patients in the effort to free hospital beds, but can encompass various schemes such as mental health, the young chronically ill and so on. It should not be regarded as a cheap alternative to acute hospital and specialist care.

Intermediate care, by definition, is not part of the current GP contract/GMS services. Although much of the medical input is provided by GPs, it does not follow that if no GP cover is available, these patients should be allocated to a GP until they are discharged from their intermediate care bed. It is envisaged that intermediate care beds will primarily be nurse managed on a day-to-day basis, and GPs would be involved from the diagnostic, management and review aspect. The role of community matrons as part of the intermediate care team is starting to be explored.

'Hospital at home' vs. hospital care in patients with exacerbations of COPD: prospective RCT
BMJ 2000; 321: 1245–8

There was no difference in readmission rates, lung function or mortality at three months when comparing hospital at home to hospitalisation.

Stroke rehabilitation at home
Age and Ageing 2001; 30: 303–10

This study looked at effectiveness and cost of rehabilitation compared to follow-up in a day hospital. In this randomised controlled trial of 480 patients, there was no difference in outcome or cost.

For intermediate care/hospital at home to be successful, it is important to set up measurements of success, and to determine the types of patients who are to be cared for and the level of care to be given, as well as determining resource allocation. A paper, *Intermediate Care and Specialist GPs*, calls for greater numbers of GPs and nurses with the necessary educational support to cope with what will be become an increased demand.

Nurse practitioners

Nurse practitioners are playing an increasingly large part in the service provision of primary care. With the ongoing struggle in some areas to fill GP posts, nurse practitioners will continue to expand their role. Their roles vary, depending upon the skills and experiences of the nurse. The main areas of input are disease prevention, health promotion, chronic disease management, immunisation (child and travel), smears, and family planning. Management of minor illnesses, triage and prescribing are areas of ongoing development, but require specific diagnostic skills' training to reduce errors in treatment and advice.

From the GP's perspective, this addition to the team will allow redistribution of workload, and it will improve access and satisfaction as well as standards of care. GPs may have more time for more challenging problems and may be able to operate with larger lists.

Possible problems include the following.

- Nurses are not regulated, so who will be accountable? Will it be us as GPs?
- Is a two-tier system being introduced, and will GP recruitment suffer further because of this, particularly in inner cities?
- GPs may lose continuity of care.
- Nurses may misdiagnose rarer but serious conditions if there is no diagnostic index of suspicion.
- GPs may start to lose their generalist role.
- Protocols and guidelines need to be developed. Who will write these – the GP? Would they then be accountable when the patient dictates a variation from the directive?
- Nurses as a body are already overloaded trying to reach targets with the nGMS contract and National Service Frameworks. Can we really expand their role further, given the current shortfall in numbers?
- Funding and training as well as interest/staffing are areas where needs have to be met.

Safety of telephone triage in general practitioner co-operatives: do triage nurses correctly estimate urgency?
Qual Saf Health Care 2007; 16: 181-4

This study used five mystery callers who telephoned four co-operatives to assess whether 118 nurses, using the telephone triage guidelines, assessed the degree of urgency accurately. In 19% of the calls the urgency was underestimated, giving cause for concern regarding safety. It would have been interesting to compare against GPs using the same scenarios.

Systematic review of whether nurse practitioners working in primary care can provide equivalent care to doctors
BMJ 2002; 324: 819–23

This review concluded that there would be greater patient satisfaction and a high quality of care. It acknowledged the different pressures of nurses and doctors. It pointed out that the trials did not look at missed diagnoses (i.e. long-term follow up, etc).

Impact of practice nurses on workload of GPs: randomised controlled trial
BMJ 2004; 328: 927–30

This was a randomised, controlled, before-and-after trial of 34 general practices in the Netherlands. Five nurses were randomly allocated to practices to undertake specific duties. Workload was derived from 28-day work diaries and measured for six months before and 18 months after the introduction of a nurse practitioner. The study found there was no significant difference in workload for GPs in this short term.

Community matrons

Community matron posts are only just being developed. They are a logical extension into the community of nurse practitioners, aimed at improving health and social care for patients with long-term complex medical problems, and at reducing hospital admissions. As yet there are no data or trials looking at the effectiveness in terms of their brief.

Their role includes the following.

◆ To avoid inappropriate hospital admissions.
◆ To optimise the health and wellbeing of adults who meet set criteria for being managed within their own home, e.g. after falls, with non-specific illness, long-term conditions, 'revolving-door' patients.
◆ They will define the category of patient, develop care plans and evaluate progress.

Nurse prescribing

www.dh.gov.uk

Since the 1990s it has been possible for nurses to prescribe independently, from limited formularies. The number of nurse prescribers is slowly increasing. It is currently around 8000, reflecting the time needed to complete training.

Prescribing by nurses falls into five different categories.

1 *Specific exemptions*, e.g. midwives, health visitors and district nurses.
2 *Patient specific directives* – a written instruction from a recognised prescriber which is patient specific.
3 *Patient group directives* – a named drug can be issued for a specific clinical

situation (all must conform to HSC 2000/026), as opposed to a clinical management plan, which is patient specific, not drug specific.

4 *Independent nurse prescribers* – who are deemed competent to assess, diagnose and make treatment decisions and may prescribe from the *British National Formulary.*

5 *Supplementary prescriber* – an independent nurse prescriber who has a voluntary prescribing contract working to clinical management plans (patient-specific, with no restriction on the condition). Some pharmacists have undertaken this role.

The benefits of nurse prescribing include the following points.

+ The prescription can be written by the clinician who sees the patient.
+ Nurses can work independently.
+ It improves patient safety since the professional seeing the patient is trained to make the decision. As a doctor signing a script, you are reliant on often-inadequate information.
+ Safety is increased by the use of electronic systems that highlight interactions.
+ The full BNF is now available for use within the practitioner's area of competence (since 2006).
+ It can free up medical time.

There are some current drawbacks.

+ A number of GP systems will not accept nursing prescribers and scripts must be a handwritten duplicate.
+ There is concern about the safety fears of many prescribers, drug safety and the necessary continuity of patient care.
+ Many nurses do not use their skills following the training, lose confidence and so are less likely to initiate scripts.
+ The Commission on Human Medicines has expressed concern over lack of monitoring of the initial objective: timely and safe access to medicines.

Developing nurse prescribing in the UK (Editorial)
BMJ 2007; 335: 316

This reviews recent papers concerning whether nurses are prescribing within their areas of competency. It considers that the 26-day theory, 12-day practical and five assignments are designed to allow rapid expansion of the prescribing force; and that it is now time to incorporate them into training by assessment to give a firmer foundation and enable a greater role.

Pharmacists

The role of the pharmacist in primary care is also increasing. Community pharmacists are an underused resource in the NHS, despite their level of training. The Government launched the first wave of its National Medicines Management Programme in October 2001. This project may help the Government go some way towards reaching its National Service Framework targets and meeting patient demand. Pharmacists can also train as supplementary prescribers in the same way as do nurse practitioners.

Following successful pilot studies, and with the new pharmacy contract, repeat prescribing for patients (along with other enhanced services such as warfarin monitoring and services for drug misusers) is to be undertaken by pharmacists and commissioned by primary care. Other areas of pharmacist management that will be considered in the future include lipid management, immunisation, diabetes and weight management.

Repeat prescribing: a role for the community pharmacists in controlling and monitoring repeat prescriptions
Br J Gen Pract 2000; 50: 271–5

This study looked at conventional repeat prescribing vs. pharmacist-managed prescribing.

It concluded pharmacist management was feasible. It identifies problems not always seen by GPs (in terms of compliance, adverse drug reactions or interactions), and could make savings (up to 18%) in the drug bill, i.e. it would outweigh the cost of the pharmacist.

Randomised controlled trial of clinical medication review by a pharmacist of elderly patients receiving repeat prescriptions in general practice
BMJ 2001; 323: 1340–3

This trial concluded that a clinical pharmacist can conduct effective consultations with elderly patients in general practice to review their drugs. These reviews resulted in changes in patients' drugs and saved more than the cost of the intervention, without affecting the workload of GPs.

The British Lifestyle Survey 2001 (conducted by consumer researcher Mintel) found that the number of people who asked the pharmacist for advice had increased by 25%. Over-the-counter analgesic sales have risen by 41% and sales for remedies for coughs and colds have increased by 10%, all over the past 10 years.

Patient group directives

These are written instructions for the supply and administration of medicines by professionals other than doctors (e.g. pharmacists, nurses, health visitors).

Their development came about following changes to the Medicines Act in 2000, the overall aim being to improve patient care. They are a recognised necessity with the advances in nurse prescribing. The process of drawing up a patient group directive (PGD) can be time-consuming, needs to be well thought out and involves a multidisciplinary team. For example, not only do pharmacists issuing emergency contraception need to be competent in assessing need and explaining related issues, but there also needs to be a way for effective reimbursement for cost of the drug.

The PGD needs to be detailed. Once it is written it must be reviewed by at least one professional advisory group prior to circulation to practices. As with any published document, it should be dated and have a plan for review.

Each directive must include the following:
+ the name of the business to which it applies
+ the date it comes into force and is due to expire
+ a description of the medicines to which it applies
+ the class of health professional who may supply or administer the medicine
+ signature of the doctor, dentist or pharmacist and appropriate health organisation
+ the clinical condition to which it applies
+ patients to be excluded
+ when further advice should be sought.

The NHS Cancer Plan

www.dh.gov.uk

The NHS Cancer Plan was introduced in September 2000 following a series of cancer guidelines, the aim being to improve cancer care and outcome in the NHS. The plan was developed by a multidisciplinary team, but for it to have any impact it needed 'local leadership and support'. Each PCT will have a cancer lead.

The Government will play its part by investing in the workforce and tackling shortages. There will be 1000 new cancer specialists. Histopathology and radiography will also be targeted.

It is hoped that the plan will be achieved by increasing capacity through new ways of working and developing opportunities, as well as by education, recruitment and retention planning. A variety of opinions have been expressed in editorials and in the letters pages, ranging from 'excellent, simple, clear, GP and patient centred' to 'a waste of money, politically motivated and barely enough investment to keep up with the increasing incidence of cancer'.

The plan has four main aims:
1 to save more lives
2 to ensure people with cancer get professional support and care as well as the best treatment
3 to tackle inequalities in health that mean unskilled workers are twice as likely to die from cancer as professionals

4 to build a future through cancer research and preparation for a genetic revolution.

There are three new commitments:
1 to reduce smoking in manual workers from 32% (in 1998) to 26% by 2010
2 to reduce waiting times for diagnosis and treatment to one month (from an urgent cancer referral to starting treatment) by 2005
3 to invest an extra £50 million in hospices and specialist palliative care.

Also discussed is the role of promoting a healthier diet, the five-a-day programme. As well as raising public awareness, children aged 4–6 years will be able to have a piece of fruit every day if they want (currently this works with fruit being offered at school instead of dessert and tuck, and having dedicated fruit tuck days where fruit is the only option).

There are plans to extend cancer screening in the following ways.
+ *Breast cancer screening* will be extended to women aged 65–70 years by 2004, and will be available on request to those over 70 years of age.
+ *Cervical screening programmes* will be upgraded and unnecessary repeats reduced.
+ *Colorectal cancer* – pilots were due for completion in 2002. If successful, population screening for those aged 50–69 years would be introduced. (This is currently on hold.)
+ *Prostate cancer* – prostate specific antigen (PSA) tests will be available to empower men to make their own choices. No formal programme is planned as too many questions remain unanswered, although trials are in progress.
+ *Ovarian cancer* screening trials are in progress.

Finally, there will be investment in research, in particular the National Cancer Research Institute. Advances in genetics will lead to a greater understanding of inherited susceptibility in the future. As things stand the cancer genetics service needs a strategic framework to develop further. The Harper Report recommended that primary care should be the principal focus for clinical cancer genetics. This in turn came from the Calman/Hine Report, which recommended networks of cancer care in research, assessment, diagnosis and treatments.

National Institute for Health and Clinical Excellence
www.nice.org.uk
NICE was launched in England and Wales in 1999 and aims to produce guidance in three areas of health in order to get the most from the resources available:
1 *health technologies* – both new and existing, including drugs, treatments and procedures

2 *clinical practice* – appropriate treatment and care of people with specific diseases and conditions
3 *public health* – promotion of good health and prevention of ill health.

It was created to produce guidelines for health professionals and must ensure its advice is based on rigorous analysis of all the available evidence, both clinical and economic. The group also seeks advice on social, ethical and moral questions from the citizens' council, a team of individuals representative of the population of England and Wales. Their decisions are advisory, not mandatory, but local health organisations are obliged to review their management against guidelines as they are published. There is a requirement to provide funding within three months for medicines and technologies recommended by NICE.

As part of NICE there is a Referral Practice Project Steering Group, which is responsible for the recently published guidelines.

Following the controversial reversal of its decision on Zanamivir, since April 2001 all evidence has to be open. However, there are still concerns that NICE may be influenced by industry or patient organisations.

Wrong SIGN, NICE mess: is national guidance distorting allocation of resources?
BMJ 2001; 323: 743–5
This article discusses the Scottish Intercollegiate Guidelines Network (SIGN) and NICE. The authors state that the way forward to remedy some of the problems is for NICE to become a recognised rationing agency. It should say no to relatively costly and ineffective new drugs. The authors suggest implementing a fixed-growth budget for new technologies, distributed to primary care trusts.

Resource allocation NICE work
BMJ 2006; 332: 1266–8
This discussion paper looks at the current position of NICE and how decisions are made. It examines some of the influences on NICE. At the time of writing there were 86 guidances and there had been 25 appeals (meaning that some subjects had been appraised several times). At the current rate there are around 20 appraisals a year, so only a minority of new treatments are covered.

The House of Commons Health Committee was conducting an enquiry into NICE in January 2002. This considered to what extent the institute had provided independent, clear and credible guidance; whether it had enabled patients to have faster access to drugs known to be effective; and whether guidance was accepted locally and acted upon. The Health Select Committee and the Consumers Association have criticised the work of NICE, as flaws have been found in guidance issued.

Many independent authors consider that it is a matter of time before NICE guidance becomes mandatory. They continue to discuss the serious concerns as to how statistical tools are decided upon and the ultimate conclusions reached.

One of the most significant human rights issues is that NICE has released a statement that in the future it recommends against treating patients for smoking-related conditions if the patients continue to smoke. Its current thought is that age and lifestyle factors that may have caused disease should not influence guidance on the use of interventions unless they are likely to affect the effectiveness of the intervention.

National Service Frameworks

National Service Frameworks (NSFs) were proposed in the 1998 White Paper: *A First Class Service: quality in the new NHS*, as part of the Government's agenda to drive up quality and reduce unacceptable variations in health and social services across the UK. They have been proposed as accompaniments to NICE and identified as priorities in *Modernising Health and Social Services: National Priorities Guidance for 1999/2000–2000/01*.

The standards will be set by NICE and NSFs delivered by clinical governance and underpinned by self-regulation and lifelong learning. The Commission for Health Improvement, the National Performance Assessment Framework and National Survey of Patients will be used to monitor the NSFs. Performance will be assessed through a small number of national milestones and high level performance indicators.

There will be advances and changes during the implementation of the NSFs. Therefore they will have to evolve if they are to stay relevant and credible in such a changing environment. Similarly, the need for learning and development (organisational, professional and personal) is recognised.

Objectives of NSFs

These are as follows:

1 to address problems that affect quality of NHS care
2 to tackle variations in:
   - agreed standards of care
   - data collection and audit
   - local provision of national services
   - funding and resources
   - involvement with non-NHS agencies.

Appraisal

www.appraisals.nhs.uk
Appraisal is a formative and developmental process. It is about identifying developmental needs as part of a personal development plan and at the time of writing does not have a performance management role. It is a yearly requirement that was introduced in April 2002.

You can register for, and access, the appraisal toolkit by logging on to the above website. You can then complete your appraisal for your appraiser online.

GP experiences of partner and external peer appraisal: a qualitative study
Br J General Pract 2005; 55: 539–43
This paper explored different views to approaches that could be adopted for appraisal. A total of 66 GPs took part in the study (46 had a partner appraisal and 20 an external appraiser). This was followed up after six months by a questionnaire, and 13 GPs were interviewed in depth.

It was felt that clarification in the role of appraisal and revalidation was needed. Given the potentially charged nature of appraisal there was a risk of collusion between appraiser and appraisee, which may lead to a superficial appraisal.

Personal development plans

The need for personal development plans (PDPs) has been recognised and evolved from the shortcomings of 30 hours of undirected Postgraduate Educational Allowance (PGEA), as well as media attention that has focused on recent medical scandals (e.g. the Bristol enquiry and the Shipman case). Revalidation will require us to demonstrate our learning, which we will have to map out according to our own individual needs. These in turn will be determined by priorities that are dictated by the influences around us, such as national expectations, primary care groups, practice and personal needs.

Good Medical Practice in General Practice, published by the Royal College of General Practitioners, states that an excellent GP:
+ is up-to-date and regularly reviews their knowledge
+ uses these reviews to develop practice and their personal development plan
+ uses a range of methods to monitor and meet their educational needs.

A First Class Service: quality in the new NHS, is a 1998 Government publication that states that lifelong learning will give NHS staff the knowledge necessary to offer the most effective and high-quality care to patients. Continuous professional development programmes need to meet the learning needs of the individual, inspire public confidence in their skills and also meet the wider developmental needs of the NHS.

The NHS Plan, published in July 2000, is about staff working smarter, not harder. All doctors employed within the NHS have been required to participate in annual appraisals and clinical audit since 2001.

The advantages of personal development plans can be summarised as follows:
+ personal satisfaction
+ personally relevant
+ more flexible than the PGEA system
+ aspirations are achieved
+ helps personal reflection
+ fulfils contract requirements
+ improved patient care
+ more cost-effective.

The disadvantages can be summarised as follows:
+ can lead to isolation
+ loss of objectivity
+ may be overwhelming
+ needs a support network or mentor
+ needs more time investment than PGEA
+ can be seen as time wasting and unnecessary by self-motivated learners
+ may be reinforcing skills that are already adequate.

Writing a PDP/Practice Development Plan

In addition to a PDP, when working in a GP setting/partnership, there will be a requirement for a practice development plan. This is based upon the same principles as a PDP.

Identifying learning needs
These represent the gap between the way things are now and the way they should be or how you want them to be in the future. Learning needs can be identified by keeping lists, reviewing referrals, conducting audits, significant event analysis, asking colleagues, i.e. 360-degree appraisal (known as the 'Johari window').

Setting learning objectives
Objectives may involve knowledge, skills, attitude, and so on. Success can be looked at by reflection, feedback, audit, assessing reduction in demand, and similar methods.

Identifying resource implications and time scales
This means that plans should be achievable.

Seeking evidence of achievement

A formal PDP is one stage of a continuous process. The evidence can be used to make a learning portfolio (i.e. a long-term record of past experience and future aspirations) containing workload logs, case descriptions, videos, audits, patient surveys, reflection, significant-event analysis and so on. This is the 'cradle to grave' idea.

Although the plan has now been formalised, conscientious doctors have been doing this for years, as it is the fundamental principle that underpins adult learning, educational theories and learning cycles. We all want to develop and work within an effective team, improve clinical care, plan constructively and provide mechanisms of accountability. PDPs are a starting point for this, which will also help us bid for resources in the future.

Revalidation: professional self-regulation and recertification

www.gmc-uk.org and www.rcgp.org.uk

Plans for revalidation have been in progress since 1998. However, the fifth report of the Shipman enquiry and recent cases (such as the Bristol case), have meant that the process of ensuring fitness to practice has become much more public.

Sir Liam Donaldson published *Good Doctors, Safer Patients* and there was a recent White Paper: *Trust, Assurance and Safety – the regulation of health professionals in the 21st century* (2007), which reinforces the Government stance on driving revalidation forward.

Revalidation will be an episodic process (probably five-yearly) to demonstrate fitness to practice to the professional regulator (the General Medical Council) and probably will start in 2009.

There will be:

◆ a relicensing process based on generic standards
◆ a recertification process that will apply to specialists or general practitioners, to show they meet standards that apply to their specialty
◆ a suspension and retraining process in the event of failure.

The responsibility of maintaining basic competence is that of the individual doctor – it always has been and always will be. There will always be other factors that allow incompetence and poorly performing professionals to be brought to our attention (e.g. prescribing data, complaints, new contract fulfilment, referral types – not specifically quantity but quality). One of the difficulties highlighted by various editorials is how to make revalidation stimulating and worthwhile for the majority of doctors, while at the same time sensitive enough to pick out those who are performing poorly.

Revalidation for Clinical General Practice was produced by a revalidation party for the Royal College of General Practitioners. It anticipates that revalidation will be related to a number of different systems, e.g. clinical governance, accredited professional development, appraisal, and GMC performance procedures.

The criteria they have identified for revalidation to work are as follows.

+ It should be understood by the public and be credible.
+ It should identify unacceptable performance.
+ It should identify good performance.
+ It should be supported by the profession and support the profession.
+ It should be practical and feasible.
+ It should not put any GPs or practices at an advantage or a disadvantage.

Revalidation should be a continuous summative process with episodic submission and assessment of fitness to practice, having been through an annual appraisal process. Evidence should be drawn from the doctor's day-to-day practice.

Where are we with revalidation/recertification?

In Autumn 2007 Lakhani published an article in *The New Generalist* about the framework of recertification. He outlines four pillars:

1 essential general practice
2 managing continuing professional development
3 modern professional practice in the specialism (performance)
4 professional standing re-licensure (standards).

There are several reasons revalidation has been postponed. The Chief Medical Officer is conducting an enquiry into the GMC's role following concerns raised by the fifth Shipman report. It is thought that initial changes may have been brought about because of the cost of revalidating 30 000 doctors a year and the duplication of current systems, with little evidence that it would stop another Shipman.

Regulation of doctors
BMJ 2007; 334: 436–7

This editorial followed the White Paper on regulation of health professionals in the 21st century. Patient safety is described as being at the centre of the proposals. The basic proposals will be based on generic standards – good medical practice – involving an annual appraisal that will contain a summative process. A 360-degree appraisal system is being piloted and will most likely form part of the process.

GMC and the future of revalidation: a way forward
BMJ 2005; 330: 1326–8

This article by Mayur Lakhani outlines ten guiding principles for revalidation. It includes the recognition that revalidation is summative, needs clear criteria, needs lay involvement, must be in addition to appraisal and clinical governance and should include local certification. It also advocates that reliability of information should be ensured; there should be alternative routes for revalidation; a tighter definition of a managed clinical environment; and that the standards should be consistent across the whole medical profession (where possible).

Clinical governance

www.cgsupport.org (clinical governance support website)

Where revalidation is a professional-based measure to ensure high standards of care, clinical governance has more of a management and quality base, being accountable to the Government through the primary care trusts. It is aimed at improving the quality of services offered in the NHS and safeguarding high standards, as well as creating an environment in which clinical excellence will flourish.

It was published in a Labour Government White Paper to highlight to the public that the NHS will not tolerate anything less than the best. This is to be achieved in a no-blame, questioning, learning culture.

In 1999, an NHS Clinical Governance Support Team was established to support the development and implementation of clinical governance. This team is now part of the Modernisation Agency. NICE will develop guidelines for standards expected of general practitioners. A recent review has found that this is no longer needed at a national level and will be done locally, the clinical governance support network being wound down over the next year.

The Commission for Health Improvement (which consists of GPs, community nurses and lay people) is a PCT-based group. Its function is to look at clinical governance in practices and to try to effect necessary change. It will visit each PCT every four years and select practices at random. It can report directly to the Health Secretary if necessary. One of the main issues for implementation is identified as being limited resources.

The Government has done for medicine as it did for teaching and created *beacon practice* status for those most worthy. These practices demonstrate high standards in access, patient care, health improvement and so on. They are paid a nominal £4000 a year and in return are expected to promote their way of working, mainly through 12 open days per year at the practice for others to learn by example.

Each GP has a responsibility to provide a high standard of care and to audit this. Patients need to be confident that their doctor is up-to-date and offering effective treatment. Clinical governance is an effective tool for monitoring and improving quality of care in general practice.

The role of clinical governance as a strategy for quality improvement in primary care
Br J Gen Pract 2002; 52 (Suppl.): S12–S17

This paper considers the process of implementing clinical governance in primary care and its impact on quality improvement. It states that success for implementation requires a multi-level approach to change (GP, PCT, NHS, etc.) and also that there are three overlapping sets of issues that enhance implementation, namely the environment (context), the leaders and the implementers or users of the change. The whole of this supplement looks at quality issues.

Making clinical governance work
BMJ 2005; 329: 679–82 (Education and Debate)

This discussion opens with the statement that clinical governance is 'by far the most high-profile vehicle for securing culture change in the new NHS'. The main points made are that:

- clinicians should be at the heart of clinical governance
- failing to take account of the scope of the clinicians' work will result in their disengagement from management
- integrated care pathways are needed for common conditions
- healthcare professionals need support and systematic evaluation of their performance.

Healthcare Commission

This is a body representing the Government to look at clinical governance at a PCG level every four years. It is made up of GPs, nurses and lay people. They can report under-performing primary care groups to the Health Secretary. They will investigate mainly organisational systems.

New proposals in the NHS Reform and Health Care Professions Bill suggest the Healthcare Commission will be able to recommend that the Health Secretary takes special measures against failing GP practices. The new bill would also create an office within the Healthcare Commission to collect and publish statistics on primary care services and give patient groups the right to inspect all GP premises.

Primary care groups

Primary care groups (PCG) were set up on 1 April 1999, working with patients and health authority representatives to develop healthcare needs in local communities following the Government's White Paper: *The New NHS: modern, dependable.*

The aim was that PCGs would ultimately develop trust status and take over from the health authority.

There were four levels of PCG, depending upon responsibility.

- Level 1 – supports the health authority in commissioning.

- Level 2 – develops budget responsibility.
- Level 3 – free-standing body accountable to health authority for commissioning (i.e. primary care trust).
- Level 4 – as for Level 3, but also covers provision of community services.

Primary care trusts

A primary care trust (PCT) is run by its board and the PCT Professional Executive Committee (PEC). The board itself comprises three heads, responsible for strategic planning:

- the chief executive, usually an NHS manager
- the PCT chairman, a lay person appointed by the Appointments Commission
- the PEC chairman, usually a GP.

There is also a medical director (who is usually not on the board), who is responsible for the day-to-day running of the clinical services.

Practice-based commissioning

www.bma.org.uk and www.dh.gov.uk

Implementing the vision was a report in 2000 by the NHS Alliance that called for multi-level commissioning (the budget having been created following the recognised need in the NHS Plan). In 2002 the Alliance published *Refocusing Commissioning for Primary Care Trusts*, and then in 2004 *Practice-led commissioning – a no nonsense guide*. They have been very keen from the outset for practice-based commissioning (PBC) to be seen as distinct from fundholding, describing it in the following ways.

- It is based on partnerships at many levels, so it encourages teamwork (there is no personal gain to be made from savings) and reinvestment for the good of all.
- The proposal is a clinical vision about what we want to achieve for our patients by improving quality of services.

As the role of planning and provision of health services is developed, practices will be expected to manage the commissioning of services, budgets, and an element of risk associated with this (although they would not be held directly responsible for any overspending, as budgets are still legally held by the PCTs). Uptake of commissioning has been described by an Audit Commission Report as being 'patchy'.

MedEconomics (April 2005) published a special edition on PBC. They have printed a ten-stage approach to PBC (page 30).

1 Find out all you can about it.
2 Discuss it with everybody.

3 Plan what you will commission.
4 Decide which services you will commission jointly.
5 Agree the budget with the PCT.
6 Sign on the dotted line.
7 Allow for patient choice.
8 Recoup your initial costs and management expenses.
9 Monitor your budget.
10 Use efficiency gains.

Dr Jenner (in *Doctor*, January 2005) discusses the new guidance and how it has moved from original thoughts in the following areas.

+ *Inevitability of PBC* – there are no targets, but by 2008 all practices will be involved in PBC.
+ *Incentives for practices* – there will be no cap (previously 50%) on the amount of savings.
+ *Accountability for practices* is to follow national priorities – national and local targets must be delivered (including Choose and Book, access, waiting list initiatives).
+ *Single practice or locality commissioning* – the new guidance tips the balance in favour of locality groups (the King's fund suggests that you need a patient population of 30 000 to manage a total healthcare budget over three years).
+ *Budget setting* – budgets will be set at 2003/4 levels of referral (to avoid the initial increase seen in fundholding, where referrals were boosted in the first year to increase budgets) and then move to a shared formula.
+ *Risk management* – practices are not financially responsible for overspends, that lies with the PCT, which can intervene if it is thought the commissioning group will be overspent.
+ *Arbitration* – the SHA can convene a panel of two GPs, one practice manager and the PCT finance director to resolve issues.

Implementing practice based commissioning
BMJ 2007; 335: 1168
This *BMJ* editorial looks at the Audit Commission's report, done in the second year of PBC, given that it is central to the Government's reforms. GPs have a better understanding of the financial consequences of their decisions following the involvement and are more engaged in managing the use of secondary care (all for a cost of around £98 million so far).

Medical error

To err is human. Individual mistakes are inevitable, but complacency will always be unacceptable.

Reducing medical mishaps is fundamental in improving quality. 'First do no harm' is part of our Hippocratic oath. Harm is done every day and it needs skill to translate these negative events into useful information. For this to happen there must be some sort of reporting to enable system changes that will improve patient safety – and for that to be successful it is recognised that there needs to be a no-blame culture. Liam Donaldson wrote that when something goes wrong, people want to know who knew what, when did they know and what did they do about it; averting your gaze or opting for a quiet life gradually loses you the respect of your peers. It is important to remain non-judgemental while making preliminary investigations, as things may not be what they seem.

Doctors tend to overestimate their ability to function flawlessly under adverse conditions such as fatigue, time pressure and high anxiety.

Aviation and other non-medical, 'hands on' industries have developed incident reporting where the focus is on *near misses*. There are incentives for voluntary reporting, confidentiality is ensured and the emphasis is on data collection, analysis and improvement rather than a punitive approach.

Gaps in continuity of care that lead to near misses or harm can be described at three levels: individual people, stages or processes.

Increasing safety can be achieved by understanding and reinforcing our ability to bridge these gaps. Despite all the defences, barriers and safeguards that are inbuilt, mistakes will continue to happen, so the aim should be on minimising the risks at each stage.

For example, system changes that would improve patient safety would include:

+ reducing complexity and having a systematic approach
+ optimising information processing with awareness of workload
+ automating wisely (i.e. using IT to support human operation rather than because it is available)
+ using constraints to restrict certain actions, and double-checking critical processes
+ mitigating the unwanted side effects of change (e.g. test on a small scale to try to predict problems and monitor the outcome)
+ training in safety issues for all staff
+ regular audit.

Examples of where this approach has been successful are seen in the pharmaceutical industry, with drugs and anaesthetic attachments.

Almost an entire issue of the *British Medical Journal* (18 March 2000) was dedicated to medical error. The 'error prevention movement' has accelerated and major changes are occurring in the way that we think about and carry out our daily work. There is an undercurrent of more slowly evolving cultural change in our learning, responsibilities and ability to admit fallibility.

For risk assessment (i.e. reporting of near misses) to be successful, incidents need to be analysed in an organisational way rather than on a personal basis. Formal protocols need to be developed to ensure systematic, comprehensive and efficient investigations. As always, training needs to be part of the developing programme if it is to be a standardised and effective tool.

Should systems reporting be voluntary?

An example of voluntary reporting is the Safe Medical Devices Act 1990. Reporting is fundamental in the broad goal of error reduction. Non-punitive, confidential, voluntary reporting programmes provide more useful information about errors and their causes than does mandatory reporting, for the following reasons.

- There is no fear of retribution.
- The depth of information is the key to understanding the problem. If reporting is forced, the primary motivation is self-protection and adherence to requirement, not to help others avoid making the same mistake.

In the *BMJ* issue referred to above (18 March 2000) a number of papers and editorials highlighted the need to move away from individual blame towards an organisational approach where we acknowledge that mistakes are inevitable. By doing this, we could build systems to prevent such events occurring and have a means of identifying them early (i.e. moving away from the *personal approach* towards a *systems approach*).

However, as things change in the future in the name of *continuous quality improvement*, it must be remembered that the person who makes the mistake needs help too – a point that is all too easy to forget and often overlooked.

Safer by design
BMJ 2008; 336: 186–8

Tonks walks us through the reasons why thousands of patients are harmed. She quotes from a Department of Health report that the NHS is 'complex, chaotic and clueless about design...the consequence being a significant incidence of avoidable risk and error'. There is the thought that we break rules to make patients' lives easier: a 'conspiracy of benevolence'. Although design skills will help reduce error they should be used with an open mind.

The World Alliance for Patient Safety

At the launch of the World Alliance in Washington in 2004, the WHO and its key partners announced a series of important actions intended to reduce harm caused to patients. These included the following.

◆ The global patient safety challenge – focusing on healthcare-associated infection.
◆ Patients for patient safety – involving patient organisations in Alliance work.
◆ Taxonomy for patient safety – ensuring consistency of concepts, principles and terminologies.
◆ Research for patient safety – promoting existing interventions and co-ordinating international efforts to develop solutions.
◆ Reporting and learning – generating best-practice guidelines for existing and new reporting systems.

The National Reporting and Learning System (NRLS) for adverse events and near misses was launched, alongside the Alliance's report to encourage healthcare professionals to report incidents on a confidential basis.

Medication and safety

Building a Safer NHS for Patients: improving medication safety was launched in February 2004. It is a paper that looks at the causes and the frequency of medication errors and sets out a framework for a common quality of care throughout the NHS (taking further steps to achieve the aims of the Chief Medical Officer's Report, *An Organisation with a Memory*). It estimates that potentially serious errors occur in between 1 in 1000 and 1 in 10 000 scripts, most of which are identified before any harm is done. The report considers medication processes generally, high-risk patient groups, high-risk drugs and organisational changes.

The Medicines Commission and the Committee on the Safety of Medicines are to be replaced by the Commission on Human Medicines which will:
◆ advise ministers on licensing policies
◆ have overall responsibility for drug safety issues
◆ advise on appointment of other professional bodies serving the Medicines and Healthcare Products Regulatory Agency
◆ hear initial appeals from drug companies when a license has been rejected.

On the trial of quality and safety in health care
BMJ 2008; 336: 74-6
A recent *BMJ* analysis considered the reasons for the slow pace of improvement as including resistance to change among health professionals, organisational structures that block improvement of care, and dysfunctional financial incentives. It reports an increase in the number of quality and safety papers being published

in lead journals and suggests that focused measures are needed to build multi-disciplinary research programmes to guide change.

National Patient Safety Agency

www.npsa.nhs.uk

The role of the National Patient Safety Agency (NPSA) is to promote an open and fair reporting culture, collecting, collating, categorising and coding adverse incidents, looking for patterns and trends, and acting on identified risks.

The NPSA was established in July 2001 to improve patient safety by running a national reporting system to log adverse clinical events and near misses, so that lessons can be shared and learned from in a blame-free way. It was brought together with the National Clinical Assessment Service in April 2005.

GPs have to report all incidents where a patient was, or could have been, seriously harmed. This follows the publication of a document entitled *A Commitment to Quality, a Quest for Excellence* in June 2001.

The NPSA document *Doing Less Harm* applies the reporting rule to all incidents, including anaphylaxis and unexpected death in the surgery (both of which are categorised as 'red'). Other incidents will be categorised as green, yellow or orange depending upon their severity.

In 2005, the NPSA introduced the *Being Open* policy, a further document encouraging healthcare professionals to be frank about their mistakes. There are three main issues to this policy.

1 The principle is that when something goes wrong you should be open, apologise, investigate, learn and provide support.
2 Patient safety investigations are disclosable if a court case results, but the benefits of being open could outweigh the costs.
3 There should be exemption from disciplinary action when reporting incidents with a view to improving patient safety.

Significant event analysis

Significant event analysis (SEA) is known by various names, including significant event audit, critical event audit or analysis, and significant event review. It can include examples of when things go right as well as wrong. It can be clinical or non-clinical and it can involve anyone in the team, the point being that such events are powerful motivators for change, and the questions that may be raised could identify a previously unidentified learning need. SEA should be felt to be a positive experience by all those involved.

How can SEA be organised?

✦ Decide who is to be involved (e.g. doctors, nurses, receptionists, administration/office staff).

✦ How are they to be organised (e.g. regular meetings, triggered by specific cases)?

✦ The time interval after the event should not be too long, otherwise momentum is lost and details are forgotten. This is especially important if new ideas are to be implemented.

✦ The meeting should be free of interruptions.

✦ A suitable environment is needed. Sometimes it is beneficial to be outside the workplace.

✦ Set ground rules (e.g. confidentiality and anonymity).

✦ Appoint a chairperson and a scribe for appropriate record keeping.

✦ The agenda may include the following points:
  - Why has the significant event been chosen?
  - What do people want to achieve by analysing it?
  - What are the facts of the case? These are often circulated before the meeting.
  - What issues are raised (e.g. care, communication).
  - What went well?
  - What went badly and how can things be improved? (Shortcomings and things that are amenable to change should be highlighted, but avoid personal attacks and keep comments constructive.)
  - What actions should be taken?
    i Formulate a plan.
    ii Prioritise points.
    iii Decide on a timescale.
    iv Consider how success can be determined.

Medical/clinical audit

Audit definitions have evolved somewhat from Maurin's 1976 thoughts (in terms of it being a general counting exercise), to the modern-day Government's definition in *Working for Patients*, which defines audit as 'the systematic critical analysis of the quality of medical care, including procedures used for the diagnosis and treatment, the use of resources and the resulting outcome and quality of life for the patients' (i.e. it is a much more active approach).

Donabedian (1982) identified three major categories:
1 audit of *structure* – delivery of care (e.g. appointments)
2 audit of *process* – how patients are treated (e.g. looking at prescriptions)
3 audit of *outcome* – what ultimately happens (e.g. mortality, morbidity).

In *Duties of a Doctor*, the GMC describes audit as an essential professional responsibility. The Royal College of General Practitioners' Information Service (No.17) published an information leaflet on medical audit in March 2001 (www. rcgp.org.uk).

Audit is a means by which we can look systematically and critically at our work – it is the final stage of evidence-based medicine. It is not research (research is done to find out what best practice is). Audit is a measure of performance against a predetermined standard. It can highlight problems, encourage change, reduce errors and demonstrate good care.

Audit is increasingly part of clinical governance and will become an integral part of revalidation. Help with audits can be found in primary care audit groups and medical audit advisory groups.

The audit cycle

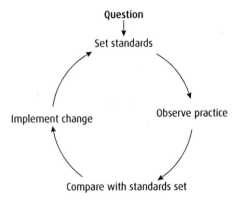

Complaints

A complaint is an expression of dissatisfaction that requires a response. The number of complaints against GPs has doubled in the last ten years. Handling of complaints has become part of the nGMS contract. Handling complaints well puts things right for the individual who has received real or perceived poor service, and it allows services to be improved. Resolving issues at an early stage is the ultimate aim. The MDU estimates that 90% of complaints are resolved at practice level.

The main complaints encountered in general practice are as follows:
- delay or failure to make a diagnosis, or an incorrect diagnosis
- failure to visit
- surgery appointment times/availability
- staff attitudes/rudeness
- inadequate examination
- refusal to refer.

If an individual wishes to make a complaint, this should be done within six months of the incident, or from finding out that there was something to complain about. The general consensus is that a complaint should be made within one year.

The *NHS Complaints Procedure* has three stages:

1 local resolution (with or without an independent lay conciliator liaising between the two parties)
2 a convenor, who can request an independent review or refer back for local resolution
3 the Ombudsman (Health Service Commissioner).

Complaints procedure in primary care

Following the Wilson Report, *Being Heard*, in 1994, the complaints procedure was revised in 1996 and is in the process of being updated again, following a response document *Reforming the NHS Complaints Procedure: a listening document* (which can be downloaded from www.dh.gov.uk). The GMC has published several booklets explaining the complaints procedure and how to raise concerns.

All practices should have a written and publicised complaints procedure explaining who patients should speak to and what to expect (required as part of our contract).

In the event of a complaint:

1 the nominated person or deputy should interview the complainant and again explain the procedure
2 complaints must be acknowledged within two working days, or at the time if verbal
3 the complainant should receive a written response within 10 working days (20 if it is a hospital complaint)
4 the response should:
   • summarise the complaint
   • explain the patient's view of the complaint
   • apologise, if appropriate
   • describe the outcome and steps taken
   • explain the next step, how to contact the health authority/PCT if the complainant is still unhappy with the outcome.

Ensure that, if the complaint is made by someone other than the patient, consent is obtained from the patient. Be clear and concise and try to avoid medical terminology. If you do have to use medical terms, ensure they are explained clearly.

Practices should:

◆ keep a separate complaints file
◆ include complaints statistics in the contract report, and for revalidation in the future
◆ hold practice meetings on complaints and how to manage them

The NHS complaints procedure is not about tackling disciplinary action; this would need to be investigated by a professional disciplinary body after having been referred by the primary care trust to a disciplinary panel. Disciplinary measures can be taken only if a GP has failed to comply with their terms of service. Furthermore, the procedure does not deal with claims for financial compensation, private healthcare treatment, or events about which an individual is already taking legal action.

The Independent Complaints Advocacy Service is the NHS body that will help patients or families who wish to lodge a complaint against the NHS.

Consent

The *Good Practice in Consent Implementation Guide: consent to examination or treatment* is a 50-page document produced by the Department of Health's Good Practice in Consent Advisory Group, which summarises legal requirements and good practice requirements on consent. Consent is a process, as you take your patients through initial examination, investigation and treatments – not a one-off event.

The *12 Key Points on Consent: the law in England* is available at www.dh. gov.uk.

The document is relevant to all healthcare professionals, including students. It briefly touches on consent issues for the use of organs or tissues after death, although this is being reviewed. It is worth noting that the law changes depending on different test cases that are brought. Also the European Human Rights Act will have some effect on English law.

The BMA ethics department published the *Consent Tool Kit* booklet (the third edition, August 2007, can be downloaded at www.bma.org.uk). It is aimed at improving understanding and the practice of obtaining valid consent. Similarly, the GMC has published *Seeking Patient's Consent: the ethical considerations*, and *0–18 Years: guidance for all doctors* (for children). Consent under the Mental Health Act is discussed early in the book.

The approach taken to consent is fundamental to the doctor-patient relationship and highlights an individual's ethical viewpoint on a patient's autonomy. Tony Hope wrote a helpful ethically-based piece on consent in *Medicine* in October 2000. He suggests a quick three-point check on legal validity.

1 Is the patient properly informed?
2 Is the patient competent to give consent?
3 Did the patient give consent voluntarily (without coercion)?

From a legal point of view, consent provides the patient with the power of veto. Without consent, a patient could successfully sue a doctor for battery. Technically, touching another person without consent constitutes battery (i.e. the patient does not need to have suffered harm). Similarly, a doctor could be found negligent if they have not given the patient certain relevant information to allow the patient to give informed consent.

The fact that a person comes to see a doctor or is admitted to hospital does not imply consent to any examination, investigation or treatment. In giving/ refusing consent it is important that the patient understands the reasons behind treatment, the associated risks and benefits, and the consequences if they refuse treatment (even the issuing of a prescription requires consent). It does not matter how the patient gives consent. It can be written, verbal or non-verbal and a signature does not prove consent is valid. Documentation of information given and of consent is important.

In UK law, the term 'informed consent' does not exist, explicit consent is required. Legal duties are defined by statute (e.g. the Children's Act 1989 and the Human Rights Act 1998) and by common law (which is general principles from specific cases). There is also guidance on the use of chaperones, which should be offered when any intimate (breast, genital or rectal) examination or procedure is to be carried out. Practices are advised to have a chaperone policy in place. This follows publication of the Ayling Report (2000) by the Department of Health.

Fraser guidelines

Confidentiality is important in all patients, but many young patients think that their parents can have access to their records, and that they have to be over 16 to see a health professional and receive treatment without their parents. This is not the case.

A young person can consent to treatment if:
- they understand the doctor's advice
- the doctor cannot persuade the young person to inform their parents, or allow the doctor to inform their parents, that they are seeking contraceptive advice
- they are very likely to begin, or continue having, intercourse with or without contraceptive treatment
- unless they receive contraceptive treatment, the young person's physical or mental health (or both) are likely to suffer.

The Bolam principle

The Bolam principle is central to understanding our duty of care as applied to consent issues (and negligence). Bolam was a patient who received ECT therapy that resulted in a fractured jaw. The patient sued (in 1957) and the outcome was such that 'a doctor is not guilty of negligence if he has acted in accordance with the practice accepted as proper by a responsible body skilled in that particular art'.

Confidentiality

The success of the doctor-patient relationship is dependent on a number of factors. Confidentiality ('secrecy and discretion') has a therapeutically significant role, and has been fundamental to our code of practice since before the Hippocratic oath. Without its assurance, patients may be reluctant to give doctors the information they need in order to provide good care. Information learned about a patient belongs to that patient (even after death) and they have the right to determine who has access to it.

Confidentiality: NHS Code of Practice

November 2003, downloadable from www.dh.gov.uk

This document is for people working in the NHS. It covers the following.

◆ Introduces the concept of confidentiality.
◆ Describes what a confidential service should look like.
◆ Describes the main legal requirements.
◆ Support tools for sharing/disclosing information.
◆ Lists examples of disclosure scenarios.

Disclosure to a third party, the Data Protection Act

A doctor's legal obligation of confidentiality is best seen as a public, rather than a private interest (i.e. the obligation is not absolute and in some situations the law allows or even obliges doctors to breach confidentiality). You are advised to discuss issues with your defence union if there is any ambiguity surrounding the need to disclose the information being requested.

Examples of circumstances where a doctor must breach confidentiality include termination of pregnancy (Abortion Act 1967), notifiable diseases (1984 Act), births and deaths (Births, Deaths and Registration Act 1953), and forms for incapacity benefit. The police can request names and addresses (but not clinical details) of persons alleged to be guilty under the Road Traffic Accident Act (1988).

Examples of circumstances where doctors have discretion to breach confidentiality include imparting information to other members of the healthcare team, a patient driving who is not fit to drive (the GMC advises informing the DVLA), and where a third party is at significant risk (e.g. the partner of a HIV-positive patient, who is unaware of the diagnosis and risk).

Consent and confidentiality go hand in hand, and it is good practice to seek the patient's consent to disclosure of any information wherever possible, whether or not you judge that a patient can be identified from the disclosure.

The Human Rights Act (1998), the Data Protection Act (1998), the Crime Disorder Act (1998) and the Common Law Duty of confidence all enable agencies to share information without consent with regard to children at risk of harm. Any person arguing that their medical information has been unlawfully disclosed is likely to argue the right to private life (Article 8(1) of the Human Rights Act).

Access to Health Records Act (1990)

A patient has the right to see medical records, obtain copies of these records and have the records explained.

Limitations include the following.

* This Act only applies to records after 1 November 1991. Records before this date are included if they are needed to understand later notes.
* A doctor can deny access to a patient's medical records if it is believed serious harm to the patient's physical or mental health will result from seeing those records.
* A doctor should ensure that the confidentiality of other individuals is maintained.

The doctor's duties in accessing health records

* The doctor should enable the patient to see the records (or copies) within 21 days, or 40 days for records that are more than 40 days old.
* The doctor may charge a reasonable fee for copying records and for time spent explaining records.
* The doctor should make corrections if the original data are incorrect.

Confidentiality and the Caldicott Report

The Caldicott Report was issued following the review of patient-identifiable information by the Caldicott committee in December 1997.

The report was commissioned in light of the publication of *The Protection and Use of Patient Information* in 1996, due to concerns about the way patient information is used in the NHS and the need to ensure confidentiality is not undermined.

There are 16 recommendations.

1 Every data flow, current or proposed, should be tested against basic principles of good practice. Continuing flows should be retested regularly.
2 A programme of work should be established to reinforce awareness of confidentiality and information security requirements among all staff within the NHS.
3 A senior person, preferably a health professional, should be nominated in each health organisation to act as a guardian who is responsible for safeguarding the confidentiality of patient information.
4 Clear guidance should be provided for those individuals/bodies responsible for approving uses of patient-identifiable information.
5 Protocols should be developed to protect the exchange of patient-identifiable information between NHS and non-NHS bodies.
6 The identity of those responsible for monitoring the sharing and transfer of information within agreed local protocols should be clearly communicated.

7 An accreditation system which recognises those organisations following good practice with respect to confidentiality, should be considered.

8 The NHS number should replace all other identifiers wherever practicable, taking account of the consequences of errors and particular requirements for other specific identifiers.

9 Strict protocols should define who is authorised to gain access to patient identity where the NHS number or other coded identifier is used.

10 In cases where particularly sensitive information is transferred, privacy-enhanced technologies (e.g. encrypting identifiers or 'patient-identifying information') must be explored.

11 Those involved in developing health information systems should ensure that best-practice principles are incorporated during the design stage.

12 Where practicable, the internal structure and administration of databases holding patient-identifiable information should reflect the principles developed in this report.

13 The NHS number should replace the patient's name on Items-of-Service claims made by GPs as soon as is practically possible.

14 The design of new systems for transfer of prescription data should incorporate the principles developed in the Caldicott Report.

15 Future negotiations on pay and conditions for GPs should, where possible, avoid systems of payment which require patient-identifying details to be transmitted.

16 Consideration should be given to procedures for GP claims and payments that do not require patient-identifying information to be transferred, which can then be piloted.

If you remember only five points from the Caldicott guidelines, try to remember that information should be:

* held securely and confidentially
* obtained fairly and efficiently
* recorded accurately and reliably
* used effectively and efficiently
* shared appropriately and lawfully.

Assuring the confidentiality of shared electronic health records
BMJ 2007; 335: 1223–4

This editorial was written following the recent loss of patient information (of 25 million people) and looks at the security issues that arise with our increasing move to centralise huge amounts of data from multiple sources. Although centralisation is thought to be advantageous from the point of view of patient safety, and for overall general security, when protecting the data there is still a great amount of concern over the NHS Care Record Service.

Medicine and the Internet

It is accepted that the Internet can improve communication and access both among professionals and with patients. One of the biggest problems with information on the net is that there is no quality control or regulation (i.e. there is no guarantee the information is reliable), which means as GPs we may need to guide our patients.

Health on the Net (www.hon.ch) is an international organisation that provides a database of evaluated health material, which you can search for information through the site. If a website offering health information displays the HON logo, it means that the site has been developed in accordance with the foundation's guidelines.

Worldwide Online Reliable Advice to Patients and Individuals (WRAPIN) has been developed to enable comparison of health/medical documents in any format through this interconnected knowledge base – another step towards the certification of quality online information.

NHS net

As part of the Government directive, all GP practices should be connected to the NHS net. It is planned that health records will be networked, thus allowing doctors 24-hour access. Appointments (Choose and Book), x-ray and pathology requests will be online, and pharmacists will accept prescriptions electronically.

Inevitably this raises data protection issues, which were addressed in the Caldicott Report, 1999.

The potential applications of the NHS net are limited only by its users. At whatever speed the NHS net is implemented, the systems it uses need to have been thought through in terms of confidentiality (patient and doctor), data protection, and litigation issues. They also need to be quick, user-friendly and accurate.

Connecting for Health

www.connectingforhealth.nhs.uk

The National Programme for IT (www.dh.gov.uk) is being implemented across the United Kingdom, its goal being to improve access to information and to develop a more traceable service activity within the NHS.

There are several major changes that should improve our ability to deliver for our patients. The main changes are listed below.

♦ *NHS Care Records Service* (NHS CRS) and the *NHS Spine* – clinical records will be available to out-of-hours doctors and will be jointly used by those professionals caring for patients (this should allow us to make better clinical decisions and reduce risk). By 2008 it is anticipated that Health Space will allow patients to read their own records (this is not yet available).

◆ *Electronic prescribing service* (EPS) – repeat prescribing will be managed by pharmacists rather than being requested through GPs. Again, this should improve satisfaction and safety. It should also reduce the number of fraudulent scripts.

◆ *Health Space* – patients will be able to book appointments online (for GP and hospital) and view a summary of their personal records. This is available in some practices. It is anticipated that access to records and email contact with health service providers will be rolled out and indeed is underway in some areas.

◆ *PACS centralised electronic storage* of images such as x-rays and scans will be available and accessible.

There will be several measures to ensure that records remain confidential.

◆ *Smart cards* – you will only be able to access the NHS CRS using a smart card.

◆ *Legitimate relationships* – only clinicians directly involved in a patient's care will be able to access the records.

◆ *Role-based access* – for example, a receptionist would have more restricted access than a GP, who would have full access.

◆ *Sealed envelopes* – patients will be able to request that certain information be withheld from the shared record.

◆ *Audit trails and alerts* – alerts would be triggered by irregular access and patients could request to see who had accessed their records. The Caldicott Guardians would be responsible for monitoring this.

Confidentiality and connecting for health
Br J Gen Pract 2008; 58(547): 75–6

This editorial has been written with the feeling that we may come under fire regarding confidentiality. There are concerns about the centralisation of health data; unlawful access to medical records; and lawful access to records (such as police wanting to see a suspect's files). As well, there is what Ross Anderson calls 'mission creep', where Whitehall plans to make use of the records once they are easily available.

A website about the issues can be found at www.thebigoptout.org.

European Computer Driving License (ECDL) Programme

This is a scheme to allow all NHS staff to train online and to be examined to ECDL standards, over seven modules of basic skills.

The scheme was developed in Finland in 1988 and is now an international non-profit-making organisation. More than 200 000 people in the UK are now registered.

Evidence-based medicine

Evidence-based medicine (EBM) was coined as a buzz phrase in the early 1990s, and has increased our awareness of research studies and improved our knowledge base within the profession as a whole. This can give our patients the confidence that we are up to date and giving them appropriate advice.

Research findings (the evidence) are almost never black and white and often look only at a specific point at the expense of other issues (e.g. resources) in a specific clinical environment. This leaves us as the clinicians (who are not the best at interpreting studies) with the dilemma of how – or indeed if – we should use certain findings.

Sources of evidence are diverse, but the gold standard is held to be a meta-analysis of randomised controlled trials. The Cochrane reviews are one point at which to access some such information, although their validity has been questioned. Following the publication of a paper in 2001, highlighting minor problems, the Cochrane collaboration took steps to improve the quality of its reviews.

Bridging the gaps in evidence-based diagnosis
BMJ 2006; 333: 405–6
This is an interesting article about making a diagnosis, and reliance on valid evidence for tests that help us reach a decision, based on many factors. It discussed the 4S test of accuracy described by Haynes, which looks at levels of organisation of the evidence from research.

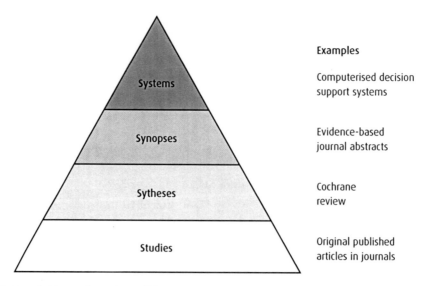

FIGURE 2.1 Evidence-based medicine.

Obviously this takes a huge amount of time. In practice, what we need in order to implement work is concise, easily-available information.

Parachute approach to evidence-based medicine
BMJ 2006; 333: 701–3

The parachute adage (i.e. you don't need a randomised controlled trial (RCT) to tell you that testing parachutes is necessary to prevent death) is expanded upon in this article from the United States. The concern is that waiting for the publication of RCTs before implementing new interventions can cost lives, because of the time it takes to get statistically significant numbers. The authors advocate taking research to the problem. In making decisions, risk, benefit, and local conditions should be taken into account, not just ideals.

Validation of the Fresno test of competence in EBM
BMJ 2003; 236: 319–21

This test was developed by the Fresno Medical Education Programme in California. It is a tool for assessing knowledge and skill (ability) in teaching evidence-based medicine and can identify the strengths and weaknesses of curricula and individuals. It has a standardised grading system and seems to be valid, although the authors point out that familiarity may have led to unrealistic scoring.

Communicating risk and evidence to patients

We communicate levels of risk to patients and colleagues throughout most of our working day, for example in prescribing medication, explaining side-effects, getting a patient's consent for a procedure, and so on. The words that we use to describe risk affect perception, which in turn may affect compliance with treatment, which in turn may affect the success of a treatment and its outcome.

Interpretation in words or figures:

Verbal	Frequency	Probability
Very common	>10%	>1 in 10
Common	1–10%	1 in 100 to 1 in 10
Uncommon	0.1–1%	1 in 1000 to 1 in 100
Rare	0.01–0.1%	1 in 10 000 to 1 in 1000

A patient's perception of risk is often very different from that of the health professional explaining that risk. Health professionals who have been trained in using decision aids (e.g. statistical aids such as percentages or probabilities, or visual aids) are able to change the context of their consultation.

1 Supporting decision making can involve several stages.
2 Clarifying the decision by explaining the problem.

3 Discussing the evidence base.
4 Acknowledging the patient's role in decision making.
5 Describing benefit and harm (avoid probabilities and try to use absolute, rather than relative, risk).
6 Understanding the patient's attitudes to the benefits described.
7 Considering how important the treatment is to the patient and how confident they are in making the decision.

When should you involve patients in treatment decisions?
Br J Gen Pract 2007; 543: 771–2

The October 2007 edition of the *BJGP* has three papers on patient involvement. This editorial reflects on various points. For true shared decisions patients must be given appropriate information about their condition, treatments, outcomes and uncertainties; and doctors must be skilled in communicating risk.

There are many tools available to help decision making (http://decisionaid. ohri.ca/ is a site from which you can download material).

The editorial concludes by emphasising the 2006 *Good Medical Practice* advice – doctors should listen to their patients and respect their preferences.

Involve the patient and pass the MRCGP®: investigating shared decision making in a consulting skills examination using a validated instrument
Br J Gen Pract 2006; 532: 857–62

This paper looks at candidates' performance compared to the OPTION (observing patient involvement) scale. Of the 252 consultations (from 63 candidates) those candidates that passed scored significantly higher OPTION scores (35.4 versus 27.3, p = 0.044). The score is based on 7 raters for 15 performance criteria, which include encouraging contribution, excluding serious conditions, using appropriate language, taking account of beliefs, seeking to confirm understanding, sharing management options and establishing a rapport. Although this was from a video submission it is easy to extrapolate the findings to the simulated surgeries of the nMRCGP®.

Freedom of Information Act 2000
www.foi.nhs.uk

This Act came into force on 1 January 2005, replacing the Open Government Code of Practice. It means that GPs (as well as members of other public services) are obliged to respond to requests for information that is held in any format, within 20 days (although this is negotiable at the time of request). A fee would not usually be charged for any work that was needed to produce the information (there is a limit of £450 per request where appropriate).

There are penalties for non-compliance and failure to produce the information.

The maximum penalty for a lead GP is two years' imprisonment. Most practices will have prepared a publication scheme prior to the Act coming into force, so that for a number of enquiries people could be referred to the website.

We in turn can use the Freedom of Information Act to benefit our patients. Dr Saul published an article in *Pulse* (September 2007 in which he used the Act to establish why a patient had been refused bariatric surgery despite meeting all the NICE criteria, and then to challenge that decision appropriately.

There are 23 reasons information would not need to be supplied that would meet the criteria for either of the following two types of exemption.

◆ *Absolute exemptions*, e.g. court records, legal prohibition, information accessible to the applicant by other means, security issues, personal information and information provided in confidence.

◆ *Public interest test*, e.g. commercial interests (this includes your private income), environmental information, health and safety, audit results, internal relations and information intended for future publication.

Chronic disease management

Chronic diseases are the main cause of morbidity and mortality in developed countries (having overtaken infectious diseases), and account for almost a quarter of a GP's workload, according to recent statistics. Managing these conditions effectively helps to reduce complications and deterioration, to avert a potential crisis, to reduce acute admissions, and to lower rates of referral to secondary care.

Meeting the needs of chronically ill people
BMJ 2001; 323: 945-6

This editorial reiterates that the best outcomes depend upon competent self-management and decision making by patients, as well as on clinical treatments. It also brings to the forefront the frequent co-occurrence of mental disorders.

Elements of a chronic-disease management programme would usually include the following:

◆ clinical guidelines
◆ patient-friendly information that is accessible
◆ continuous quality improvement and clinical audit
◆ access to specialist care
◆ resource management techniques and systems
◆ case management
◆ patient education and counselling

◆ tracking systems
◆ national disease registers.

Chronic disease morbidity registers allow the audit of standards such as compliance and prescribing. This in turn enables better planning of services and the making of necessary changes. The data extracted are dependent on accuracy of diagnosis and coding. A number of chronic diseases form part of the specific indicators in the new GMS contract.

Further issues
◆ Care must be organised. If a system is methodical it reduces the risk of error. The use of computers is very helpful, both in terms of speed (once the data have been input) and for audit when trying to improve quality. Protocols need to be in place, but flexible enough to allow for patient-dependent factors.
◆ The patient should be the most important member of the team. It is their life and in essence we are there in an advisory capacity.
◆ Ethical issues arise when giving the patient a diagnosis of a chronic disease and then motivating them with regard to management and compliance, when they still consider themselves to be a 'normal healthy adult'.
◆ Economic and political issues arise in funding screening programmes and chronic disease clinics in an evidence-based way (medical care, equipment, administration, audit).
◆ No doctor or other member of the primary healthcare team should make the mistake of underestimating the psychological impact that a chronic disease can have on a person's life. It should not be trivialised, but wherever possible we should help that person to keep things in perspective.

Monitoring chronic disease: a rational approach
BMJ 2005; 330: 644–8 (Clinical Review)
This is an interesting review, taking the reader through the phases of monitoring in chronic disease and the importance of measuring the correct marker (for predicting clinical outcome, detecting changes in risk early). Monitoring should be reliable and affordable. The review considers monitoring a patient for both benefit and harm (in response to treatment) and the fact that although we always try to monitor progress, this may not always be beneficial to the patient.

Labelling chronic disease in primary care: a good or a bad thing
Br J Gen Pract 2004; 54: 932–8
This discussion paper specifically considers osteoarthritis. It considers that diagnostic labels are useful when symptoms relate to pathology (which in turn can help with decisions on effective management), but emphasises that labels

have limitations and overstate a problem, which may misdirect a patient's perception.

Support for self care for patients with chronic disease
BMJ 2007; 335: 968–70

Self care is defined as actions taken 'to lead a healthy lifestyle; to meet their social, emotional and psychological needs; to care for their long-term condition'. The Department of Health has a three-tier approach: case management, disease management and self-care support. A critical part of the support is the expert patient programme.

Effectiveness of the diabetes education and self management for ongoing and newly diagnosed (DESMOND) programme for people with newly diagnosed type 2 diabetes: cluster randomised controlled trial
BMJ 2008; 336: 491–5

This paper, with an accompanying editorial, looked at 824 adults and looked at a six-hour educational community programme compared to usual care. In the intervention group haemoglobin A_{1C} reduced by 1.49% as compared to 1.2% in the control (not a significant difference). Weight loss significantly improved (95% confidence interval −3.45 to −2.41, p = 0.027 at 12 months). There was also a positive association in perceived personal responsibility and in weight loss in the intervention group.

The Expert Patient: A New Approach to Chronic Disease Management in the 21st Century, published in 2001, proposed that every PCG should have a lay-led training course in self management for chronic diseases for patients. For the pilot schemes and to mainstream the programmes through the NHS by 2007, £2 million is being invested.

The gold standard for this was a six-session group intervention led by lay people who have the disease, or experience of it, to help improve skills and confidence of other patients.

Although people have needs specific to their individual disease, they have a core of common requirements:

+ knowing how to recognise and act upon symptoms
+ dealing with acute attacks or exacerbations of the disease
+ making the most effective use of medicines and treatment
+ understanding the implications of professional advice
+ establishing a stable pattern of sleep and rest and dealing with fatigue
+ accessing social and other services
+ managing work and using the resources of employment services
+ accessing chosen leisure activities
+ developing strategies to deal with the psychological consequence of illness
+ learning to cope with other people's response to their chronic illness.

How effective are expert patient (lay-led) education programmes for chronic disease?
BMJ 2007; 334: 1254–6

This analysis reflects on four randomised controlled trials. Although the programmes increase patients' confidence they are unlikely to reduce significant targets such as admission. They are not recommended over other programmes at this stage.

Guidelines

Guidelines are defined as systematically developed statements to assist practitioner and patient in making decisions about appropriate healthcare for specific clinical circumstances (Field and Lohr).

The aims of producing guidelines usually include the following:
- to assist decision making
- to improve quality of care, effectiveness and outcome
- to standardise medical practice.

Guidelines need to be produced in an evidence-based way that acknowledges limitations such as resources, staffing and the local population for whom the guidelines are intended. They are thought of as a simple way to get evidence out into practice, improving quality of care in an equitable way. Despite this, there are so many guidelines, changing so frequently, that even when looking at NICE guidance in isolation a *BMJ* article found that one in six trusts were not adhering to them.

Guidelines in practice, considering their role
Are they useful?
- Are they relevant in a clinical context?
- Are they user friendly?
- Are they evidence based?

Appraisal of guidelines takes place through the NHS Appraisal Centre for Clinical Guidelines prior to national implementation.

Implementation
- The people who will be using the guidelines should have a sense of ownership, and should preferably be involved in the development (if not, then they should be involved in auditing and making amendments at a later stage).
- Local facilitators should help with the process of implementation.

Legal implications
+ Guidelines can be used in court by an expert witness (but not in place of the witness) to demonstrate standards of care.
+ Non-compliance with clinical guidelines does not mean that care is sub-standard.

Compliance
It can be difficult to comply with guidelines, as they are not written for individual patients, but rather they reflect a consensus opinion based on the current evidence without making it apparent that they take into account uncertainties, and ethical or cultural issues that may arise in clinical management.

Potential benefits of guidelines
Benefits for patients include the following:
+ improved consistency of care
+ empowerment to make informed choices.

Benefits for healthcare professionals include the following:
+ improved quality of clinical decisions (although to a variable degree)
+ guidelines are evidence based so they increase knowledge, highlight gaps and, through audit, improve quality of care.

Benefits for healthcare systems include the following:
+ efficient use of resources
+ distributive justice (i.e. ethical issues relating to rationing)
+ improved public perception of equality.

Potential drawbacks of guidelines
+ They may be incorrect/flawed/biased or conflict with those of other professional groups.
+ They can be time consuming to implement.
+ They are written for populations, not individuals.
+ They will increase the overall resources needed (e.g. statins in cardiovascular disease).
+ They need regular review to keep them up to date and usable.
+ They do not address the complexity and uncertainties of medical practice.
+ There are a vast number in use that we must be familiar with.

Quality of care of older patients with multiple co-morbid conditions: implications for pay for performance
JAMA 2005; 294: 716–24
This paper looked at following guidelines for major conditions (hypertension,

ischaemic heart disease, diabetes, COPD and osteoarthritis) in a hypothetical case. It found that although the hypothetical patient would be eligible for 12 medications, none of the guidelines modified their directives or discussed issues relating to co-morbidity.

Developing clinical guidelines: a challenge to current methods
BMJ 2005; 331: 631–3 (Education and Debate)
This is an interesting discussion of the drawbacks of the current publication of guidelines (lack of consensus, transparency and failure to make clear the level of resources we have in the health system). It explains the three most commonly used methods of developing guidelines (nominal group technique, the Delphi survey and a hybrid of the two) and suggests a way forward that would enhance transparency by having explicit guideline goals, providing information on reasons for disagreement and including information on the strength of support for the recommendation.

Thou shalt versus thou shalt not: a meta-analysis of GPs' attitudes to clinical practice guidelines
Br J Gen Pract 2007; 57: 971–8
Adherence to guidelines is variable. This meta-analysis looked at 17 qualitative papers. It found that guidance was followed to differing degrees depending upon whether it was prescriptive (encouraging a certain type of behaviour and innovation) or proscriptive (discouraging certain treatments or behaviours, which, in rationing, may affect the relationship with our patients). Another reason identified was differing patient needs (see the paper discussed above and the lack of consideration for co-morbidities that was noted in most guidelines).

Screening
Wilson's criteria (1966) can be briefly summarised as follows.
1 The condition must be:
   - common
   - important
   - diagnosable by acceptable methods.
2 There should be a latent period where effective interventional treatment is possible.
3 Screening must be:
   - cheap/cost effective
   - continuous
   - safe
   - repeatable
   - non-invasive
   - acceptable to patients

- such that the test for screening must have a high positive predictive value.
4 Treatment must be available.

Technically, screening is a form of secondary prevention, i.e. it involves identifying pre-symptomatic disease before significant damage is done. Examples of primary prevention would include immunisation and water sanitation. Tertiary prevention is about limiting complications (e.g. in diabetic care).

When establishing a screening programme you need to consider the ethics of not just the test but the implications of positive and false-positive results. Increasing numbers of studies are looking at the negative effects of screening. For example, a normal cholesterol result may mean that a patient's diet subsequently lapses because they feel justified in indulging more often. Another example would be the psychological implications of being given a false-positive result in, say, *Chlamydia* screening.

The UK National Screening Committee is responsible for advising the Government on the merits of screening for a particular disease and health problems. It published the first report in 1998 and the second in 2000. In the final section of the report it set out recommendations for eight common conditions: aortic aneurysms, diabetic retinopathy, vascular disease, osteoporosis, hypertrophic cardiomyopathy, ovarian cancer, prostate cancer and syphilis.

Gaining informed consent. Is difficult – but many misconceptions need to be undone
BMJ 1999; 319: 722-3 (Editorial)
The author discusses some of the detrimental effects of screening, such as anxiety, false alarms, false reassurance, unnecessary biopsies and associated risk, over-diagnosis and over-treatment. Because of these implications the issues around gaining consent, emphasising the importance of sharing decision making and a patient's autonomy, are all of paramount importance and should be considered.

Death certification
Death certification provides legal evidence of the fact and cause(s) of death, which then allows the death to be registered. It has been a statutory obligation in England since the 1830s. It is important to be as accurate as possible. A mode of dying is not acceptable as a cause of death.
Terms that imply a mode of dying include the following.

Asphyxia	Asthenia	Brain failure
Cachexia	Cardiac arrest	Cardiac failure
Coma	Debility	Exhaustion
Hepatic failure	Renal failure	Respiratory arrest
Shock	Syncope	Uraemia

Old age can be used as a cause of death only if the person is over 70 years of age and a more specific cause of death cannot be given, although with reforms this may become less acceptable unless a patient is older.

Duties of the medical practitioner of the deceased include the following.

+ If you were in attendance in the deceased's last illness you are required to certify the cause of death, if you are able.
+ You are legally responsible for the delivery of the death certificate to the registrar. This may be done personally, by post or by a relative (or other person).
+ You should also complete the notice to informant (attached to the death certificate) and the counterfoil in the book for your records.

There are three kinds of certificate.

1 Medical Certificate of cause of death (Form 66) – any death after the first 28 days of life.
2 Neonatal Death Certificate (Form 65) – any live-born death within 28 days of birth.
3 Certificate of Stillbirth (Form 34) – any death of an infant after 34 weeks of pregnancy that showed no signs of life after delivery from the mother.

When to refer to the coroner

There is no statutory duty to report to the coroner (this would otherwise be done by the registrar) but voluntary reporting where suggested avoids unnecessary delay and anxiety for the relatives.

A death should be referred if:

+ the cause of death is unknown
+ the deceased has not been seen by the certifying doctor either after death or within 14 days before death
+ death was violent, unnatural or was suspicious
+ the death may be due to an accident (whenever it occurred)
+ the death may be due to self-neglect or neglect by others
+ the death may be due to industrial disease or related to the deceased's employment
+ the death may be due to an abortion
+ the death occurred during an operation or before recovery from the effects of an anaesthetic
+ the death may be suicide
+ the death occurred during or shortly after detention in police or prison custody.

Death certification and doctors' dilemmas: a qualitative study of GPs' perspectives
Br J Gen Pract 2005; 55: 677-83

This paper gives a good introduction to the additional uses of death certification:

◆ to monitor trends and patterns of disease
◆ to guide health promotion, resource allocation and service planning
◆ for research and epidemiology
◆ for the settlement of estates, welfare and pension entitlements.

Inaccuracies of death certification are thought to range from 20–65%. When looking at determining influences on the recording of a cause of death it was found that clinical uncertainty and the role of the deceased's family were the two main factors.

The Shipman Inquiry
www.dh.gov.uk

The Shipman Inquiry was set up in January 2001 following the conviction of Harold Shipman for the murder of 15 of his patients. Its purpose was to investigate the extent of Shipman's unlawful activities, enquire into the activities of statutory authorities and other organisations involved, and to then make recommendations on steps needed to protect patients in the future.

Five reports have been published by Dame Janet Smith and her team. The first three examine the extent of Shipman's criminal activities (looking into the care of more than 800 patients), the police investigation, and death certification. The fourth report (*The Regulation of Controlled Drugs in the Community*, published in July 2004) gives a detailed report on prescribing, dispensing, storing and disposing of controlled drugs. The fifth report (*Safeguarding patients: lessons from the past – proposals for the future*, published in December 2004) looks at revalidation and monitoring of GP performance, the role of the GMC, disciplinary procedures, whistle blowing and the handling of complaints.

Recommendations for death certification include the following.

◆ A coroner's office would be notified of all deaths.
◆ The officer would examine two forms before certifying the cause of death.
  • Form 1: completed by a health professional recording the facts surrounding the death, including the persons present at the time of death.
  • Form 2: to be completed by the doctor who last treated the patient; relevant sections of the patient's notes could be attached.

A practical method for monitoring general practice mortality in the UK: findings from a pilot study in a health board of Northern Ireland
Br J Gen Pract 2005; 55: 670-6

Monitoring mortality rates was recommended in the Baker Report, following the Shipman case. This would pose several challenges. The data would need to be of high quality, and be linked to general practices. It is not clear how easy it would be to distinguish variations in mortality and, if any variation was identified, to decide what should be done with the information. This pilot study looked at cross-sectional and longitudinal mortality rate variations and assigning variation reasons (e.g. nursing homes, levels of deprivation, age/sex profiles). The ultimate aim of data collection in the pilot was to improve quality of care. There was a consensus of apprehension about the release of any such data to the public and how it might be incorrectly interpreted.

Recommendations for revalidation include the following.

- A mandatory knowledge-based test at least every seven years; every five years if the clinician is over 50 years of age.
- It should include a folder of mandatory evidence (e.g. prescribing data, complaints record, evidence of continuing professional development).
- Primary care trusts would be able to issue warnings to, and impose financial penalties on, underperforming GPs

Concerns raised about the GMC include the following.

- There has been a failure to lay down clear policies governing fitness-to-practice procedures.
- There has been a failure to take into account the difficulties faced by complainants.
- There has been a failure to investigate complaints.
- There has been a tendency to preserve a doctor's privacy against the legitimate public interest.
- There is a concern over determination to undertake a sufficiently thorough investigation.

Learning from tragedy, keeping patients safe

This is an overview of the Government's action programme that was set up in response to the Shipman Inquiry.

Although the report considers all aspects, the following are specific points regarding death certification.

- Medical certificates for cause of death would be checked by an independent medical examiner attached to clinical governance teams.
- If not satisfied with the cause of death, this can be referred to the coroner.
- The medical examiner would have full access to the medical records and would be allowed to discuss the death with the doctor signing the certificate and with the family.
- All unexpected deaths would be treated as significant events and followed up by a clinical audit team.

A medical examiner would have at least five years of full registration. A draft bill is currently being looking into. Certification by a single doctor in burial cases would cease, as would payment for cremation certificates. Instead a fee would be payable to the medical examiner service in all cases.

There is some concern that, after death, a body may not be seen by a healthcare professional and the responsibility would be with the Ministry of Justice.

Advance directives (living wills)

In medieval times a good death was a prepared death. Advance directives are statements (usually written and formally witnessed) by a person about the medical care that they do and do not want if they become incompetent in the future. They can be compared with an advance statement, which explains your general wishes and views.

Is there such a thing as a life not worth living?

BMJ 2001; 322: 1481–3

This article debates the practical difficulties of measuring, and ethical issues associated with determining, the quality of life in situations where a life has been judged to have no quality. Patients who are dying may find some quality in life even when it has been assessed by current measures as being abysmal. The use of proxies is touched on as a problem for similar reasons, namely the disparity between an observer's assessment and the patient's own evaluation.

Legally, the whole subject of advance directives is complicated. At present there are six types of advance statements:

1. a requesting statement reflecting an individual's aspirations and preferences
2. a statement of general beliefs and aspects of life that an individual values
3. a statement naming proxy
4. a directive giving clear instructions relating to some or all of treatment
5. a statement specifying a degree of irreversible deterioration after which no life-sustaining treatment should be given
6. a combination of all of the above.

An advance directive should not preclude the provision of basic care, defined as maintenance of bodily cleanliness, relief of sustained pain and provision of oral nutrition and hydration.

The current legal situation in the UK

- The person must be competent at the time of declaration (Mental Capacity Act 2005).
- The person must be informed in broad terms about the nature and effect of treatments and procedures.
- The person must have anticipated and intended the refusal to apply to the circumstances that subsequently arise.

◆ The person must be free from undue influence when issuing the declaration.

Adherence to advance directives in critical care decision making: vignette study
BMJ 2003; 327: 1011–14

This article raises the point that advance directives are open to widely varying interpretation, partly due to the ambiguity of a directive's terminology, and partly due to the willingness of health professionals to make value judgements concerning quality of life.

A GP is likely to be involved with advance directives in one of two ways.

1 Advising patients when advance directives may be appropriate and advising on the phrasing of the directive (visitors to the Age Concern website, www.ageconcern.org.uk, can obtain information on advance directives and a pack to help draw up a directive).

2 As a repository of the advance directive, which could be forwarded to the appropriate department on request.

An advance directive has been legally binding on a doctor in common law since 1994 and has been endorsed by the British Medical Association since 1995 and the legal professions. Most experts believe that directives should be reviewed periodically, e.g. every five years.

Formatted versions are available from either the Terrence Higgins Trust (0171 831 0330) or the Voluntary Euthanasia Society (0171 937 7770).

Medic Alert is allowed to engrave bracelets advising that the patient has a living will. They can also keep a copy and fax it to the appropriate department, or read it to the paramedics.

Withholding and withdrawing life-prolonging treatments: Good practice in decision making
General Medical Council August 2002, www.gmc-uk.org

This publication looks at guiding principles and our ethical obligations to show respect for human life, dilemmas of starting and stopping treatment, a framework of good practice, and areas of special consideration.

Assisted dying and euthanasia

Both assisted dying and euthanasia involve medical assistance. Providing a patient with the means to end life (e.g. medication) is termed 'physician-assisted suicide', while ending life if a patient is physically unable to do so themselves is termed 'voluntary euthanasia'. Both are illegal in the UK, and a World Medical Association resolution has condemned the practice as unethical.

On the sanctity of life

Br J Gen Pract 2007; 57(537): 332-3

Weingarten writes an interesting article about length versus quality; the difficulties doctors and religious people have; and the perception that this would be a killing. In both medical science and religious doctrines there are circumstances where the duty to save life is not absolute: for example, when it is no longer possible to use life for its God-given purpose it loses its state of holiness. The final thought is that the term 'sanctity of life' confuses the debate.

Moral dimensions

BMJ 2005; 331: 689-91 (Education and Debate)

The author considers the following three moral principles.

+ *Deontology* – the view that some kinds of actions are unconditionally prohibited; the doctrine of the sanctity of life is often the argument against euthanasia.
+ *Basic (negative) moral rights* – meaning that individuals are free to do as they see fit with themselves. With this view we have no positive right to receive help when we are in distress.
+ *Utilitarianism* – an action is wrong if, and only if, an alternative is available with better consequences.

Although many doctors and politicians oppose legalised euthanasia, this article concludes that in limited circumstances it may be beneficial.

Taking the final step: changing the law on euthanasia and physician assisted suicide

BMJ 2005; 331: 681-3 (Education and debate)

This is written from a legal perspective and opens with a profound statement: doctors in the UK can accompany their patients every step of the way, up until the last. The law stops them helping their patients take the final step.

The proposed legislation under the Assisted Dying for the Terminally Ill Bill would allow a competent adult (who has lived in the UK for at least one year), who is suffering unbearably as a result of a terminal illness, to receive medical assistance to die at his or her request. The bill includes various safeguards to protect both the patient and the physician. Current public opinion is 82% in favour of allowing assisted dying.

Many concerns are discussed following the above paper. They look at the Oregon model of assisted suicide, legalisation in Sweden, and the need for our own patients to travel when they are at one of the most vulnerable points in life (for themselves and their family), often in pain. Similarly, the worries doctors would have if they were to consider undertaking such a role, and the impact on their own personal and religious beliefs. Although the Bill may go some way to addressing these concerns and providing a legal framework, the issues will continue to be debated at length.

The House of Lords Select Committee has been recently asked to consider the Assisted Dying for the Terminally Ill Bill, and the US courts have recently concluded that doctors can lawfully withdraw hydration and nutrition from a patient in a vegetative state. This, and the fact that we have increased our life span (through public health and improved medical care), and increased knowledge of human rights and the limitations of modern technologies, means that interest in assisted dying, in the media and in society, has increased.

General practitioners' workload

The Royal College of General Practitioners printed its updated information sheet on GP workload in 2004. Its findings are briefly summarised below.

* There has been an increase in the number of part-time contracts in general practice, from 5.4% in 1990 to 22.3% in 2003.
* Length of a consultation increased from 9.36 minutes in 1997 to 13.3 minutes in 2004 (data from the Audit Commission).
* Ninety-seven per cent of patients were able to see a GP within two working days.
* Ninety-eight per cent of patients were able to see a healthcare professional within one working day.

How should hamsters run? Some observations about sufficient patient time in primary care
BMJ 2001; 323: 206–8

This article states that GPs in the UK and the US believe they have less time for each patient, although statistically this is not the case. Doctors feel stressed because there is now more that can be done within a consultation and for a particular problem, patient's expectations are higher, and there are more external forces impinging on their practice.

There is little evidence to support that doctors are 'running faster' in terms of both patient management and administration, despite the fact that doctors complain more. Reasons areas of workload have increased include the following.

* The population has increased by 3%, to 58.4 million (but the birth rate is lower, so much of the increase is from immigration).
* Life expectancy has doubled over the last 150 years:
  * there has been a 9% increase in the geriatric population in the last decade

- there has been a 13% increase in the number of people aged over 75 years in the last decade.
- Infant deaths have decreased.
- Divorce affects one in two marriages (with associated social morbidity).
- Families are more spread out (so there is a decreased support network).
- Single-parent family numbers have increased.
- Preventative healthcare has added 23% to the workload.
- It is now more acceptable to present with mental health problems.
- Most consultations are minor; 15% are life threatening and need to be identified.
- Overall knowledge has increased (the *Oxford Textbook of Medicine* now runs to three volumes).
- There is increased accessibility (telephone and email) to healthcare and surgeries.
- GPs are accountable for practice nurse roles, etc.
- There have been advances in information technology.
- There are greater numbers of part-time GPs.

Derek Wanless (a former NatWest Bank chief executive) has published his final report, *Securing our Future Health: Taking a Long-Term View* (the Wanless Report). The main points can be summarised as follows.
- The current method of funding healthcare, through general taxation, is fair and efficient so should not be tampered with.
- Around 70% of the work currently done by doctors could be done by nurses and other healthcare professionals.

The Wanless review
BMJ 2007; 335: 572-3
This editorial summarises NHS performance since 2002. On the positive side there are greater numbers of staff, and there is less waiting time. There is improved provision for high-priority areas (such as cardiology and cancer). On the negative side there has not been an improvement in productivity (in real terms) and new contracts have come at high cost.

The editorial focuses purely on 'before and after', without detailed insight into the collated information, and recognises that more funding is necessary to deliver further improvement.

The new GMS contract (2004) was sold partly as a way GPs could control their workload. There are, however, significant penalties for doctors choosing to limit certain services. There are many initiatives that try to decrease workload, such as electronic prescribing, nurse practitioners and prescribers, and reviews of nursing management for chronic disease. Similarly, there are many issues that will demand an increase in our workload in the future, such as Choose and Book, practice-based commissioning, and keeping ourselves up to date. A person's personal work ethic and their time management skills are always important in managing workload.

Stress and burnout

There are four levels of human functioning: emotional, mental, behavioural and psychological.

Burnout is the end-stage response to excessive stress and dissatisfaction. No one is immune to stress. You don't have to be overworked to struggle with stress, and you need to find a work pressure level that is constructive, not destructive. To do this, you need to be self-aware and to recognise how stress affects you. How you then manage will depend on whether you think the level of stress is a good or a bad thing. It should be actively managed with your own personal survival plan to prevent burnout in the long term.

Stress is also a physiological response to an inappropriate amount of pressure. Noradrenaline levels increase and this, via the medulla, increases adrenaline production. This in turn increases ACTH levels and hence steroid production, which we all know improves immunity and ability to deal with stress. When you stop working, or go on holiday, all this falls down and you develop a cold.

People heading towards burnout go through four stages: overwork, frustration, resentment and finally depression (with burnout). It has always been acceptable to complain about stress, but it has not been acceptable to have symptoms, as these are interpreted as a sign of weakness. As GPs we need to be aware of the wellbeing of our employees and ourselves.

Causes of stress

These include the following:
+ escalating workload
+ frequently imposed change
+ patients' expectations
+ fear of litigation
+ conflict (e.g. between career and family life)
+ lack of career structure.

Predisposing features

In the doctor, these include the following:
+ Type A personality, obsessional personality
+ conscientiousness, high personal standards
+ reluctance to decline work
+ reluctance to delegate
+ competitive nature
+ fear of failing to match colleagues' achievements.

In the practice, they include the following:
+ single handed, or dysfunctional partnership
+ professional isolation
+ repeated interruptions
+ unpredictable work
+ long hours, out-of-hours cover
+ lack of variety, no challenge
+ lack of peer recognition.

In society, predisposing features include the following:
+ increased patient expectations
+ shift of work from secondary care
+ increasing litigation and complaints
+ imposed change and political agendas.

Signs of stress and burnout to look out for include the following:
+ poor time-keeping and decision making
+ sick leave
+ increasing frequency of mistakes
+ strained relationships.

What can we do for our employees?
+ Understand that inappropriate pressures lead to stress; differentiate between pressure and stress.
+ Conduct staff appraisals/personal development plans to identify problems.
+ Hold practice development sessions:
  • review attitudes to stress
  • audit – establish a base line, make the issue less confrontational, measure effectiveness of any strategy
  • develop skills at dealing with pressure – assertiveness (not aggression) and increase resilience – by creating a balance and developing your own strategy for dealing with pressure; time management
  • look at neuro-linguistic programming – this technique helps you understand the structure of how you think and behave; it uses specific techniques to make your thinking and behaviour more resourceful.
+ Be vigilant, observe individuals.
+ Develop your own helping skills.
+ Useful websites:
  www.mindtools.com
  www.employersforwork-lifebalance.org.uk.

What can we do to avoid burnout ourselves?

Br J Gen Pract 1993; 43(376): 442-3

Although published some time ago, this article remains relevant. It recommends the following.

+ Trainees should be given realistic expectations of general practice
+ Choose the right job
+ Develop practice support systems as well as personal ones (e.g. groups outside work).
+ Be assertive.
+ Develop time-management skills.
+ Be aware of your own response to stress.

Other considerations

Delegate, prioritise, keep up to date, audit, develop practice policies, balance your life (maintain outside interests), and make sure you have a plan for dealing with stress.

Organise your workload with realistic targets. Also take time out to exercise and for other hobbies (i.e. strike a professional/personal balance).

Make time to exercise and for sleep. And beware caffeine!

Speaking to your trainer and other colleagues often helps get things in perspective and gives solutions you may not have considered. Primary care trusts usually have dedicated counsellors who can assist staff.

How you manage pressure, stress or burnout is up to you, but make sure you do manage it, otherwise someone will take it in hand and you will be 'managed' as someone else deems appropriate – not a comfortable situation.

The difficult patient

This is an inevitable problem for us all, and it happens for different reasons (doctor, patient and/or external factors). 'Heartsink' patients form a different group of people from frequent attenders. They have been defined (by Groves, 1978) as patients who most physicians would dread having to treat as they engender negative feelings.

As early as 1951, Groves defined four types of difficult patient.

1 *Dependent clinger* – grateful, but seeking reassurance for minor ailments.
2 *Entitled demander* – complaining about imagined shortcomings in the service provided.
3 *Manipulative health rejecter* – has symptoms that the doctor cannot improve.
4 *Self-destructive denier* – refuses to accept that their behaviour modifies their illness, and will not modify their habits.

Heartsink patients are often over-investigated or referred unnecessarily, particularly if they are seeing several GPs and no one doctor takes responsibility for that patient. It is important, for your own sanity (as well as being in the patient's best interest) to develop coping strategies and a sensible, thorough approach to heartsink patients.

Coping strategies

* Recognise your own feelings.
* Accept that heartsinks will occur.
* Review patient's notes.
* Set goal limits for the patient.
* Assume ownership of a problem and review regularly.
* Set limits for the patient (e.g. when you expect to see them again).
* Challenge inappropriate demands.
* Hold peer group meetings/Balint groups with other doctors.
* Consider alternative sources of therapy (for your patient).

Heartsink patients: a study of their general practitioners
Br J Gen Pract 1995; 45(395): 293–6

Mathers looked at the heartsink patients' GPs and found that GPs who had a low level of job satisfaction and no post-graduate qualifications reported more heartsink patients. It is important to recognise this association – for our own self-preservation. If we are stressed, our coping mechanisms start to fail and we start heading towards burnout.

Angry patients

We come across patients who are angry in many ways and for many reasons: a patient may have had difficulty getting an appointment, feel someone has been rude to them or that there has been a mistake or shortfall in the service provided. Anger may come in the form of a letter, in a consultation, or across the reception desk; it may be anticipated, but it may also be totally unexpected. Although anger is mainly expressed verbally, sometimes there may be a physical element to it.

For the current examination, the most likely way you will have to deal with anger will be in the simulated surgery. Practise dealing with anger in your training practice and consider using the following ideas to try to defuse the situation. Remember, patients get angry for many reasons and respond differently to techniques to calm things down, so feel your way gently.

Handling aggressive patients
BMJ Careers 12 August 2006

This article by Anita Houghton looks at non-violent communication to deal with anger and considers three main rules.

1 Resist your instinctive responses (the fight or flight mechanism) – try not to be defensive or confrontational.

2 Remain calm – manage your own mental and emotional state.

3 Be curious about the patient's feelings and needs.

In the simulated surgery cases there is further discussion around a specific problem, with tips. In your own surgery a number of such cases will be expected before they happen and your team will have ways of checking that all is well, such as a well-timed phone call or interruption – and there are always the alarm bells if you find yourself in a dangerously aggressive situation.

Integrated/alternative medicine

Complementary medicine (which focuses on health and healing) and conventional medicine (which focuses on disease and treatment) have traditionally been distinct from one another, but recently they have become increasingly integrated. This means complementary medicine will have to be subject to similar clinical, scientific and regulatory standards to those applied to conventional healthcare.

The *ABC of Complementary Medicine* estimates that 30% of the UK population use alternative medicines and 40% of GPs offer access to complementary treatment. Furthermore, most review articles feature herbal remedies to some degree, as they are becoming an increasingly used method of self-treatment, despite lack of evidence as to their effectiveness. Public awareness of complementary medicines has meant that their use has increased dramatically over the last 10 years, although many practitioners of complementary medicine remain unregulated.

Regulating herbal medicines in the UK
BMJ 2005; 331: 62–3 (Editorial)

This editorial discusses the use of a specific committee to help consumers distinguish between unproven herbal therapies as compared to more pharmaceutical treatments proven to have an effect. Currently in the UK, the Medicines and Healthcare Products Regulatory Agency is consulting on a proposal for a herbal medicines committee.

Perceptions about complementary therapies relative to conventional therapies among adults who use both: results from a national survey
Ann Intern Med 2001; 135: 344–51

A total of 831 people in the USA who use alternative/complementary medicine were surveyed.

* Around 80% thought the combination of complementary and conventional medicine was superior to either alone.
* Most saw a conventional doctor first.
* Around 70% did not subsequently disclose they were seeing a complementary therapist as it was not thought to be any of the doctor's business, rather than this information being withheld for fear of criticism.

Acupuncture

www.medical-acupuncture.co.uk

On the basis of current evidence, acupuncture is effective in treating nausea and vomiting, back pain, dental pain and migraine. The incidence of adverse reactions to acupuncture is relatively low. It is the most popular form of complementary therapy among GPs (used by 47%). This popularity has only emerged in the UK over the last 20 years, although the technique has been used for many thousands of years in Chinese medicine.

Non-medical acupuncturists should be members of the British Acupuncture Council, which has strict educational criteria and a code of practice. Physiotherapists may belong to the Acupuncture Association of Chartered Physiotherapists, and doctors usually choose to belong to the British Medical Acupuncture Society (link given above).

Adverse events following acupuncture: prospective survey of 32 000 consultations with doctors and physiotherapists

BMJ 2001; 323: 485–6 (there is an accompanying editorial)

This study found that no adverse events were reported after 34 407 acupuncture treatments from data collected over a four-week period. It did not look at patients' experiences of adverse events, but it is nevertheless encouraging and reassuring research.

Herbal remedies

The Traditional Herbal Products Directive came into force in October 2005. It means that all unlicensed herbal remedies sold in the UK will be regulated by 2011. Companies will have to prove that new products have a traditional use and have accompanying safety data.

Popularity in the UK means sales are increasing by 20% a year. The users often have the belief that 'herbal equals natural', and that herbal is both safer and cheaper than conventional medicine, with no side effects. However, many herbal products do have side effects and can interact with other drugs.

As there is little legislation for control, doses of preparations can vary widely, even in the same product. Some products may also contain conventional medicines (e.g. one eczema cream was recently found to contain high doses of dexamethasone, although it had been advertised as a natural product).

* *Ginseng* – this is teratogenic, increases the international normalised ratio (INR), and may also increase blood pressure. It also interacts with digoxin. There are several varieties. The active ingredients (ginsenosides) are antioxidants and enhance nitrate production.
* *St John's Wort* – this is a weak SSRI and antiviral drug. It is a liver-enzyme inducer, so may reduce the concentrations of digoxin, carbamazepine, warfarin and the oral contraceptive pill. It also interacts with several drugs.

◆ *Ginkgo biloba* – this is used to delay clinical progression of dementia. It is a potent inhibitor of platelet-activating factor so can increase the risk of bleeds (including intracerebral bleeding) in patients on aspirin or warfarin.

The herbal advice line is staffed by members of the National Institute of Medical Herbalists (www.nimh.org.uk). They can give advice on remedies, interactions, and use of herbal products in children and pregnancy.

Homeopathy

This needs to be distinguished from herbal remedies. Homeopathic remedies contain minute or non-existent amounts of the original substance and are prepared by successive dilutions.

Although to our knowledge there are insufficient randomised controlled trials to advocate the use of homeopathic treatments in specific conditions, many people report having benefited from them.

Are the clinical effects of homeopathy placebo effect? Comparative study of placebo-controlled trials of homeopathy and allopathy

Lancet 2005; 366: 726–32

This meta-analysis of 110 trials concluded that their results were not compatible with the hypothesis that the clinical effects of homeopathy were completely due to placebo effect. There was weak evidence for a specific effect of homeopathic remedies, but the findings were compatible with the notion that the effect was that of placebo.

Homeopathy – A Guide for GPs (from the Faculty of Homeopathy) describes a range of NHS services that are now available and gives details on how GPs can refer patients.

The Glasgow and London Homeopathic Hospitals are the two leading bodies in research in this field, but funding is severely lacking. The Faculty of Homeopathy website (www.trusthomeopathy.org/faculty) is a good source of information.

Antioxidants

These include ginseng, β-carotene, vitamin C and E, minerals such as zinc and copper, flavonoids, etc.

Most of the evidence available is in the form of cohort studies. As yet there seems to be insufficient evidence that taking antioxidants offers much in the way of benefit to healthy people.

Mortality in randomised trials of antioxidant supplements for primary and secondary prevention: a systematic review and meta-analysis

JAMA 2007; 297: 842–57

This analysis considered 68 trials of 232 606 patients and found that there was a significant increase in the risk of mortality, especially with β-carotene, vitamin A and vitamin E. Vitamin C and selenium had no effect on mortality.

Medical ethics

> Understanding the law helps us deal with disputes, a proper understanding of medical ethics will help us work in true partnership with our patients.
>
> (Dr Cox, 8 November 01)

This is a source of anxiety for many, especially when approaching exams like the MRCGP®. The Hippocratic oath first outlined an ethical approach to medicine, and the General Medical Council requires that medical ethics be a core subject in the medical curriculum. Try not to be daunted by the subject. Most of what you need you already know, but it is now a case of formulating a way of thinking and talking about ethical principles, using an ethical model that you can apply to a given situation.

Medical ethics applies to all areas of medicine, including end-of-life decisions, medical error, priority setting, biotechnology, education, consent and confidentiality.

Ethics and communication skills
Medicine 2000; 28
This provides an excellent narrative, not just on ethics but on communication skills as well. I have summarised some of the discussion on ethics below.

Questions on ethical values cannot be solved by simply applying an algorithm. If we are to practise medicine in a way we think right we must:
+ clarify what value judgements are relevant in a specific clinical situation
+ be aware of the relevant issues
+ subject our views to critical analysis to ensure they are logical and consistent
+ adapt or change our views in the light of such analysis.

In addition, we must practise medicine in a legal framework.

The Four Principles approach
+ Respect for *autonomy* (self-rule) – help patients to make their own decisions and respect those decisions even when you do not agree with them.
+ *Beneficence* (do good) – this entails doing what is best for the patient, but who is the judge of what is best? This may conflict with autonomy.
+ *Non-maleficence* (avoiding harm) – in most cases this does not add anything to the principle of beneficence.
+ *Justice* – this incorporates time and resources.

Revising and implementing the Tavistock principles for everybody in health care
BMJ 2001; 323: 616-20

The Tavistock group published their original five principles in 1999. The principles are not evidence based but are meant to serve as an ethical framework for those working to improve medical error.

The ethical concepts of the Tavistock group

These can be summarised as follows.

- *Rights* – people have a right to health and healthcare.
- *Balance* – care of individual patients is central, but health of the population is also our concern.
- *Comprehensiveness* – in addition to treating illness we have an obligation to ease suffering, minimise disability, prevent disease and promote health.
- *Co-operation* – healthcare succeeds only if we co-operate with those we serve, each other and those in other sectors.
- *Improvement* – improving healthcare is a serious and continuing responsibility.
- *Safety* – do no harm.
- *Openness* – being open, honest and trustworthy is vital in healthcare.

The Declaration of Helsinki (revised for the fifth time by the World Medical Association) was adopted in 1964 and sets out widely accepted ethical principles for medical research involving human subjects. It is not clear whether this declaration has any real legal standing, or whether it is just to serve as a guide. The UK Clinical Ethics network is there to offer educational and practical support for clinical ethics groups.

Part 3

Consultation models and critical reading

Consultation models

The consultation – you can't ignore it; it is central to what we do every single day and has always been important. To be an effective doctor, communication skills are of paramount importance, and for these to be evident there has to be an inclination to engage with your patient. Harry Brown described the consultation as a 'complex series of interactions that have to be analysed and assessed quickly'. Although we become accustomed to doing this rapidly, it is in itself a huge area of risk.

Once you are familiar with the different models you can use the frameworks to help structure consultations in a positive way, especially if you feel that your usual style isn't working.

What I have tried to do in this section is give a brief summary of several models. Of course, this is no substitute for reading the original texts from cover to cover, but this is probably a little easier to digest.

It is worth noting that the formal, history-taking part of clinical management, if used prematurely, can stifle the patient's agenda. A patient's initial narrative is an important part of the consultation. It has been proved that, contrary to popular belief, the majority of patients will not go on to talk indefinitely, but will usually stop within one minute. Allowing patients to get their problem off their chest uninterrupted greatly increases satisfaction on all sides.

Getting it right in the consultation
Getting it right in the consultation: Hippocrates' problem; Aristotle's answer
Dr John Gillie, Occasional Paper 86, The Royal College of General Practitioners

This paper considers many thoughts and approaches to medicine, decision making, ethical values and philosophies that have developed, mainly over the last 50 years, but drawing on work 2000 years old (given the understanding that human nature has changed little over that time).

Among others, Gillie considers Toon's analyses of several models of general practice, and McWhinney's (1996) description of the four main ways general practice differs from other specialties. These can be briefly summarised.

+ General practice defines itself in terms of relationships, especially the doctor-patient relationship.
+ We tend to think in terms of individuals rather than to generalise.
+ We have an organismic approach (i.e. consider the whole) rather than mechanistic (i.e. consider the part).
+ It is the only major field that transcends the division between mind and body.

This will in no way be a quick read, but it will be worthwhile.

Communication skills
Everything you were afraid to ask about communication skills
Br J Gen Pract 2005; 55: 40–6

This discussion paper, by Skelton, starts by citing the Toronto consensus statement on communication: effective communication is a central clinical function that largely determines the patient's satisfaction and compliance, and positively influences health outcomes. It looks at the teaching of communication skills and their place in the curricula, posing the philosophical question that rather than teaching communication skills perhaps the focus should be on attitudes, in the belief that this would generate the appropriate communication skills.

Doctor-patient relationship
Reflections on the doctor-patient relationship: from evidence to experience (MacKenzie lecture)
Br J Gen Pract 2005; 55: 793–801

Moira Stewart considers general practice 'whole-person medical practice' and gives this lecture with the understanding that doctor-patient relationships evolve over time and with shared experiences (with a common goal of diagnosis and cure).

The six interactive components of the patient-centred methods discussed are summarised as:
- exploring disease and the patient's illness experience
- understanding the whole person
- finding common ground
- incorporating prevention and health promotion
- enhancing the patient-doctor relationship
- being realistic.

The paper concludes that without general practice there would be more confusion, fear and doubt.

Balint model

This is a psychological model of the doctor-patient relationship. The understanding that doctors have feelings and that these have a function within the consultation form part of the model.

Balint explains that a patient's problem will have psychological and physical components and that these will be interlinked. Indeed, psychological problems may manifest themselves clinically. Individual doctors vary in their awareness of these points, but they can be trained to be more sensitive and aware.

Important features of Balint's model include:
- the doctor as a drug
- the fact that the child of a patient may be brought with a trivial problem for

the patient to make contact (i.e. the child as the presenting complaint)
+ elimination by appropriate examination
+ collusion of anonymity
+ 'the Flash'.

Berne's transactional analysis
The Games People Play
Berne (1968). Penguin Books: London
This model looks at the roles that patients and doctors take within the consultation, and identifies three ego states.
+ Parent – critical or caring.
+ Adult – logical.
+ Child – dependent.

This is a useful model for analysing why consultations go wrong. Often a doctor will flit between adult and parent state, and the patient will flit between adult and child (and parent to a lesser degree). Imagine a consultation in which both the doctor and the patient assumed the role of 'child'. I'm sure you would agree it is likely to be dysfunctional.

There are many variations on Berne's ego states. Peter Tate considered how people perceive themselves with a health belief model and identified three types of patients: the internal controller (a person in charge of their own health); the external controllers (they do not believe they are in control); and the powerful others (who do not believe they are in control, but are not fatalists either).

Stott and Davis model
Stott and Davis (1979) published a four-part model that would probably be the way many of us deal with a consultation.

Management of presenting problem	Management of continuing problem
Management of health-seeking behaviour	Opportunistic health promotion

Neighbour's model: the inner consultation
This is a popular checkpoint model. It consists of the following steps.
1 Connecting – establishing a relationship; this needs rapport-building skills.
2 Summarising – 'What I am hearing is . . .'; this needs the ability to listen, and skills to facilitate effective assessment.
3 Hand over – responsibility is given to the patient. This needs good communication skills to hand over the responsibility for management, as it involves negotiating and influencing (to a certain extent).
4 Safety netting - 'Have I missed anything?' and instructions for follow-up if

imp.

necessary. It needs predictive skills to suggest contingency plans for the worst-case scenario.
5 House keeping – 'Am I fit for the next patient?' You need to be self aware, to be able to file one consultation so there is no effect on the next.

Pendleton model *for use in CSA !*

Otherwise known as the 'social skills model', the Pendleton model has seven tasks.
1 To define the reason for the patient's attendance including:
  - the nature and history of the problems
  - their aetiology
  - the patient's ideas, concerns and expectations
  - the effects of the problem.
2 To consider other problems:
  - continuing other problems
  - at-risk factors.
3 To achieve a shared understanding of the problems with the patient.
4 To choose with the patient an appropriate action for each problem.
5 To involve the patient in the management of their case and to involve them in acceptance of appropriate responsibility for it.
6 To use time and resources appropriately.
7 To establish or maintain a relationship with the patient that helps in the achievement of other tasks.

Byrne and Long model (1979)

This is a six-point 'time-sequence model' (i.e. it is based on the observed sequence of events).
1 The doctor establishes a relationship with the patient.
2 The doctor attempts to discover the patient's reason for attendance.
3 The doctor conducts a verbal (and physical) examination.
4 The doctor (with or without the patient) considers the problems.
5 The doctor (with or without the patient) makes a further plan (e.g. investigation, treatment etc.).
6 Consultation is terminated, usually by the doctor.

Middleton agenda model

This is a four-point dynamic model where the patient's agenda is paramount. It is not task orientated.
  - Patient's agenda: this includes the ideas and reasoning that underlie the problems presented.
  - Doctor's agenda: this includes risk factors, continuing problems, public health agenda, partnerships and personal agendas.

- Communication skills: these can be chosen to reconcile the agendas (e.g. facilitation and negotiation).
- Negotiated plan: this includes management of problems and health promotion.

Triaxial model

This looks at a patient's problems in physical, psychological and social terms.

Calgary-Cambridge guide

This model (1996) can be summarised as follows.

1 Initiating the session:
   - establishing a rapport
   - identifying reasons for consultation.
2 Gathering information:
   - exploration of the problem
   - understanding the patient's perspective
   - providing structure for the consultation.
3 Building the relationship:
   - providing the correct amount and type of information
   - aiding accurate recall and understanding
   - achieving a shared understanding
   - shared decision making
   - negotiating a management plan.
4 Closing the session:
   - final summary.
5 Contracting: establish a plan or contract with the patient.
6 Safety netting: similar to Neighbour's model.
7 Final check: before moving on.

BEST

BEST: a communication model

BMJ Careers 22 July 2006

BEST is a model that is explained as improving communication within a consultation rather than for analysis of the consultation.

- Begin with non-verbal clues.
- Establish information gathering with informal talk.
- Support with emotional channels.
- Terminate with a positive note.

A fusion
Philosophy, understanding and the consultation: a fusion of horizons
Br J Gen Pract 2008; 546: 58–60

Clark explains that an understanding happens when our present understanding or horizon is moved to a new understanding or horizon by an encounter; thus the process of understanding is a 'fusion of horizons'. Doctors and patients run similar processes in a consultation: pre-understandings, openness to meaning, language and imagination. Within this is a circle of understanding with fluid movement between the whole and the part.

Critical reading

At the risk of sounding like a secondary-school teacher, I will point out that your ability to assess the quality of the work published will improve only if you practice. If you decide to take the nMRCGP®, critical appraisal will form part of the applied knowledge test (MCQs).

It is well recognised that we are clinicians, not skilled statisticians, and although it is important, for day-to-day journal reading, to have a simple critical appraisal template that you can apply to articles, it is usually not necessary to appraise articles from scratch. There are some excellent books on appraisal of research, but since the written part of the MRCGP® is no longer, this has probably less of a specific focus. I have included here some basics (from first principles) on reading a paper and statistics, which you will hopefully find of help.

READER
READER: an acronym to aid critical reading by general practitioners
Br J Gen Pract 1994; 44: 83–5.

Items to consider are the following.

R Relevance:
- to general practice
- to your environment
- general awareness.

E Education:
- behaviour modification
- challenges to practices and beliefs.

A Applicability:
- own environment
- generalisability.

D Discrimination:

- quality of the study
- type of study: descriptive/randomised controlled trial
- sample size
- selection
- controls
- bias
- results
- statistics
- conclusions.

E Evaluation: reflection.

R Reaction: implementation

Remember to always try to first be positive about a study.

Template for critical appraisal

1 Summary
   Concise statement of topic and conclusions.
2 Introduction
   Is there a clear outline?
3 Methods and design
   Are the selection and sample size appropriate?
   Strengths, limitations.
4 Results
   Is presentation clear?
   Are results both clinically and statistically significant?
5 Discussion
   Are statements true?

Keele University model

This method will help you get the important information from each section (i.e. summarise the paper). This provides the basis for evaluating it.

1 Is it of interest?
   Look at the abstract, title, authors, etc.
2 Motivation: why was it done?
   Look at the introduction; is it clear? Who funded the research?
3 Design: how was it done?
   Look at the methods: sample, recruitment, numbers, collection of data.
4 Measurements: are they valid/reliable? Analysis: what statistics were used?
   Any ethical problems, or bias?
5 Results: what did it find?
   Look at the results; is data described; do the numbers add up? Was statistical significance assessed? Were all the data used?

6 Conclusions, what are the implications?

7 Look at the discussion. Has anything been overlooked? Are the findings relevant?

8 Anything else of interest? For example, references.

Appraisal of a paper

+ Is the hypothesis clearly described?
+ Are the outcomes measured, clearly described? If these are first mentioned in the results section then the answer to this is no.
+ Are the characteristics of groups (e.g. inclusion/exclusion criteria) clearly described?
+ Are the interventions clearly described?
+ Are the main findings clearly described?
+ Does the study provide estimates of random variability in the data for the main outcomes?
  • If the data are non-normally distributed, the inter-quartile range should be quoted.
  • If the data are normally distributed, the standard error of the mean, standard deviation and confidence intervals should be used.
+ Have important adverse events been reported?
+ Have the characteristics of patients lost to follow-up been reported?
+ Have actual probability values been reported (e.g. $p = 0.04$ rather than $p < 0.05$)?

External validity
+ Were the subjects representative of the population?
+ Were the staff and facilities representative of the treatment that most patients would receive?

Internal validity, bias (think selection and information)
+ Was the study blinded?
+ Were the statistical tests used appropriate (e.g. non-parametric tests used for data that are not normally distributed)?
+ Was compliance with the intervention reliable?
+ Were the main outcome measurements to be used, reliable?

Implications of the study (the final part of appraisal of a paper)
+ What is the general importance in light of other research?
+ Can you extrapolate from the study group to general practice?
+ Is the size of the result observed important? The answer may be no, even if the results are statistically significant.
+ If you conclude that the results are important, what are their implications?

- For patients.
- For general practice:
  - i workload
  - ii financially
  - iii education
  - iv resources
  - v other members of the primary health care team.
- Wider issues: ethics, right to choice.

Qualitative research

The approach is similar to quantitative appraisal.

- Focus on methods (e.g. interview techniques and settings, source of internal bias), as well as the role of the researchers and their qualifications.
- Look at the quality control measures used (e.g. content analysis, grounded theory).
- In qualitative research the conclusions and discussions are not usually separate.

Part 4

Statistics

Statistics

Statistics is about gathering, communicating, analysing and interpreting information.

In medical statistics we tend to use *inferential statistics*, in that we draw conclusions from a sample drawn from the population.

When critiquing papers, or embarking on research or audit yourself, you need to have a fundamental understanding of the basics. Although this section is rather functional, I will attempt to put the theory in very simple terms and explain things that may otherwise be somewhat unclear. It is then a matter of reading the statistical analyses in papers to gain further understanding.

Since first writing this I have discovered Dr Chris Cates (www.nntonline.net). There have been several articles published in the press in bite size chunks.

Types of data

There are two distinct types of data.
+ Qualitative data give descriptive information.
+ Quantitative data give numerical information.

Quantitative data can be either *continuous* (e.g. 0.1 kg to 44 kg – all values within the span are possible), or they can be *discrete*, usually obtained by counting (e.g. 0, 1, 2, 3 ... – such as the number of moles on the skin, or shoe size).

Bar chart

A bar chart is a graphical representation of values/numbers.
+ The height of the column is proportional to the frequency it represents.
+ Each column should have the same width.

Pie chart/pie diagram

This is a circle divided into sectors at angles that are proportional to the frequency of the data they represent.

Measures of location

Mode

This is the MOst commonly occurring value. It assumes that the modal class is divided into the same ratio.

Time taken to critique a paper (minutes)	Number of people
0–9.9	4
10–19.9	7
20–29.9	9
30–39.9	6
40–49.9	5
50–59.9	3
60–120	9

The mode is time 20–29.9 minutes, *not* 60–120 minutes, as this modal class is longer.

There can be more than one modal class.

Median

This is the middle value of data once it has been placed in numerical order.

> e.g.   3 4 5 6 7 $\underline{7}$ 8 8 8 10 15
> The '7' that is highlighted is the median.

> e.g.   0 1 2 4 5 5 6 7
> The median is half way between 4 and 5, so is 4.5.

Mean

This generally means the average.

$$\text{mean} = \frac{\text{sum of the values}}{\text{number of values}}$$

The mean and median are a measure of symmetry, or lack of it.

In a normal (Gaussian) distribution the mode, median and mean all have the same value.

Positively skewed

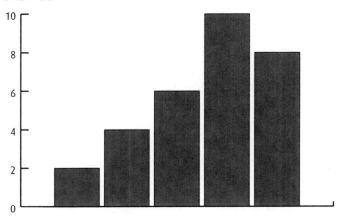

Negatively skewed

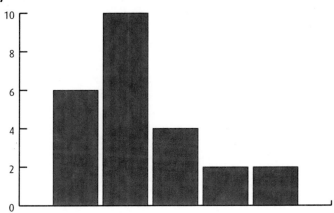

Measures of dispersion
Range
This is the difference between extremes (i.e. the largest and the smallest). It does not take into account anything about the distribution of the data.

Quartile spread
- The median is halfway through the data.
- The point halfway between the lower extreme and the median is the *lower quartile.*
- The point halfway between the median and the upper extreme is the *upper quartile.*
- The difference between the upper and lower quartile is the *interquartile range.*

Standard deviation

Whereas range and interquartile range relates to the median, standard deviation relates to the spread about the mean. The standard deviation uses all values and is therefore sensitive to outliers (i.e. extreme values).

SD = square root of the variance

$$\text{Variance} = \frac{\text{sum of the square deviations from the mean}}{n}$$

In a normal distribution:
+ 65% of values lie within 1 SD
+ 95% of values lie within 2 SD
+ 99% of values lie within 3 SD.

Probability

'Probability' indicates the degree of likelihood of an event happening, or the uncertainty of an event occurring.

$$\text{Probability of an outcome} = \frac{\text{number of events in the outcome}}{\text{total number of possible events}}$$

For example:
+ the probability of rolling a 6 when throwing a dice is $^1/_6$
+ the probability of throwing a 6 followed by another 6 is

$^1/_6 \times {}^1/_6 = {}^1/_{36}$
i.e. probability of a *and* b then *multiply*

+ the probability of throwing a 6 or a 4 is

$^1/_6 + {}^1/_6 = {}^2/_6 = {}^1/_3$
i.e. probability of a *or* b then *add.*

Errors

There are two types of error.
+ Random error: the sample mean deviates from the true mean despite the sample being representative.
+ Systematic error: the sample is not representative (i.e. there is bias).

Hypothesis test and *p*-value

This is a test of significance.
1 First step is the statement of null hypothesis, e.g. 'there is no difference

between the two groups under study'. (That is, postulate the hypothesis that the intervention will have no effect.)

2 Second step is conducting a test of statistical significance based on the null hypothesis:
   - *t*-test
   - chi-squared test.

3 Third step is the production of a *p* value from the statistical tests.

The *p* value is the probability of the result occurring by chance if the null hypothesis was true. If the *p* value is small, it is unlikely to have occurred by chance (i.e. it is a significant result). Usually $p < 0.05$ indicates a significant result. If $p < 0.01$, the result is highly significant (likely to have occurred by chance in < 1% of cases).

It is important to appraise a study before taking the *p* values as meaningful, as it may be irrelevant in the following circumstances:

- poor design of trial
- bias
- trial affected by confounding factors.

If there is a small sample size, the statistical analysis may be unable to detect a significant difference when there may be one. This is referred to as the power of the study.

Confidence intervals

Confidence intervals (CI) are another way of assessing the effects of chance (c.f. *p* value). CI is a way of communicating the level of uncertainty, and it can be calculated for various statistical analyses (e.g. odds ratios, relative risks, risk difference, sensitivity, specificity).

- There is an upper and a lower value and, assuming the study was not biased, the true value can be expected to lie between these two values.
- Most studies use 95% CI or 95% confidence limit – this is usually two standard deviations either side of the mean.
- The wider the range of the CI, the less certain/significant the results are. The more people there are in the study, the smaller the interval will be.
- If the CI range includes zero, the result is not statistically significant.
- If the results are expressed as a ratio, a CI including 1 is not statistically significant.
- The results are visual.

Risk
Measure of risk
New cases = incidence

Existing cases = prevalence

$$\text{Incidence} = \frac{\text{new illness episodes}}{\text{population at risk during a specific period of time}} \times 10^a$$

$$\text{Prevalence} = \frac{\text{no. of individuals with existing disease}}{\text{population size during specific time period}} \times 100\%$$

Measures of association

Risk is calculated by comparing what happens to different groups of people. It runs from zero to 1.

Consider a population split into two sub-populations:

- population 1 = population exposed to risk factor
- population 2 = population not exposed.

Both populations have an associated risk of disease.

$$\text{Probability of disease/death} = \text{Risk (R)} = \frac{\text{no. with the disease}}{\text{no. at risk of disease}} = \frac{d}{n}$$

$$\text{Risk difference (RD)} = \text{Risk1} - \text{Risk2} = \frac{d1}{n1} - \frac{d2}{n2}$$

$$\text{Relative risk (RR)} = \frac{R1}{R2} = \frac{\frac{d1}{n1}}{\frac{d2}{n2}} = \frac{d1 \times n2}{d2 \times n1}$$

$$\text{Absolute risk (AR)} = \frac{R1 - R2}{R2}$$

Absolute risk and relative risk are figures used to assess the strength of a relationship between a disease and any factor that might affect it. Relative risk is relatively meaningless. Absolute risk is more important to understand, so we can impart meaningful information to our patients.

Absolute risk

$$\text{Absolute risk} = \frac{\text{the number of events that occur in the (treated or control) group}}{\text{number of people in that group}}$$

The absolute risk reduction (ARR) is the difference between the control group and the treated group: ARR = ARC − ART.

Relative risk

Relative risk (or risk ratio) in randomised controlled trials and cohort studies, or relative odds in cohort or case controlled studies, is the ratio of the absolute risks of the disease between the two groups.

◆ RR < 1, then intervention reduces the risk of the outcome being studied.
◆ RR = 1, then the treatment has no effect on the outcome being studied.
◆ RR > 1, then the intervention increases the risk of the outcome being studied.

Odds

i.e. ratio of people who have pos. to people who do not. Ratio of number of people when people.

Odds are a way of representing probability in a different way to risk. They are defined as the ratio of the probability of an event happening to that of it not happening (i.e. risk). Values run from zero to infinity.

used in case-control studies

Odds ratio (OR)

This is a measure of the effectiveness of a treatment; an estimate of relative risk.

$$OR = \frac{\text{ODDs in the treated group}}{\text{ODDs in the control group}}$$

◆ OR < 1, effects of the treatment are less than those of the control treatment.
◆ OR = 1, effects of the treatment are no different from the control treatment.
◆ OR > 1, effects of the treatment are greater than the control treatment.
   The effects can be good or bad.

Diagnostic testing

	Disease +ve	Disease −ve	Total
Test +ve	a	b	a + b
Test −ve	c	d	c + d
Total	a + c	b + d	a + b + c + d

$$\text{Sensitivity} = \frac{\text{no. test positive and disease positive}}{\text{no. disease positive}} = \frac{a}{a + c}$$

$$\text{Specificity} = \frac{\text{no. test negative and disease negative}}{\text{no. disease negative}} = \frac{d}{b + d}$$

Positive predictive value is the probability that an
individual diagnosed test positive will be true positive $= \dfrac{a}{a + b}$

Negative predictive value is the probability that an
individual diagnosed test negative will be a true negative $= \dfrac{d}{c + d}$

Number needed to treat (NNT)

This is the number of people you would need to treat with a specific intervention (e.g. aspirin for people having a heart attack) to see one occurrence of a specific outcome (e.g. prevention of death).

$$NNT = \dfrac{1}{\text{absolute risk reduction}}$$

This value can be multiplied by 100 if using a percentage.

So, the smaller the ARR, the higher the NNT

Cates' website (www.nntonline.net) allows you to produce a visual representation of NNT if you have basic statistical information.

The number needed to screen - an adaptation of the number needed to treat
Journal of Medical Screening 2001; 8: 114-15.

This paper suggests that estimates of NNT should carry a health warning. The concept of preventing one event should be compared with the more likely probability that several people will benefit by having an event delayed by a few years. For example, an antihypertensive drug that reduces the incidence of stroke by 30% can be interpreted in two ways: the drug prevented 30% of strokes (with no effect on the other 70%); or that all strokes in the treatment group were delayed by three years.

Other statistical terms
Bias
This is the deviation of the results from the truth, a one sided inclination of the mind.
- *Publication bias* is seen where studies with positive results are more likely to be published.
- *Selection bias* is where there are systematic differences between sample and target populations.
- *Information bias* is where there are systematic errors in measurement of outcome or exposure.

Hazard ratio

Hazard ratio is the statistical term used to describe the relative risk of complication due to treatment, based on a comparison of event rates.

Heterogeneity

This term is used when there is no overlap of the trials used in a meta-analysis.

Homogeneity 'similarity'

This term is used to state that all trials on the plot have an overlap of confidence intervals (i.e. in a meta-analysis).

Meta-analysis

This is a statistical method for looking at a number of original research papers in an attempt to answer a question by combining results of several studies. The methodology of the search (e.g. not confined to English; using more than one search engine; including unpublished trials) is a good indicator as to the validity of the results.

Validity

This refers to how rigorous a study is.

◆ *Study validity* is the validity with respect to internal and external bias.
◆ *Internal validity* is the degree to which conclusions internal to the study are legitimate.
◆ *External validity* is the degree to which conclusions generated from the sample could be generalised to the target population.

Study designs

Experimental

These consist of *randomised controlled trials* – a minimum of two groups, to which patient allocation is random. One of the groups is the control (i.e. non-experimental group).

Observational

◆ Cross sectional survey:
  • sample frame is observed at one particular time
  • gives prevalence estimates
  • cause and effect are difficult to establish.
◆ Cohort study:
  • longitudinal follow up of two or more cohorts (groups) with recorded exposure to a risk factor
  • provides comparative incidence estimates between exposed groups and non-exposed

- there can be surveillance bias.
- Case controlled study:
  - used to compare two groups when prevalence is low
  - ODDs ratios are used for analysis.

Forest plot

This is a pictorial representation of ODDs ratios in the form of horizontal lines. They represent the 95% CI of each trial, with a vertical line representing the point where the study intervention would have no effect (if the horizontal line crosses the vertical line, the result is not significant).

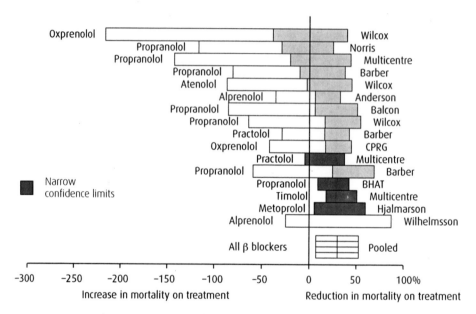

FIGURE 4.3 Forest plots: trying to see the wood and the trees. *BMJ.* 2001; 322: 1479–80.

Funnel plot

This is a graph where each study is represented by a dot, the position of which depends on the size of the effect of the intervention (on the horizontal axis) and the study size (on the vertical axis).

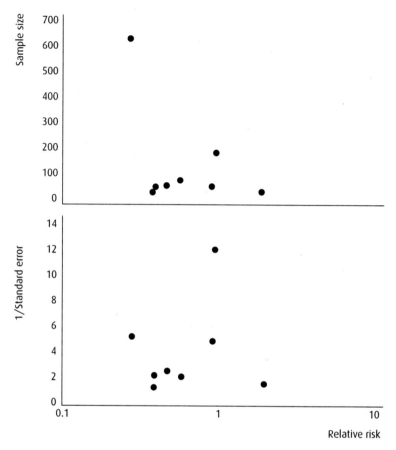

FIGURE 4.4 Effect of measure of precision (plotted on y axis) on appearance of funnel plots. The case of the misleading funnel plot. *BMJ*. 2006; 333: 597–600.

Part 5

Practice for the nMRCGP®

Practice for the nMRCGP®

The final part of this book is all about the final hurdle – the exam. The new MRCGP® exam tests an incredible range of knowledge, clinical and communication skills as well as professional attitudes (a key point to remember is that despite your personal feelings and beliefs, you are taking this exam in a professional capacity).

It is important to read and understand the current regulations for each module at the time of application (www.rcgp.org.uk). There is a curriculum published on the website (www.rcgp-curriculum.org.uk) that ought to be considered essential reading and that can be used as a checklist. It is described as a guide – it by no means includes everything.

The Postgraduate Medical Education and Training Board (PMETB) agreed that the Royal College exam should be the only route possible to allow entry into general practice. You know that you are fully fledged when you receive your Certificate of Completion of Training (CCT). The alternative to the nMRCGP® is the Interim Membership by Assessment of Performance (iMAP), which is a portfolio-based assessment.

The current nMRCGP® consists of the following.

The exam
- Applied Knowledge Test (AKT) – the three-hour multichoice test.
- Clinical Skills Assessment (CSA) – the thirteen station OSCE.
- Workplace-based Assessment (WBA):
  - Case-based Discussions (CbD)
  - Consultation Observation Tool in primary care/mini Clinical-Examination (COT/mini CEX) – either video or joint surgery
  - Multi-source feedback (MSF) – from the team.

Other tools
- Patient Satisfaction Questionnaire (PSQ)
- Eportfolio – you have to register with the college to get this started.

The nMRCGP® describes 12 competency areas:
- communication and consultation skills
- practising holistically
- data gathering and interpretation
- making a diagnosis/making decisions
- clinical management
- managing medical complexity and promoting health
- primary care administration and IMT

+ working with colleagues and in teams
+ community orientation
+ maintaining performance, learning and teaching
+ maintaining an ethical approach to practice
+ fitness to practice.

When you are working for the exams I would encourage you to consider topics in isolation (either individually, in a study group – this might help you focus to get the work done and would be a good forum for discussions – or with work colleagues), before thinking about doing exam papers. As you come towards sitting the exam try working the sample papers (against the clock is a must for at least one of the papers). The core curriculum is there as a solid guide and is a useful checklist of most issues you will come across in general practice. It can be downloaded from www.rcgp.org.uk. Get involved in your training practice and take on the tricky cases. There really is nothing to beat experience at ground level for helping you to learn and remember, even when it doesn't go according to plan!

Applied Knowledge Test (AKT)

www.rcgp-curriculum.org.uk/nmrgcp/akt.aspx
This is a three-hour, computer-based multiple-choice examination where around 80% of questions will be on clinical medicine, 10% on critical appraisal and evidence-based medicine and a further 10% on health informatics and administration (with a total of around 200 questions). It is important to read the college information as this information may change. The sample paper provided on the website gives you a stem for which you have to select the single best answer; extended matching questions; flow charts; and picture spots to identify.

   You can view the exam format at www.pearsonvue.com/rcgp/.

   The questions below are a mix of these aspects, as well as true/false questions (testing you on every step rather than just the process of elimination). Although they have not been validated to the extent that the Royal College would validate its questions, they are factually correct at the time of printing.

   When you are revising, remember that ENT, ophthalmology, dermatology and other specialties will feature in the exam.

   For AKT (MCQ) exams, it is important to know how to interpret certain phrases. The following definitions are from the college guidelines, but you will find almost identical definitions in most MCQ books.

+ *Diagnostic, characteristic, pathognomonic and in the vast majority* – implies that the feature would occur in 90% of cases.

- *Typically, frequently, significantly, commonly and in a substantial majority* – implies that the feature would occur in 60% of cases, or more.
- *In the majority* – implies that the feature would occur in 50% of cases, or more.
- *In the minority* – implies that the feature would occur in less than 50% of cases.
- *Low chance and in a substantial minority* – implies that a feature may occur in up to 30% of cases.
- *Has been shown, recognised and reported* – all refer to evidence found in authoritative medical texts.

It is good practice both here and with other AKT books to set aside a time period to simulate the exam (I estimate that these questions should take around one hour) as your concentration may be quite different when doing a paper this way as compared to dipping in and out. Whatever approach you decide to take, practice as many questions as you can (not forgetting the sample questions on the Royal College site and the GP papers).

Practice questions

Unless otherwise stated answer True or False for each of the following.

1 There are various treatment options in cognitive impairment and associated behavioural changes. Which of the following statements would be appropriate management decisions?

   a Antipsychotic medication is useful for behavioural changes in dementia with lewy bodies (DLB).

   b Acetylcholinesterase inhibitors (such as donepezil) should be considered for treatment of moderately severe Alzheimer's disease (MMSE score 10–20).

   c Following the initiation of acetylcholinesterase inhibitors patients should have their response assessed by their GP after six months.

   d After assessing a patient with dementia who has developed agitation but is not delirious, alternatives to pharmacological management would include aromatherapy, animal-assisted therapy, and multi-sensory stimulation.

   e Alzheimer's disease is associated with an increased risk of cardiovascular disease and modifiable risk factors should be addressed.

2 In assessing a patient's degree of cognitive impairment and competence consider the following statements.

   a If a patient lacks competence you should automatically discuss his/her condition with the next-of-kin.

   b Whatever his/her degree of understanding, your patient has the right to expect the medical information to be held in confidence.

   c Disclosure without consent is justified if failure to do so may expose the patient or others to serious harm.

    d No one can give or withhold consent to treatment on behalf of a mentally incapacitated patient.

    e If an unwise decision is made this should be viewed as lack of capacity.

    f A person can appoint a Lasting Power of Attorney to act on their behalf if they should lose capacity in the future.

3 Parkinson's disease (PD) guidelines were published by NICE in June 2006. Pharmacological intervention and manipulation of symptoms can be tackled in various ways. Consider the questions below.

    a When using Levodopa for tremor in early PD it is wise to use the lowest possible dose to control symptoms.

    b When starting treatment it is not necessary to use adjuvant therapy with Levodopa.

    c Hypersexuality and pathological gambling are recognised as an uncommon disorder known as dopamine dysregulation syndrome.

    d If a patient is getting side effects there is no significant risk to withdrawing treatment.

    e If a patient is struggling to control late symptoms in PD, oral apomorphine may help, although its use would be directed by specialist units.

4 Testamentary capacity is dependent on a number of factors that in our role as General Practitioners we are often called upon to confirm given that an increasing number of wills are contested after a testator's death.

    a If a person is suffering from delusions they are automatically considered incapable of testamentary capacity.

    b A testator must be able to understand both the effect of making a will and the extent of his or her estate.

    c The 'golden rule' should always be observed no matter how straightforward matters may appear.

    d It is important for a medical practitioner to review all wills where a person has made serial wills over the last years of their life.

    e Answers should be recorded verbatim in the medical records when assessing testamentary capacity.

5 In the prescribing of antidepressants:

    a Features that characterise serotonin syndrome include: confusion, delirium, shivering, sweating, myoclonus and changes in blood pressure.

    b It is acceptable to use venlafaxine as a first line antidepressant.

    c Sertraline would be the drug of choice when starting treatment following a myocardial infarction.

    d A QT interval of 0.44 seconds would be reassuring when starting a tricyclic or venlafaxine.

    e With the exception of fluoxetine 20 mg daily, it is unwise to stop antidepressants abruptly if a patient has been taking them for six weeks or longer.

6 The following could be considered safe antipyretic interventions in a feverish child.
   a Having a cold bath.
   b Antipyretic drugs such as paracetamol or ibuprofen.
   c Tepid sponging.
   d Keeping a child well wrapped up to sweat out the fever.
   e Keeping the child completely stripped off.
7 Consider the following statements on potential unwanted outcomes experienced by women using treatments for heavy menstrual bleeding and match them to the appropriate stem. (Common 1 in 100 chance, less common 1 in 1000, rare 1 in 10 000, very rare 1 in 100 000)
    i Common problems would include irregular bleeding over 6 months.
   ii Rare problem of indigestion and peptic ulceration. Worsening of asthma may be seen in some women.
  iii Mood changes, headaches and breast tenderness are common side-effects. Deep vein thrombosis and heart attack are seen rarely.
   iv A less common effect seen is loss of bone mineral density.
    v Common effects would be menopausal-like symptoms such as flushing and vaginal dryness.
   a Combined oral contraceptive pills.
   b Levonorgestrel-releasing intrauterine system.
   c Gonadotrophin-releasing hormone analogue.
   d Injected progestogen.
   e Non-steroidal anti-inflammatories.
8 Eclampsia and pre-eclampsia can occur in 2–8% of pregnancies. Consider the information below.
   a The diagnosis of these conditions is antenatal rather than postnatal.
   b It is unsafe for syntometrine to be used for the active management of the third stage of labour.
   c Foetal growth restriction is a recognised finding that often pre-dates pre-eclampsia.
   d Patients should be started on antihypertensives, preferably an ACE inhibitor or diuretic, if the systolic blood pressure is over 160 mmHg.
   e Of the 18 women who died in 2003–5 with eclampsia, a significant number of deaths were linked to major substandard care.
   f Magnesium sulphate reduces the risk of an eclamptic seizure by 87%.
9 Staging of prostate cancer helps categorise the disease to allow individualised discussions on treatment, as there is no clear consensus on optimum management at different stages. Consider the following statements.
   a A Gleason score is extrapolated from a biopsy and looks at glandular differentiation, relationship of glands to stroma and differentiation (Grade 1 = well differentiated; 5 = poorly differentiated).

   b In localised disease, high risk would be classified as Gleason grade 8 or more.

   c In advanced metastatic disease from prostate cancer, radical prostatectomy would be an effective first line treatment.

   d Low-dose rate (LDR) brachytherapy is as effective as external beam radiotherapy for patients with localised disease.

   e Active surveillance with yearly PSA testing may be suitable for some men with low-risk localised disease.

10 Consider the following statements on treatment of erectile dysfunction with phosphodiesterase type 5 (PDE) inhibitors.

   a Only 19% of men take PDE inhibitors correctly.

   b Sildenafil and vardenafil should be taken with food.

   c Starting dose for sildenafil is 25 mg.

   d Alpha-blocker doxazosin is known to have a synergistic effect with sildenafil.

   e The effects of tadalafil last for up to 36 hours.

11 Consider the following ophthalmological problems and choose the most appropriate answer for the stems below. Each answer can occur once, more than once or not at all.

   i Pingueculum

   ii Scleritis

   iii Dendritic ulcer

   iv Blepharitis

   v Pterygium

   vi Conjunctivitis

   a Would be seen as wing shaped fibrovascular tissue arising from the conjunctiva and extending onto the cornea.

   b The lid margin is seen to have scaling and some crusting, there may be some thickening of the eye lid.

   c Prominent features include severe pain and exquisite tenderness on palpation of the globe of the eye.

   d Is seen with acne rosacea and seborrhoeic dermatitis.

   e Would present as a painful, red, photophobic eye, often associated with herpes simplex (type 1).

12 Obesity is an ever increasing public health concern. Consider the following stems, as applied to adults, when answering the questions below. Each stem may be used once, more than once or not at all.

   i Healthy weight

   ii Overweight

   iii Obesity I

   iv Obesity II

   v Obesity III

vi Waist circumference 94–102 cm

vii Waist circumference more than 102 cm

viii Waist circumference 80–88 cm

ix Waist circumference more than 88 cm

a Which would be representative of a BMI 30–34.9?

b For a male classified as Obesity I what waist circumference would equate to a high risk?

c Using the classification for obesity, what would be the advised earliest point at which you could start drug treatment in a patient with hypertension?

d For a female classified as overweight what waist circumference would equate to increased risk?

e In a patient with no co-morbidities, at what level (assuming other measures have been unsuccessful) would you consider a surgical opinion?

13 Based on current guidelines, which of the following would be considered appropriate in the management of a chronic obstructive airways disease patient who smoked and has mild persistent symptoms such as breathlessness and sputum production?

a Short acting bronchodilator.

b Forced Expiratory Volume (FEV1) every three years to assess progression.

c Low-dose inhaled corticosteroids to reduce exacerbations.

d The need for pulmonary rehabilitation.

e Smoking cessation advice.

14 Considering long term oxygen therapy:

a Therapy reduces secondary polycythaemia.

b Arterial blood gas measurements should be made as soon as possible following the identification of hypoxaemia.

c It is important that patients use only the amount of oxygen they feel they need.

d Blood gas measurements should be made on at least two occasions, three weeks apart.

e If a patient has end stage COPD and is using LTOT it is acceptable for her/him to continue smoking as long as the oxygen is turned off whilst smoking.

15 Consider the following scenarios and the requirement/current advice for BCG vaccination for tuberculosis (TB). Answer True if they should be vaccinated; False if they should not be vaccinated.

a Contacts of TB who have no evidence of vaccination and are Mantoux negative.

b New entrants to the UK with no evidence of previous vaccination, who are younger than 65 years of age.

c A booster vaccination for healthcare workers working with people with active TB, where their original vaccination was more than 20 years previous.

d All school children (unless contra-indicated) at the age of 14 years.

e Rural police officers clearing road kill such as badgers.

16 Considering chronic kidney disease (CKD):

a Patients with an estimated glomerular filtration rate of 52 should be referred for a renal assessment.

b A CKD 4 patient with a haemoglobin of 10.5 g/dL and ferritin of 110 mcg/L would not benefit from iron supplementation.

c Other pathologies than CKD should be considered in all patients as a cause for anaemia.

d Iron deficiency anaemia is diagnosed with a ferritin of less than 100 mcg/L in CKD 5.

e Erythropoietin management is a secondary-care specialty and should not be prescribed in primary care.

17 The risk of colorectal cancer can be reduced in many ways. From the options below select those answers where there is known evidence of a reduction in mortality.

a Hormone replacement therapy for the menopause.

b Aspirin 75 mg daily.

c Screening using faecal occult bloods.

d Screening using flexible sigmoidoscopy.

e Proton pump inhibitors.

18 Which of the following statements are correct concerning Barrett's Oesophagus?

a 65% of people affected with this condition are male.

b The main symptom at presentation is dysphagia.

c A known risk factor for developing Barrett's oesophagus is cigarette use of more than 10 a day.

d Regular endoscopy surveillance is recommended after diagnosis.

e Treatment of Barrett's oesophagus should include a proton pump inhibitor for life.

19 Consider the following statements in relation to ischaemic stroke.

a Each year there are 249 000 new cases of stroke diagnosed in England and Wales.

b Following a stroke, 23% of people die within 30 days.

c Following a stroke, 60% of people are alive after three years.

d It is recommended that patients should take modified-release dipyridamole (200 mg) and aspirin (if tolerated) as a life-long treatment.

e Clopidogrel is contraindicated in patients who have had an anaphylactic reaction to aspirin.

20 Although behavioural therapies are important in smoking cessation, pharmacological therapies are also used first line. Consider the following statements and match them to the options below.

  a This nicotine receptor partial agonist has been developed from a laburnum seed extract.

  b Although effective for smoking cessation it is not licensed for this use.

  c Is known to lower seizure thresholds and should not be prescribed with antidepressants.

  d May cause hypoglycaemia, so should be avoided in diabetics.

  e Would be the best choice in pregnant women.

  f Extending the use may be effective at preventing relapse.

    i Varenicline

    ii Nicotine replacement therapy

    iii Buprenorphine

    iv Nortriptyline

21 The effect of smoking has many permutations. The following statements are either true or false.

  a 80% of long-term smokers will die of smoking related diseases.

  b Smokers are twice as likely to suffer fatal heart attacks as non-smokers.

  c In a practice of 9000 patients routine brief advice may result in an extra 50 patients giving up in a year.

  d Nicotine patches have been shown to achieve a better quit rate than gum.

  e Motivational interviewing achieves results by promoting changes in addictive behaviour.

22 Select the most appropriate choice of antihypertensive from the options below for each scenario in a hypertensive patient.

    i Candesartan

    ii Felodipine

    iii Doxazosin

    iv Atenolol

    v Ramipril

    vi Bendrofluazide

  a A 58-year-old Caucasian male patient.

  b A 52-year-old Black female with a blood pressure of 162/94 mmHg.

  c A 64-year-old female with newly diagnosed angina and hypertension.

  d A 72-year-old patient on amlodipine with inadequately controlled blood pressure.

  e A 45-year-old diabetic patient with blood pressure 146/92 mmHg.

  f A 50-year-old patient with hypertension, intolerant of perindopril.

23 The following are known terminologies or side effects from cocaine drug use.

  a Smoking 'free base' cocaine or crack is associated with gum disease.

  b Long term use is known to cause dehydration.

    c Injecting cocaine can increase the risk of endocarditis.

    d Anorexia.

    e 'Speedballing' is when amphetamines and crack are used together.

24 Consider the following points regarding red-flag symptoms in primary care.

    a Macroscopic painless haematuria has a positive predictive value (PPV) of 3.4% for cancer in men.

    b The PPV of haemoptysis in men is 7.5%, lower than expected because it is frequently associated with chest infection.

    c Dysphagia is a recognised alarm symptom associated with Barrett's oesophagus.

    d Rectal bleeding in a patient over 45 years of age with haemorrhoids should always be investigated.

    e Data from the GP Research database has shown that new onset of alarm features such as haematuria, haemoptysis, dysphagia or rectal bleeding in men over 65 years of age is associated with an increased risk of cancer.

25 The following are correct procedural elements of the UK Resuscitation Council guidelines.

    a On finding a patient in an out-of-hospital cardiac arrest immediately perform two rescue breaths.

    b Current compression:ventilation ratio is 20:2 for adults.

    c After assessment, initial management would be 30 chest compressions.

    d In securing the airway it is important to remove any debris, including false teeth.

    e If you are in doubt whether the person is breathing normally after 10 seconds, take some time to assess for a further 10 seconds.

26 Regarding the NHS colorectal screening programme:

    a All patients aged 45–70 years will be invited to take part.

    b It will be a three-yearly rolling repeat of the test.

    c The stool will be tested for a CEA antigen.

    d It is estimated that four people in 100 will have an uncertain result needing a repeat test.

    e Of patients needing colonoscopy, one in 10 will be found to have a cancer.

27 Consider the following statements relating to coeliac disease.

    a Anaemia, depression and diarrhoea are known to be linked with a coeliac disease diagnosis.

    b It is common in that there is a 1% prevalence of the disease.

    c Antibody serology has now become the gold standard test.

    d There is a 15% increased risk of malignancy if left untreated.

    e Because coeliac patients are known to have a degree of splenic atrophy, it is wise that they receive penicillin prophylaxis for invasive procedures.

28 Concerning febrile convulsions:
   a Febrile convulsions are seen in 1–3% of children aged 0–8 years.
   b The fever is usually at least 40 degrees centigrade.
   c 60% of children will have recurrent febrile convulsions.
   d There is a 1% increased chance of developing epilepsy after a febrile convulsion.
   e It is important to rapidly reduce the temperature to gain control of the seizure.

29 Consider steps 1 to 5 of the British Thoracic Society Guidelines for Children aged 5 to 12 years and select the correct response from the options below.
   i Inhaled sodium cromoglycate
   ii Inhaled beta agonist
   iii Leukotriene receptor antagonist
   iv Referral to paediatrician
   v Inhaled steroid 400 mcg/day
   vi Inhaled steroid 800 mcg/day
   vii Inhaled steroid 1000 mcg/day

30 The following are known causes of cough in children.
   a Pertussis.
   b Atrial septal defect.
   c Laryngomalacia.
   d Norwalk virus.
   e Cystic fibrosis.

31 Eczema in children and adults can be successfully treated to reduce symptoms. Consider the following options.
   a Atopic eczema is the same as atopic dermatitis.
   b By the age of 12 years there is a lifetime prevalence of 23%.
   c Using steroid cream under occlusion is contraindicated because of the risk of steroidal side effects.
   d Patch testing is important to determine whether there is an allergic component to creams and perfumes if a child is not responding to hydrocortisone and emolient treatments.
   e Eczema herpeticum is where zoster infects an area of eczema giving rise to systemic symptoms.

32 Acne is a chronic skin condition affecting 80% of adolescents at some point. Apply and consider the following statements.
   a Three in 10 teenagers have acne that needs to be treated.
   b In deciding on appropriate treatment it is important to assess the psychological impact of the condition.
   c Benzoyl peroxide use may reduce antibiotic resistance.
   d Dianette, the licensed oral contraceptive, is useful when treating females with acne.

    e It is acceptable to use Roaccutane in primary care so long as the patient understands the risks of pregnancy and possible side effects.

33 The following are recognised as alternative names for rubella.
    a Epidemic roseola.
    b German measles.
    c Infectious rubellosis.
    d Liberty measles.
    e Erythema infectiosum.
    f Three day measles.

34 The following would be appropriate treatments for the conditions stated.
    a Erythromycin for pertussus.
    b Co-trimoxazole for anthrax.
    c Immunoglobulin for post-exposure prophylaxis of rubella in non-immune pregnant women.
    d Rifampicin for post-exposure prophylaxis of suspected meningococcal meningitis.

35 The following are requirements when a person dies of Hepatitis C.
    a By law the GP must inform undertakers.
    b The body must remain in a sealed body bag in the coffin.
    c You must complete a notification-of-disease form for the CDSC (Communicable Disease Surveillance Centre).
    d Body bags should be labelled *biohazard* with tape or tags.
    e All bodies must be cremated (burial is not permissible by law).
    f Coffins must be hermetically sealed, e.g. lid soldered shut.

36 The following are differential diagnoses of gynaecomastia (breast tissue growth in males).
    a Chronic liver disease.
    b Puberty.
    c Treatment with frusemide.
    d Zoladex treatment for prostate cancer.

37 The following are known risk factors for osteoporosis.
    a Maternal vertebral fracture at the age of 62 following a fall down stairs.
    b A bilateral salpingo-oophorectomy at the age of 42.
    c Coeliac disease.
    d Hypothyroidism.
    e Ulcerative colitis.

38 The questions below relate to shingles (*Herpes zoster*) infection.
    a *Herpes zoster* typically affects a single dermatome, crossing the midline.
    b Antivirals are effective only if started within 24 hours of the appearance of the blisters.
    c Classically there is a prodrome of pain and paraesthesia before the appearance of the rash.

d Use of steroids early in treatment is known to reduce post-herpetic neuralgia.

e Tricyclic antidepressants are useful only for the chronic pain of post-herpetic neuralgia.

39 Haemochromatosis can be either secondary or genetic. Consider the following points.

a Venesection as a form of treatment is used only when the patient is symptomatic.

b It is a known cause of diabetes.

c If undergoing venesection it is sensible to take an iron supplement to guard against inadvertent iron deficiency.

d In haemoglobinopathies such as β-thalassaemia intestinal absorption of iron may lead to a secondary haemochromatosis.

e Hook osteophytes are a known association.

40 Paget's disease is a condition of increased bone turnover causing pain.

a The risk in the UK is rare under the age of 40 years with an overall prevalence estimated at 5%.

b Bone biopsies are essential in correctly diagnosing Paget's disease.

c Classical problems include tibial bowing and spontaneous fractures.

d Raised calcium and alkaline phosphatase are usually seen.

e There is an increased risk of developing osteosarcomas in Paget's.

41 Consider the options below and match to the most appropriate answer. Each answer can appear once, more than once or not at all.

   i Melanoma

  ii Squamous cell carcinoma

 iii Actinic keratosis

  iv Bowen's disease

   v Basal cell carcinoma

a This would be an important differential to a cutaneous horn.

b This would be seen mainly on the lower leg of women.

c A person with a large number of benign melanocytic naevi would be at increased risk of developing this.

d Usually a slow growing, locally destructive tumour.

e May respond well to diclofenac sodium gel.

42 In relation to statistical analyses of significance:

a The 'null hypothesis' is the test proving there is no difference between two groups.

b The p value is a measure of significance generated from tests such as t-test.

c p values are unaffected by trial design.

d A confidence interval of 97% is based on results that are two standard deviations from the mean.

    e A confidence interval expressed as a ratio that includes zero, is
       statistically significant.

43 Choose the correct answer from the list of options below.

	Screening test positive	Screening test negative
Problem present	29	42
Problem absent	64	364

   i 29/93
   ii 29/71
  iii 42/71
  iv 42/406
   v 64/93
  vi 64/428
  vii 364/406
 viii 364/428
  ix 29
   x 42
  xi 64
  xii 364

Choose the most appropriate answer:
a Positive predictive value
b Negative predictive value
c Specificity
d Sensitivity
e False negative

44 In the diagnosis of altered bowel habit select the most likely cause of the
   problem from the list of options below.
     i Carcinoma of the colon
    ii Irritable bowel syndrome
   iii Campylobacter enteritis
   iv Giardiasis
    v Crohn's disease
   vi Ischaemic colitis
  vii Pseudomembranous colitis
 viii Laxative abuse
   ix Chronic pancreatitis
   a An 18-year-old girl has been amenorrhoeic for six months, has lost
     a lot of weight and has developed loose stools, going at least four times
     a day.
   b A 28-year-old female patient has recently been made redundant. She has

started with episodic diarrhoea with small volume stools and a feeling of incomplete defaecation. There is abdominal pain and bloating.

c A 22-year-old student has returned from Russia with episodic loose stool and passing offensive wind.

d A 48-year-old man with a family history of polyposis coli defaulted from the surveillance programme some years ago. Over the last three months he has developed altered bowel habit and has lost a little weight. There has been one episode of rectal bleeding.

e A 36-year-old business man has completed a two-week course of cephalexin. He has now developed a fever, diarrhoea and cramping abdominal pains.

45 For each of the questions choose the most appropriate answer from the list of options below.

   i No precautions needed
  ii 7
 iii 14
 iv 5
  v 19
 vi 21
vii 3

a A patient needing post-coital contraception has presented too late for Levonelle-2. If she has a regular 28-day cycle, up to what day is it acceptable to use an IUD?

b Cerazette (a progestogen-only contraceptive) is started on day 1 of your patient's period. How many days should you advise that she use additional contraception?

c A patient is four hours late taking her Loestrin-20 contraceptive pill. How many days are extra precautions required?

d Your patient is changing from a combined contraceptive pill to Noriday, without a break between pill packs. How many days are extra precautions required?

e Your patient is breast-feeding and needs contraception. How many days post partum can the POP Femulen be started?

f If your post partum lady wanted to start Micronor (her usual POP), from when can this be started?

g Within how many days (after unprotected sexual intercourse) should Levonelle-2 be taken to be effective as post-coital contraception?

h A patient calls having missed two of her Microgynon pills (day 10 and 11 in her pill pack). How many days does she need to use extra precautions for?

46 The conditions listed below are known causes of jaundice.

a Gilbert's disease.

    b Beta-thalassaemia.

    c Carbimazole.

    d Thyrotoxicosis.

    e A bilirubin of 30 mmol/L.

47 A 42-year-old schoolteacher with known haemochromatosis and associated arthritis develops an intermittent dilated left pupil with a weakness and intermittent patchy paraesthesia affecting her limbs. Which of the following below is the most likely diagnosis (select only one)?

    a Diabetes.

    b Myasthenia gravis.

    c Horner's syndrome.

    d Multiple sclerosis.

    e Holmes-Adie pupil.

For questions 48–50 below select the most appropriate answer from the list.

    a Med 3

    b Med 4

    c Med 5

    d Med 6

    e RM 7

    f Self certificate

48 This can be issued if a patient has been in hospital for a knee arthroscopy for three days and comes to see you one week post discharge requesting a note to cover that time.

49 This can be used to cover the period of absence from work for a patient who has taken four days off for gastroenteritis.

50 A patient requesting a note because of diarrhoea and vomiting (having been off for one week and not having previously seen a doctor) to be backdated to the day before the appointment for a further week as they are still convalescing.

51 A 78-year-old lady being treated on the medication below develops swollen ankles and, since the swelling started, itching over her lower limbs. Which of the medications is the most likely culprit?

    a Aspirin E/C.

    b Simvastatin.

    c Ramipril.

    d Felodipine.

    e Bendrofluazide.

52 A four-year-old child weighing 20 kg is having an acute exacerbation of asthma (viral trigger); pulse is 110/minute and respiratory rate 36/minute. There are no life threatening features. Which prednisolone regime below would be the most appropriate?

a 40 mg for 5 days
b 10 mg for 3 days
c 10 mg for 5 days
d 20 mg for 3 days
e 20 mg for 5 days

For questions 53–55 select the most likely diagnoses. Each answer can apply once, more than once or not at all.
a Testicular tumour
b Testicular torsion
c Varicocoele
d Epididymitis
e Epididymal cyst

53 A painful scrotum with swelling and positive Prehn's sign.
54 A 10-year-old boy with a painful, swollen scrotum.
55 A 24-year-old man with a painless lump that transilluminates with a pen torch.
56 The following problems are seen with HIV infection. (True/False)
a Pneumocystis carinii.
b Persistent lymphadenopathy.
c Pityriasis versicolor.
d Seborrhoeic dermatitis.
e Diarrhoea.
57 Consider the following statements regarding tuberculosis in the UK. (True/False)
a The recent increase in TB is due to improved air travel and foreign holidays in third-world countries.
b The Mantoux test is diagnostic of TB.
c 14-year-olds are routinely offered the BCG vaccination (earlier if at risk).
d Only pulmonary TB is highly contagious.
e With supervising the taking of medication, drug resistance in TB is much less of a problem.
58 Effective teamwork requires the following. (True/False)
a Information systems.
b Professional divisions.
c A blame culture to get to the bottom of problems and understand shortcomings.
d Goals and objectives.
e Appropriate leadership.

For questions 59 and 60 consider which would be the most appropriate measure.

  a Case fatality
  b Prevalence
  c Incidence
  d Mortality
  e Median survival
59 A measure of the number of new cases of TB within one year in the UK.
60 The number of patients in your practice with CHD who died within six months of stopping clopidogrel.

Applied Knowledge Test (AKT) answers

1 This is a question structured around treatment options from the NICE/SCIE Dementia guidelines 2006.
  a F Antipsychotics can cause severe adverse reactions in DLB.
  b T
  c F This should be assessed by the specialist clinic at 2–4 months.
  d T These could be delivered by either health or social care staff, or family.
  e T Such as smoking, alcohol excess, obesity, hypertension and hyperlipidaemia.
2 This question covers the Mental Health Act 2005 as well as consent issues.
  a F See the GMC and NICE guidelines on consent issues.
  b T Even after death.
  c T
  d T Even if that person has Lasting Power of Attorney, consent is valid only if it is informed, competent, uncoerced and continuing.
  e F
  f T A Lasting Power of Attorney is also able to make decisions on health and welfare.
3 Review of Parkinson's is necessary as it can crop up in many guises in the nMRCGP®.
  a T Starting treatment early used to be avoided; new theories are that it may slow progression.
  b F It is recommended as adjuvant therapy reduces off-periods.
  c T This also includes stereotypic motor acts and is difficult to manage.
  d F They may suffer with acute akinesia or neuroleptic malignant syndrome.
  e F Apomorphine would only be useful as subcutaneous injection because of first pass metabolism if taken orally.
4 Regarding testamentary capacity
  a F Only if the delusion influences the testator in making a particular decision.
  b T

   c T This is where a will is witnessed by a medical practitioner, having satisfied himself of the capacity and understanding of the testator.

   d T Time consuming though this may be, it may reveal impairment of memory, judgement and even delusions.

   e T

5 a T This may be seen when combining two serotonergic antidepressants.

   b F This is known to have more side effects and be more difficult to discontinue.

   c T It has the most evidence for safe use in this situation.

   d F In adults this is normally 0.33–0.44 seconds; anything longer increases the risk of arrhythmia, especially with use of this medication.

   e T As there is increased likelihood of withdrawal symptoms and cardiac arrhythmias with tricyclics. Fluoxetine is less likely to be a problem due to the long half-life.

6 This question is taken from the NICE guidance on management of fever in children.

   a F This can vasoconstrict and cause core temperature to shoot up, hence increasing the risk of fits.

   b T Recommendation is to alternate dosing.

   c F

   d F

   e F

7 This question uses data from the NICE guidance on heavy menstrual bleeding and pharmacological treatments.

   a iii

   b i

   c v

   d iv

   e ii

8 The answers to these questions are based on the RCOG guidelines and the confidential enquiry into maternal deaths.

   a F Up to 44% of cases have been reported to occur postnatally.

   b T Syntometrine should not be used if a mother is hypertensive.

   c T

   d F They should be started on treatment, labetalol is recommended.

   e T Substandard care was stated for eight of the 18 deaths.

   f F MAGPIE found it to reduce the risk by 58% (95% CI 40–71%).

9 This question is taken from the cancer back-up site.

   a T

   b T Maximum would be 10.

   c F In advanced disease hormone therapy to cause androgen deprivation (usually with an LHRH analogue) would be first line.

    d T Shown to be as effective as EBRT and radical prostatectomy up to T2a.

    e F Active surveillance may be suitable but would involve three-monthly PSA testing, re-imaging and biopsy at 12–18 months.

10 These questions are taken from the *BMJ* article 'Treating erectile dysfunction when PDE5 inhibitors fail' (*BMJ* 2006; 332: 589–92).

    a T 81% of men do not take their tablets correctly (41% will have a better effect if re-educated).

    b F Food delays absorption (tadalafil is not affected); they should be taken 30–60 minutes before intercourse.

    c F Recommended 50 mg.

    d T Doxazosin has a weak erectogenic effect.

    e T

11 a v Pingueculum is often similar in appearance but does not involve the cornea.

    b iv

    c ii Dendritic ulcers would not have such a painful globe.

    d iv

    e iii

12 This question applies to adults and is taken from the NICE guidance on obesity.

    a iii

    b vi More than 102 cm would be very high risk.

    c ii Hypertension is classified as a co-morbidity. Starting treatment at a BMI of 28 is recommended; this would be 30 (Obesity I) if there were no co-morbidities.

    d viii A waist circumference of more than 88 would be high risk.

    e v You could consider this first line if the patient had a BMI of 50, where considered appropriate.

13 This question is taken from the BTS and NICE Guidelines for COPD.

    a T

    b F This is recommended yearly with FVC.

    c F Inhaled steroids are recommended for moderate to severe COPD.

    d T Although, logistically, this is not routinely available.

    e T

14 This question is from the BTS and NICE guidelines for COPD.

    a T

    b F Only once over an exacerbation or on maximal therapy.

    c F LTOT should be used for at least 15 hours a day.

    d T

    e F Although realistically this will happen, the risk of burns to themselves and of fire are significant. They are unlikely to get any benefit if they continue smoking.

15 This question is taken from the Green Book and NICE guidance on TB.

   a T

   b F Either under 16 or 16–35 from sub-Saharan Africa or a country with a TB incidence of 50 per 100 000.

   c F Only if no evidence of previous vaccination, younger than 35 years and Mantoux negative.

   d F This schedule was stopped in 2005.

   e F

16 This question is taken from the NICE guidelines on anaemia management in CKD and the clinical guidelines from the renal association www.renal.org.

   a F This is usually straightforward to investigate, manage and protect the kidneys in primary care.

   b F They would; you should aim for a serum ferritin of 200–500 mcg/L.

   c T This is true, although especially so if the eGFR is >60.

   d T Also CKD 3 and 4.

   e F Shared care protocols allow for a robust primary/secondary care interface.

17 This question on colorectal cancer is taken from the Drugs and Therapeutics Bulletin 2006; 44(9) and the NHS screening information.

   a F It is known to reduce the risk of colorectal cancer but not yet mortality.

   b F Aspirin 300 mg daily is known to prevent and reduce recurrence of adenocarcinomas.

   c T

   d F Neither flexible sigmoidoscopy nor colonoscopy is known to reduce mortality although they are excellent methods for investigation and screening.

   e F

18 These questions on Barrett's oesophagus are taken from 'Dilemmas in managing Barrett's oesophagus' 2006; 44(9): 69–72.

   a T

   b F This is a late symptom; usually dyspepsia is the only symptom.

   c T

   d T Not great evidence for this; different units differ on recall (usually two-yearly).

   e F Although there are suggestions this reduced the risk of carcinoma of the oesophagus there is insufficient conclusive evidence; treatment should be directed at symptom control.

19 This question is taken from information in the NICE guidelines: National Institute for Health and Clinical Excellence. *Clopidogrel and modified-release dipyridamole in the prevention of occlusive vascular events: NICE technology appraisal guidance 90.* London: NIHCE; 2005. www.nice.org.uk/nicemedia/pdf/TA090quickrefguide.pdf

    a F 110 000 cases of stroke and 30 000 of TIA.

    b T

    c F 30–40% are alive at three years.

    d F Recommended for two years after the most recent event, then step down to aspirin.

    e F

20 This question is adapted from the *BMJ* article (2007; 335: 37) on managing smoking cessation and the BNF.

    a i

    b v Has been shown to be effective in meta-analyses.

    c iii

    d iii

    e ii There is a theoretical risk that nicotine may harm the baby. This has not been shown in three meta-analyses.

    f ii Too early to know in buprenorphine and varenicline.

21 a F 50%

    b T British Heart Foundation (BHF).

    c T BHF

    d F No form of NRT is better than another.

    e T There are four principles:
- empathise using reflective listening
- look at discrepancy between patient's beliefs and current behaviour
- sidestep resistance with empathy (do not confront)
- encourage by building the patient's confidence to change.

22 These answers are taken from the joint BHS and NICE guidance table on pharmacotherapy.

    a ii Although calcium-channel blockers or diuretics are options.

    b ii Felodipine is the best choice in these two questions.

    c iv Beta-blockers are essential treatment for coronary heart disease.

    d vi

    e v

    f i

23 a T Smoking cigarettes is also known to cause this problem.

    b F A risk with each use, there is an increased energy level and body temperature.

    c T The risk is higher with poor hygiene and groin access.

    d T Nausea and anorexia are recognised with heroin use.

    e F Cocaine and heroin.

24 This question is taken from 'Alarm Symptoms in early diagnosis of cancer', recently published in the *BMJ* (*BMJ* 2007; 334: 1040).

    a F This is the figure for women, it is 7.4% in men.

b T

c F Associated with oesophageal cancer, Barrett's is premalignant.

d F If concerned that there is other pathology, work out the history and risk.

e T This was a cohort study of 762 325 patients over six years.

25 This information was taken from the UK Resuscitation Council (www.resus.org.uk).

    a F Call for help and assess the safety of the area.

    b F 30:2

    c T

    d F Teeth help give form to the mouth, meaning you will usually get a better seal.

    e F Treat as if they are not breathing normally.

26 This question is based on www.cancerscreening.nhs.uk/bowel/.

    a F 60–70 years of age.

    b F Every two years by post.

    c F It will be tested for faecal occult blood.

    d T 2 in 100 will need colonoscopy, 4 in 100 will need a repeat.

    e T 5 in 10 will be normal, 4 in 10 will have a polyp and 1 in 10 will have cancer. Two in 1000 people screened will have a colorectal carcinoma discovered.

27 This information is taken from the Primary Care Society for Gastroenterology guidance on coeliac disease.

    a T

    b T

    c F Endoscopy and biopsy remain the gold standard.

    d T There is also a risk of osteoporosis, anaemia and autoimmune diseases.

    e F Although it is wise to consider pneumococcal, Hib and influenza vaccines.

28 a F Seen in 3–8% of children six months to six years.

    b F By definition at least 38 degrees.

    c F 30%.

    d T Normal risk is 1.4%, risk after a febrile convulsion is 2.4%.

    e F Care needs to be taken as peripheral vasoconstriction may increase core temperature. Using ibuprofen and paracetamol would form part of the ongoing management, but, if fitting, the child will be unable to take medication.

29 See www.brit-thoracic.org.uk.

    a ii

    b v

    c iii

d vi

e iv

30 a T

b F

c F   Although if associated with reflux, it may.

d F   This causes gastroenteritis.

e T

31 a T

b T

c F

d F   Patch testing can be considered; usually if there seems to be a deterioration with certain creams.

e F   *Herpes simplex* infection giving clusters of blisters and possibly systemic symptoms.

32 a T   Although it affects 80%, most respond to self management.

b T   This can be done using the Acne Disability Index (ADI) or the Acne Quality of Life Scale (AQOL).

c T   It has antibacterial, anti-inflammatory and keratolytic properties, helping reduce resistance of *Propionibacterium acnes.*

d F   Yes it is useful, but it is not a licensed contraceptive.

e F   This is really a specialist drug. Because of the implications, it is important to ensure other avenues have been fully explored prior to use.

33 Alternative names for rubella.

a T

b T

c F

d T

e F   This is fifth disease, parvovirus.

f T

34 a T   As an alternative to penicillin.

b F   Penicillins.

c F   This does not confer a benefit; varicella-zoster IG is recommended in similar circumstance if exposed to chicken pox or *Varicella zoster.*

d T

35 Requirements when a person dies of Hepatitis C.

a T   Cannot embalm the body.

b T   Implications on viewing the body, no clothes or makeup for burial.

c F   Should have already been done.

d T

e F

f T

36 The following are differential diagnoses of gynaecomastia (breast tissue growth in males)
  a T
  b T Usually regresses.
  c F With spironolactone.
  d T All gonadorelin analogues.
37 These answers are taken from the references documented in the osteoporosis part of this book.
  a F This would be classed as a traumatic fracture, as more than body height.
  b T If the patient had used HRT until she was over 45 then this would be F.
  c T This is classed as a malabsorptive problem.
  d F Hyperthyroidism is, so would over-treatment for a prolonged period of time with thyroxine
  e T
38 Answers for this question are taken from a recent review article in *BMJ* 2007; 334: 1211)
  a F It does not usually cross the midline.
  b F Meta-analyses have shown that if started within 72 hours they reduce pain severity and duration.
  c T
  d F This is not the case. It is worth considering to reduce pain from the acute attack in elderly patients.
  e F There is some evidence that used in the acute phase it may reduce neuralgia.
39 These answers use the *Oxford Textbook of Medicine* coupled with experience from the first patient I diagnosed and became involved in helping manage. I have included this question as it is the type of diagnosis that requires clinical suspicion and awareness as, like amyloidosis, it can present in many varied ways.
  a F
  b T As iron accumulates in the B-cells of the pancreatic islets.
  c F The body is absorbing and storing more iron than it needs without this.
  d T Due to iron overload.
  e T Seen on x-ray, arthritis can affect any joint but it is usually the metacarpophalangeal joints.
40 These questions are developed from a clinical review article in *GP* (March 2008) written by Dr Rod Hughes.
  a T The risk of developing the disease doubles every 10 years in those over 50 years of age.

b F   Useful to distinguish between Paget's and malignancy.

c T   Stress fractures occur because pagetoid bone is weaker than normal bone, and skull bossing and jaw changes are often seen.

d F   Raised calcium is usually only seen if the patient is bed-bound/ immobile.

e T   Especially if untreated or long standing.

41 a ii

b iv

c i

d v

e iii   Although may make the skin quite sore.

42 As statistics questions come up in the comics, Pulse, Update, etc., practice as many as you can.

a F   It is the hypothesis that there is no difference, that you then go on to disprove.

b T $p < 0.01$ is highly significant.

c F   May be irrelevant, depending on the design (e.g. if a sample size is too small).

d F   This would usually be a 95% confidence interval.

e F   A ratio could not include zero. If the ratio is greater than 1 then the result is not significant.

43 a i

b vii

c viii

d ii

e x

44 a viii

b ii

c iv

d i

e vii

45 These answers are taken from the Faculty of Family Planning Guidance and the BNF.

a v

b i

c i

d i

e ii

f vi

g vii

h i

46 These are textbook answers.

a T Especially at times when the body is stressed, e.g. with infection.

b F Not unless associated with liver disease such as haemochromatosis.

c T And propylthiouracil. Treatment with these drugs needs monitoring.

d T Can cause a hepatocellular dysfunction.

e F Usually appears when serum bilirubin is greater than 35 mmol/L.

47 The correct answer is (d) multiple sclerosis.
    Haemochromatosis may lead to diabetes but pupillary changes are unlikely.
    Horner's syndrome is not in itself a diagnosis; there is usually a cause.
    Similarly, Holmes-Adie pupil (not syndrome) is an observation.

48 c Med 5

49 f Self certificate

50 a Med 3

51 d This is a known side effect of calcium-channel blockers.

52 d In children 2–5 years, 20 mg for three days; in children older than 5 years,
       30–40 mg for three days (from the BTS guidelines).

53 d Prehn's sign is pain relieved on elevating the scrotum.

54 b

55 e

56 a F This would be AIDS.

    b T

    c F

    d T

    e T Also weight loss, oral hairy leukoplakia, shingles, arthralgia.

57 a F Due to immigration from Eastern Europe, sub-Saharan Africa and
          Asia.

    b F Generally unhelpful. Chest x-ray is a better investigation.

    c F This is no longer routinely done.

    d T Spread by droplets from coughing.

    e F Drug resistance is still an increasing problem.

58 a T Communication lines are important.

    b F Professional divisions usually create obstacles.

    c F

    d T

    e T

59 c As incidence is the measure of developing a condition in a period of
       time.

60 a Case fatality is the death rate in people who already have a condition
       defined in a period of time.

Clinical skills assessment

This will form an OSCE style of exam. You will be assigned a consulting room at the exam centre and have thirteen ten-minute consultations (12 of which are assessed and one of which is a test case). The cases will assess the following main areas.

◆ Primary care management – common problems.

◆ Problem solving skills – more complex data gathering and interpretation.

◆ Comprehensive approach – the ability to manage risk and co-morbidities.

◆ Person-centred care.

◆ Attitudinal aspects.

◆ Clinical practical skills – looking at practical skills.

All other instructions as to what you are allowed to take in with you and what will be provided are on the Royal College website. Make sure you read this, even if you have sat the exam before.

During your training you will be doing video work and joint surgeries that will help you focus on your consulting style and critique yourself, as well as enabling you to gain advice from your trainer. Although videos can be uncomfortable to watch at times, they allow you to constructively analyse your consulting style, foibles and acumen in line with how the Royal College will mark your ability in the CSA.

The difficulty in writing the assessment tasks in this book in a way that ensures that you direct the role play in the direction needed (which is the best way to practice these skills), means there is probably more information given here than you will receive in the exam itself. From the point of view of practising for the exam, it will be more worthwhile if the person being tested does the role play with the minimum amount of information.

Do not forget to introduce yourself in every case!

SIMULATED SURGERY: CASE 1

Freda Jones is 65 years old.

Past medical history: polymyalgia rheumatica.

Current medication: prednisolone 9 mg daily.

Her symptoms to date have been controlled by prednisolone use (monitored with ESR and CRP alongside her symptoms, both of which have been normal for the last four months), but you have been able to reduce the dose only slowly and she is currently on 9 mg/day of prednisolone.

She is on no other medication and has no other significant medical history (including fractures).

You may ask the lady any questions you feel are relevant, as you would in your own surgery.

This is very clearly going to be a case about primary prevention and risk assessment for osteoporosis; but start with the niceties and recap any PMR symptoms and how they have improved.

Glucocorticoid induced osteoporosis
Royal College of Physicians Guidelines 2002
These guidelines give a good overview of the risks and treatment in this group of patients. There is no safe dose of prednisolone and doses as low as 2.5 mg/day can affect bone mineral density. The guidelines advise that all patients older than 65 years committed to glucocorticoid treatment for at least three months should be started on bisphosphonates.

Further assessment of this patient's osteoporosis risk should include the following.

⬧ Smoking history (if she is a smoker you can assess the need for and acceptability of intervention at this point).
⬧ Alcohol use (should be less than 14 units a week).
⬧ Family history of maternal hip fractures.
⬧ Exercise undertaken – is it increasing since PMR symptoms were controlled? It is recommended that patients should undertake 20 minutes bone-loading exercise three times a week. The improvement in muscle tone helps with balance but there is no evidence that walking, alone, reduces falls.
⬧ Diet (1200 mg calcium/day is recommended in those over 51 years of age). It is difficult to assess this just from a review conversation; it may be worth considering a food diary to look at in more detail (i.e. the patient could drop it in for you to look at and call her back if she needs calcium supplements).
⬧ Falls prevention (it would be a real bonus if you could find the time to incorporate). If the patient has fallen in the past you need to try and assess further:
  • do they know why they fell/was there LOC?
  • are there *environmental elements*? – if so consider occupational therapy
  • was the patient able to *get up*? – if not consider physiotherapy
  • are the falls *recurrent or unexplained*? – consider specialist falls referral
  • *don't forget to review Rx and BP*
  • consider glucose test when next doing ESR and CRP.

If you are doing well, or if the consultation is also looking at how you deal with confrontation, the patient may challenge you as to why this wasn't discussed with her in the first instance. The fact it wasn't is not ideal, but it isn't necessary to condemn her previous physicians. This advice is only just coming through in NICE guidelines; she was being started on steroids that may have upset her stomach and it is not always ideal to start everything at the same time – focus first on getting things right. There are lots of sensible reasons you can advance why this may have been put on a back burner.

You need to be conscious of time and think what needs to be tied up in bringing the consultation to a close:

* the PMR – timing of the next dose reduction and bloods
* the need for bisphosphonates with or without calcium whilst on the steroids, if willing to take
* health promotion to reduce risk of falls and osteoporosis
* what time period you will set for a review – telephone consultation with the next blood results or follow up in surgery?

References
* NICE
* Help the Aged – national falls campaign each June
  www.helptheaged.org.uk
* Age concern – provides services funded by local councils aimed at reducing isolation
  www.ageconcern.org.uk
* Later Life Course – gait and balance training (lists of qualified instructors, download balance exercises)
  www.laterlifetraining.co.uk
* The British Geriatrics Society – section on website dedicated to bone health
  www.falls-and-bone-health.org.uk
* The College of Occupational Therapists – helpful information on environmental assessments
  www.copt.org.uk

SIMULATED SURGERY: CASE 2

Catherine Reid is a 53-year-old lady with no significant history.

This lady is well presented and articulate, comes to see you to discuss the menopause. There is no significant past history on her files, she consults infrequently and there is no repeat medication.

This consultation shouldn't faze you. It could quite easily cover similar principles if it was a simulated case on general contraceptive advice.

History
First, the history is important, starting with a general opening question to under-

stand the reason for the visit. This will form the basis for the rest of what will hopefully be a successful consultation.

+ Full history should include gynaecological history and current symptoms of the climacteric (flushing, mood changes, concentration, memory, sleep, menstrual problems, libido, vaginal dryness and an assessment of continence).
+ Family history, especially enquiring about venothromboembolism, breast or gynaecological cancers, coronary heart disease.
+ Medication history focusing on what over-the-counter remedies may have been tried and for how long in each case.
+ Lifestyle (alcohol and smoking history, caffeine intake and dietary assessment looking at calcium intake as well as calories).
+ Contraception – it is important to ascertain what method is being used.

Examination
You would expect the examination to be straightforward blood pressure and weight. It is unlikely in this instance that you would be required to perform a urogenital or breast examination (you may want to allude to it or even discuss mammogram screening).

Investigations
Investigations may or may not be necessary depending on the history from the simulated patient. It is important to realise that some of the symptoms experienced may be indicative of thyroid disease. At this age a follicle-stimulating hormone (FSH) test to confirm someone is going through the menopause is not going to add to management. Cardiovascular risk assessment may be warranted and is increasingly done as a routine base line.

Management
Management discussion will be focused around the issues raised in the consultation.

+ Lifestyle measures to improve menopausal symptoms and also to help prevent future problems such as cardiovascular disease, osteopenia/ osteoporosis (including dietary changes, smoking cessation and alcohol advice, weight-bearing exercises) with a suggestion about seeing your practice nurse.
+ Herbal options such as red clover, sage, Menopace, soya – with suggestions to seek advice from the herbalist in a reputable outlet.
+ Other non-pharmacological options. For example, if lubrication and urogenital symptoms were problematic Sylk or other lubrication may be appropriate – make sure, if condoms are a preferred method of contraception, that your suggestions are not oil-based. Another option available on prescription is Replens.

◆ Pharmacological options would mainly focus on HRT preparations (patches, tablets, gels and creams), although other treatments such as clonidine or antidepressants may be considered.

If the consultation follows an HRT prescribing route then it will be important to discuss all the risks and preparations; and to have a suitably timed follow-up (such as three months in the first instance).

There are other practical issues.

◆ Try not to forget contraception. It is recommended that contraception is used for two years after the last menstrual period if that is before the age of 50; and for one year if over 50. Complete loss of fertility is assumed at 55 years.

◆ If the consultation has followed a health promotion route, it is similarly important to have a follow-up plan, even if it is an open plan leaving the responsibility with the patient.

If you are doing well you may be challenged more on risks associated with HRT, specific questions about contraception or through more of a psychological overlay, with relationship problems. As you know, information comes to us in all sorts of ways. Use the cues the patient may give you.

SIMULATED SURGERY: CASE 3

Trudy Franks is a 68-year-old lady.

Current medication: Ramipril 10 mg and aspirin 75 mg daily.

This lady is coming to see you with waterworks' problems. She is leaking with coughing.

She is a diet-controlled diabetic and hypertensive. Both of these conditions are well controlled; blood tests and chronic disease reviews have been done recently by the practice nurse and are satisfactory.

In role playing this you can alternate between stress, urge and mixed incontinence pictures. This case was written with stress incontinence in mind.

One in six people over 40 years of age are incontinent several times a month. Effective treatment is possible in 70–80% of cases.

Feedback from your opening question may well give you the whole answer here, but it is important to go through the checklist in your mind.

History

Identify the following.

◆ What the problem is, how long it has been a problem, when the lady is leaking (is it just with sneezing or is it with walking, bending), if sexually active, is this causing problems (for example with orgasm or just being inhibitory)?

- Is the loss purely with stress events or is there a degree of urgency? Similarly, has there been any faecal incontinence?
- Have there been any recent precipitating factors such as an upper respiratory tract infection?
- Are there any other issues indicative of malignancy/pelvic mass, constipation or prolapse?
- Are pelvic floor exercises routinely being done or have they been in the past?

Questions must be asked about fluid intake and voiding pattern, especially if there are symptoms of an overactive bladder.

You need to try and draw out any psychological impact this is having, such as whether it is stopping social events, whether there has been overflow despite pads, generally how it may be affecting quality of life.

Past gynaecological and obstetric history is important to clarify (although this would routinely be in the records in real life, I doubt many of us would have looked that far back prior to seeing a patient for a first encounter).

Similarly it is important to clarify past family history.

Examination

In a real situation you would want to examine the abdomen, pelvis (including an internal examination) to look for masses (including signs of retention), prolapse, atrophy and to assess the integrity of the pelvic floor.

You would also assess for any neurological features/saddle paraesthesia depending on the history.

While it is unlikely you will be doing this in the simulated case, you may be presented with information or alternatively you may be presented with a lady refusing to be examined.

Investigations

Urine is the only real investigation (to check for urinary tract infection (UTI) and haematuria; protein should have been checked at the previous routine review).

Urodynamics and ultrasound are unlikely to be necessary at this stage (see the NICE guidance reference below).

Management

Management depends on the type of incontinence. Assume you have not identified any reasons for referral.

- Three-day bladder diary.
- First line management includes pelvic floor exercises for at least three

months. You would need to explain the process of doing these (eight contractions at least three times a day, although 10 times daily for treatment is better). Depending on the patient's understanding you may need physio input and biofeedback.

♦ Medication would not be necessary first line. Duloxetine may be offered as an alternative to surgical treatment.
♦ You would hope to avoid surgical intervention. If you were asked about this you could talk around urethral tapes, intramural bulking agents with or without prolapse repairs.
♦ Considering District Nurse or Health Visitor input for support, assessment and supply of pads may be necessary (Tena Lady are expensive).

References
♦ National Institute for Health and Clinical Excellence. *Urinary incontinence: the management of urinary incontinence in women: NICE clinical guidance 40.* London: NIHCE; 2005. www.nice.org.uk/nicemedia/pdf/ CG40NICEguideline.pdf
♦ The Continence Foundation www.continence-foundation.org.uk/
♦ Wellbeing of Women, The Big Squeeze www.wellbeingofwomen.org.uk

SIMULATED SURGERY: CASE 4

James MacBurney, 46 years old and previously fit and well.
    James, a Caucasian, is a retired banker who is coming to see you because he wants the blood test for prostate cancer.

Feasible opening statements might be that a friend or family member has recently been diagnosed with prostate cancer, his partner may have been encouraging him to come or he may just have been reading the Daily Mail.

Assessing risk factors
♦ Family history – it is thought that there may be a 5–10% risk of inheriting a genetic cause. It is important to ask about family history, including ages, as a slight increase in risk is seen if close relatives (father, brother) have had prostate cancer under 60 years. There is also thought to be a link with female members of the family who have had a breast cancer when under 40 years of age.
♦ Diet – a diet high in animal fats, including dairy products, and high in calcium (possibly linked to dairy) contributes to a higher risk. A diet low in fruit and vegetables is similarly linked. If people eat a lot of tomatoes

(including ketchup) there is a protective effect from the lycopene. Selenium may be protective if taken as a supplement.

⬥ Ethnicity – Afro-Caribbean men seem to be at higher risk; whereas Asians seem to have a reduced risk.

Alongside enquiry into the risk factors, asking about symptoms (using the IPSS) is important.

Be aware of the argument that 'Surely it is better to know, then we can make an informed decision about what we are dealing with' and the 'What would you do?' question.

The rest of the consultation will be a discussion about risk. Note the following.

⬥ There is no evidence that screening healthy men for prostate cancer reduces mortality. It may do more harm than good (of 100 men with a raised PSA, 30 will have a prostate cancer).

⬥ In the USA screening is suggested for men over 50 who have a 10-year life expectancy.

⬥ The results of trials (ProtecT, ERSPC and PLCO) are awaited to clarify whether there is a benefit from screening, as well as the role of early treatment.

⬥ PSA will be normal in one in five men with prostate cancer (i.e. false negatives would be falsely reassuring).

⬥ Biopsies as part of assessing a raised PSA may lead to bleeding or infection of the prostate gland.

⬥ Prostate cancers grow very slowly and investigations and treatments may be worse than the cancer.

If the patient has no family history and is under 50, you should probably be encouraging them to go away and think about things. Possibly suggest downloading the leaflet from the NHS cancer screening website (in short, discourage him without saying no).

www.cancerscreening.nhs.uk/prostate/faqs.html

Another useful website you could direct him to is the National Cancer Institute (www.cancer.gov/), where he can select 'prostate cancer' for further information.

SIMULATED SURGERY: CASE 5

Mr A Fugax is a 64-year-old gentleman who comes to see you following loss of vision in his right eye three days previously. The vision returned after a few minutes.

There have been no consultations with this gentleman over the last couple of years and he is on no medication.

This would be an ideal case for simulated surgery, as you would expect to find nothing abnormal on examination in a live case, so there would be nothing to simulate.

History

The history is one of sudden loss of vision in a quiet eye. You will be thinking of differentials as you ask the questions (arterial and retinal vein thrombosis being the two main ones with your brief, although keep an open mind).

Description of the visual loss (including pain, diplopia and current level of vision), past occurrences and family history of vascular disease need to be ascertained.

Examination

In writing this, I anticipate the story to be one of amaurosis fugax (the vision disappears as though there is a blind or a veil being pulled across it). This sort of event should be considered as a transient ischaemic attack.

Examine the eyes – fundoscopy for vitreous haemorrhage and papilloedema.

Cardiovascular examination would include blood pressure, pulse rhythm, heart sounds and carotid artery auscultation.

Cranial nerves (depending on time) might be a useful base line, even if you only manage ii, iii, iv and vi.

Investigations

Blood tests – fasting glucose and cholesterol. You may wish to consider an ESR if you think there may be temporal arteritis – this will be unlikely in these cases.

ECG – looking for atrial fibrillation and left ventricular hypertrophy

Any further investigation, such as carotid Doppler studies, echocardiogram or brain imaging would, in most areas, require referral to the Transient Ischaemic Attack (TIA) clinic.

Further management

Management would be structured around limiting cardiovascular risks. Explaining amaurosis fugax as a TIA/mini-stroke of the eye might be enough for the patient to understand the logic. You may get more pressing questions about how and why it happened.

Diet, alcohol, exercise and smoking advice should be as per the guidelines (British Hypertensive Society or Heart Foundation).

Blood pressure would need to be less than 140/85, 130/80 if it was a diabetic situation.

Aspirin treatment 75 mg daily, clopidogrel or dipyridamole could be considered.

Driving – with a TIA you are unable to drive for a month. You do not need to notify the DVLA but you should inform your insurance.

Future management would include review of results and consideration of pneumococcal and influenza vaccines.

SIMULATED SURGERY: CASE 6

Mrs Jean Smith, a 36-year-old lady (who has never smoked), comes to see you for the results of her oral glucose tolerance test (which is normal). You had previously requested her glucose, as she was more thirsty than usual, and on two occasions the fasting results were 6.4 and 6.7.

Her body mass index is 32.1 and previous blood pressure was 148/94 mmHg.

Her lipid profile from the same bloods:

- total cholesterol 5.9
- HDL cholesterol 1.2
- total cholesterol:HDL ratio 4.9
- triglycerides 2.4

ECG did not show any left ventricular hypertrophy.

This case would move the balance from full history-taking skills to you taking the lead, imparting information and to a certain extent motivational interviewing without being confrontational. It is important to understand where she is and some of the history before coming out with ideas and plans. To be successful, a patient will need to want to achieve weight loss, have a long-term view and it will need to be at the right time.

Clarify that it is just the results she has come back for (you never know!). Although there were reassuring factors, you need to focus primarily on lifestyle with regards to the weight (as this will have an impact on the blood pressure, lipid profile and glucose as well as other health issues).

You will note there is no waist circumference above so you may want to check this along with a further blood pressure before moving on.

Assessing lifestyle, co-morbidities and willingness to change

- Ask about diet (including alcohol) and physical activity (explore this, walking the dog twice a day or going to the gym doesn't mean they are getting enough exercise).
- Look at eating behaviour and psychosocial stress.
- Environmental, social and family factors need to be explored.
- Explore understanding of the potential for weight loss to improve health.
- Determine the motivation behind change, given the real future risk of diabetes and hypertension.

Planning and goals

This will depend on the conversation so far. Be very careful not to get frustrated with any answers. In all probability you will be sitting opposite a character who has yo-yo dieted and who has tried everything seriously, with initially good effects – but then motivation will have slipped. Boredom, tiredness and lack of motivation at the end of a working day should be tackled with the issue of weight.

- Consider a food diary, with further advice and regular support from the practice nurse (a dietitian is probably not necessary at this stage).
- Healthy eating, avoiding snacks and processed food. Look at the 5-a-day approach and changing the balance of food in the day. Salt may be brought up. There is not usually a need to be too restrictive but setting the scene for normal portions and calories is often adequate (this isn't a quick fix so you have to try to keep your patient on side).
- Look at physical activity and explore where she feels this may be increased (walking to school if she has children, using the stairs, exercise DVDs, avoiding TV in the evenings, tourist information for local free walks for the weekends).
- Aim for 30 minutes exercise on five or more days a week.
- Discuss eating behaviour (if eating is used as comfort or because of boredom), speed of eating, using water instead of juice or carbonated drinks.
- Discuss setting sensible weight loss goals, such as a maximum 0.5–1.0 kg a week
- Plan for follow-up, either with yourself or your practice nurse/someone who the patient can develop a rapport with. Give her the option.

Further issues

- Medication – at this early stage it shouldn't be necessary, although it might be seen as an answer. The old guidelines of needing to lose 2.5 kg no longer apply, but jumping in to medication without dealing with diet, lifestyle and the psychosocial issues just sets you up to fail before you've started. Promise to come back to it.
- Other agencies – may be needed, depending upon revelations in the consultation: for example counselling, job centre input, dietitian, relate (you never know what might come into the consultation).

References

- National Institute for Health and Clinical Excellence. *Obesity: the prevention, identification, assessment and management of overweight and obesity in adults and children: NICE clinical guidance 43.* London: NIHCE; 2006. www.nice.org.uk/nicemedia/pdf/CG43niceguideline.pdf

♦ Obesity Care Pathway 2005
www.nationalobesityforum.org.uk

SIMULATED SURGERY: CASE 7

Mr Andrew Marks is 65 years old.

He comes to see you having had a three-month history of altered bowel habit (loose stool three times a day). There has been no blood (other than on one occasion where he had developed a small pile which has now resolved) or mucus.

There is a family history in that his father died of rectal carcinoma aged 54.

He is a non-smoker, has a diet rich in meat and processed foods and drinks around 30 units a week.

This is the sort of situation where you would have little other than a name and age to go on and your skill at covering all points within the history and discussing further management options will be judged.

History

Check the above history and determine exactly what is meant by a change in bowel habit, whether there is a suggestion of infective cause (asking re travel, other illnesses and systemic features).

A review of systems – including assessment of any weight loss, possible iron deficiency anaemia and (thinking along the lines of bowel cancer) suggestion of metastases.

Examination

Full abdominal examination would be expected, starting with the hands and mucous membranes and ending with PR (do not forget inguinal and cervical nodes). It is unlikely that you would need to perform a PR unless there is a dummy model.

Discussion

It is likely that you will have encountered this situation several times in your training practice. The need to determine the underlying cause through referral to a 14-day wait clinic (or equivalent cancer initiative in your area) is ultimately the most important point to get across and agree upon in a sensitive way.

Allow the discussion to be led by the patient before jumping in with leading questions about whether they have any specific concerns.

Broach the subject of endoscopy carefully (you never know quite how it will be received). Although for referral to such a clinic you would need to talk about cancer as a positive differential, it is important to remember other differential diagnoses and the reason for the urgent clinics is as much about exclusion as it is about early diagnosis at a more treatable stage.

Other investigations

Consider full blood count, urea and electrolytes, liver function tests specifically. Thyroid function, ferritin and CEA along with stool samples could also be considered.

Safety netting

Many surgeries will have an audit trail of urgent referrals to ensure that patients have been seen and managed appropriately. From the patients' point of view they should have been seen within two weeks. Suggest that if a patient has not been seen in that time, they contact you/your office staff so you can chase things up.

Agree on a follow-up after the investigations, allowing time for letters to come through, and what to do if the situation gets worse or there are abnormalities in the blood tests.

SIMULATED SURGERY: CASE 8

In this case you have a name and age, and no other information from which to start the consultation: Jayne Pickham, aged 24 years.

Jayne is a 24-year-old accountant who has come with headaches. They have been happening on a monthly basis (not related to periods and she has not been prescribed the oral contraceptive pill from elsewhere), usually towards the end of the month.

The headache usually lasts for 48 hours and causes a blurring of her vision (doesn't wear glasses and a recent eye check has been fine). It does not cause vomiting and usually settles with rest.

So far she has not used any treatment other than an occasional paracetamol.

Headaches account for almost 5% of GP consultations and a clear history is the key to a diagnosis.

The history above reflects a clear common migraine history (month end being significant as it is usually the busiest time of the month for accountants, especially those working in a VAT-registered business) but it is important to assess several things before making the diagnosis.

History

Find out the story:
* When, where, how long, relieving or exacerbating factors, are there any auras? Make sure there is only one type of headache occurring.
* Has this happened before?
* What does she mean by an occasional paracetamol (check usage of ibuprofen as well).

Ask specifically about worrying features: headache on waking or with coughing and sneezing (suggesting raised intra-cranial pressure), or other neurological symptoms or signs.

Is there a smoking or significant family history?

Examination
This needs to include blood pressure, weight (thinking laterally about benign intra-cranial hypertension) as well as a full neurological examination.

Cranial nerves (you will only be able to ask about sense of smell but nerves ii–xii should be tested, including corneal reflex). Pupillary reflexes and papilloedema are unlikely to be forgotten if done at this stage.

Look for cerebellar signs – nystagmus, past-pointing (ataxias), dysdiadochokinesis, speech problems and tremor.

Investigations
Unless there are specific queries raised it is unlikely that you would need to arrange any investigations at this stage.

Management
Avoidance tactics – if there is a relationship with specific triggers such as tiredness, stress, caffeine, alcohol, etc.

Simple analgesia – dissolvable paracetamol and aspirin in the first instance (with or without an antiemetic, for example Migraleve). Encouraging the patient to take medication early, at the start of the attack, rather than braving it out, is usually effective.

Review – it is important to arrange a review to judge effectiveness of treatment, Explain that there are many treatment options, depending on response. If headaches are happening monthly it is unlikely you would need prophylaxis (although if anxiety was a trigger that could be discussed for PRN use). Triptans such as sumatriptan (50–100 mg after onset of the attack) or zolmitriptan (2.5 mg at the onset of a headache, repeating the dose after two hours if there has been no response, to a maximum of 10 mg in 24 hours) would probably be discussed next.

Other issues
There is a global campaign to reduce the burden of headache worldwide. See 'Lifting the Burden', which discusses headaches, types and management: www. l-t-b.org. This is a useful site for a headache overview, as is the BNF.

Other health promotion issues may be relevant, again depending on time and other revelations (smoking, alcohol, and sexual health – she is as yet too young for smears) would all be part of a holistic approach. But again, these are add-ons. Do not use them to detract from the problem about which the patient has come to see you.

If you are doing well for time, questions may be asked about outcomes and further management or why she hasn't been offered the screening talked about in the press. Be careful not to lose all the valuable points you have clocked up, and if you run out of time suggest you pick up on those important points at her next visit.

SIMULATED SURGERY: CASE 9

Mr Payne is a 68-year-old gentleman.

He has a past history of hypertension and osteoarthritis.

Current medication on repeat: aspirin 75 mg, perindopril 4 mg and co-codamol 8/500.

This gentleman is coming in with worsening of his osteoarthritis over the last two years.

He has had physiotherapy in the past and, although having to resort to using a stick, is still fairly mobile, walking his dog and looking after his wife (she has no medical problems specifically).

He is using the co-codamol six tablets a day with some relief, although his sleep is sometimes disturbed because of the pain on turning over. The only side effect is constipation, for which he uses senna from the chemist.

The main issue here is assessing pain and mobility accurately to determine the most appropriate and useful management to help this gentleman.

The answer is based on the NICE guidance on osteoarthritis. National Institute for Health and Clinical Excellence. *The care and management of osteoarthritis in adults: NICE clinical guidance 59.* London: NIHCE; 2008. www.nice.org.uk/nicemedia/pdf/CG59NICEguideline.pdf.

History

+ Clarify mobility – how far he is walking the dog; how far can he walk on the flat; can he manage stairs, etc?
+ Exercise – having seen the physiotherapist, has he managed to continue doing the exercises to help local muscle strength? Was it helpful for him before and is it a referral worth revisiting?
+ Review of systems – to assess the development of any other pathologies, and to determine whether you are still dealing with osteoarthritis affecting the same joints.
+ Pain – assess the degree of pain both practically and using pain intensity scales. It is unlikely you will have a pain scale in your bag, but you could ask him to grade the intensity verbally and assess what he has modified in his day to day life.

Examination
Look at the musculoskeletal system and the impact on the affected and surrounding joints (whether there is some developing compensation).

Management
This needs to be a shared decision making approach to the problem.

Consider analgesia changes (working up the pain ladder) and treatments to prevent side effects.

Consider the role of steroid injections, depending upon the site of pain.

Non-pharmacological options – heat (care and advice with hot water bottles), TENS machines, physiotherapy referral (for stretching, exercise, heat treatment, acupuncture, etc).

Appliances – this gentleman already has a stick but it may be worth an occupational therapist assessment to determine whether he would benefit from further aids.

Referral – from the above history this gentleman is fairly fit. Although you would be making non-surgical suggestions at this point, it might be worth broaching referral as an option looking towards joint replacement if you are unable to afford him more comfort with the above suggestions.

Other issues
Follow-up – be sure to arrange follow-up to assess response to treatment.

Consider other co-morbidities (his hypertension review) and his home circumstances, why he looks after his wife (does she need to see you or do they need social service input)?

SIMULATED SURGERY: CASE 10

You are asked to take an urgent telephone call for a four-year-old child with a rash and temperature. The mother is asking for advice and possibly an urgent visit.

The history from the parent includes the recent onset of a blotchy red rash (yes it does blanch) mainly on the chest, a temperature for three days following a cold, and the recent development of diarrhoea but no vomiting.

The child has been otherwise fit and well, is a little off food but tolerating fluids well.

Remote assessment and triaging of patients in a way that is safe and makes best use of time available in the day is an important part of our day to day work. The idea behind this consultation is that it is a simple self-limiting illness that does not require a visit or appointment.

History

The history includes a rash, upper respiratory tract infection and diarrhoea. You will need to assess hydration status. It is important to determine what has been used for the temperature (possibly paracetamol or ibuprofen). The caller may use brand names. If you are not familiar with these names, either a trip to the chemist in your registrar year or simply asking the caller to read the drug name from the side of the box will allow you to clarify what has been used. If medication has been used then assess the response and its duration.

Ask about mottling and whether the patient is alert (although likely to be tired, it should still be possible to engage their child).

Examination

As you will not be able to perform a specific examination looking for the traffic-light approach advised in the NICE guidance (www.nice.org.uk/nicemedia/pdf/CG47QuickRefGuide.pdf), you can ask about urine output and dry mouth to assess hydration.

Management

Temperature management, hydration and safety netting are the key points here.

Regarding raised temperature, tepid sponging is no longer recommended because of the fear of causing a peripheral vasoconstriction, which in turn may increase the core temperature and increase the likelihood of a febrile convulsion.

Explain that the parent should not over- or under-dress the child (wearing socks is a good idea).

Regular fluids and antipyretics will help to minimise symptoms.

You may want to discuss the future need to take stool samples or suggest if things have not resolved within a week it would be worth making an appointment (assuming they get no worse in the meantime).

It is important to consider nursery exclusion (if applicable) because of the diarrhoea.

Safety netting

Give advice concerning signs that should make the parent call the surgery again. These include:

◆ development of a non-blanching rash
◆ if parents are concerned (especially if the child is worse than when they last received advice)
◆ if there is a fit – fit is difficult to drop into conversation without it sounding alarming. If you have talked about temperature control and have explained that one of the reasons it is important is because young children sometimes fit with very high temperatures, then it is easier to include at this stage.

Conclude by asking whether there are any other queries or concerns, and by checking the parent is happy and understands the advice. Even though you may have suggested signs that should cause the parent to contact the surgery, it is nice to end the conversation in an open way so that the parent feels able to contact you if there are increasing concerns.

SIMULATED SURGERY: CASE 11

Holly is a 14-year-old coming to see you by herself.

She would like the vaccination to protect her against cervical cancer and although they are doing it at school her mum hasn't signed her consent form.

She is otherwise fit and well.

The Gillick test is the means by which you can judge whether a child under 16 is mature enough to understand what treatment involves, including the risks. It shows that a child is competent to consent to treatment (such as contraception and vaccinations). The Gillick test is in accordance with the Fraser guidelines:

- the child understands the doctor's advice
- the doctor cannot persuade them to involve their parents about the matter on which they are seeking advice
- unless they receive treatment their physical or mental health is likely to suffer.

The fact that Holly is here discussing it with you today doesn't necessarily mean she has the understanding to consent. It may be purely peer pressure, in that all her friends are having it done and she doesn't want to be left out. The discussion needs to be around all factors.

Given how the research stands at the moment, there is little in the way of risk and a huge amount to gain in vaccinating young women.

It would be important to explore:

- why her parents haven't signed the form for school (is it a case of a lost form, are there misunderstandings, religious or cultural reasons)
- is there a reason Holly has decided to come by herself?
- can she encourage her parents to be involved in this decision so you can all discuss the benefits together? Would it be easier if you were to broach the subject with them?

Vaccinating her would certainly be in her best interest (whether she is sexually active or not) but there is no rush to do it there and then (most surgeries would need to order the vaccine in prior to administration) and encouraging an open frank discussion is the ideal solution. If this is not going to be possible and she understands the pros and cons, there is no reason not to offer the vaccine.

Other issues

Sexual health and other lifestyle choices can be easily included and make this a tight, thorough consultation.

SIMULATED SURGERY: CASE 12

John Humphries. Aged 47.

Has a past medical history of back pain.

Discectomy 2004 (L4/5).

Medication on repeat prescription: co-codamol 8/500 2 tablets qds prn 100.

The history is a recent acute exacerbation of his back pain, with some right gluteal pain and spasm (no specific trigger but his work is quite physical).

He is having difficulty walking and getting from sitting to standing but has no red flags.

He needs a sick note as he works as a plumber and would be unable to do his job and has self-certificated this last week.

History

Although this is relatively straightforward, you must go through a thorough history of triggers, thinking about minimising the risk in the future.

A basic descriptive pain history in relation to this event is needed.

You have to go through the check list of red flags: is he able to pass water and open the bowels without difficulty (if there is difficulty clarify whether this is different to usual); are there any specific neurological features; have there been any night sweats (and if so how do they relate to the pain); and has weight been stable.

You need to be as sure as you can be from the history that this is not an acute emergency (cauda equina or infection) or metastatic bone pain.

Clarify medication use (are there any additional OTC preparations) and whether a physiotherapist, chiropractor or acupuncturist has been used in this instance.

Examination

Look at mobility, straight leg raise and degree of spasm. A quick neurological examination including reflexes and sensation at S1 would be worthwhile.

Management

Medication will depend on what is negotiated. If there is a lot of spasm a short course of diazepam may be needed.

Co-codamol – if the current dose is already maximised then you could step up to 30/500.

Anti-inflammatories – if needed.

Sick note – he will need a Med 3 for one to two weeks in the first instance.

Planning further review/management (one to two weeks or sooner) with a view to physiotherapy if his symptoms don't improve or get worse is important, alongside brief advice about mobility and exercise (he may still have his old exercises memorised).

Exams and courses to consider while doing your training

Whilst going through your hospital you will have a study allowance and grants that can be used for different courses (relevant to general practice, not necessarily the subspecialty you may be doing as part of the rotation at that time).

Use the study leave time and money wisely, bearing in mind that if you want to go on revision courses this will use a lot of your registrar allocation and that certain courses will be free in certain posts (e.g. advanced life support).

Diplomas to consider
DRCOG (Diploma of the Royal College of Obstetricians and Gynaecologists)

This is not necessary for general practice, but if you look at job advertisements some practices stipulate that they would like applicants to have the diploma. This diploma is now a three-hour paper, in two parts.

If you want to give it a go, request the information from the college early. If you can time it with your obstetrics and gynaecology attachment, you will probably find it easier to be motivated, and get significantly more out of the teaching on rounds from your seniors.

> RCOG, 27 Sussex Place, Regent's Park, London NW1 4RG
> Tel. 020 7772 6200
> www.rcog.org.uk

DFFP (Diploma of the Faculty of Family Planning)

This, again, is not essential to be a GP unless you want to do Family Planning sessions or fit coils and implants. You can do ad hoc family planning sessions once you have the diploma, while you are still doing either hospital posts or GP registrar year, which may help keep your skills up-to-date.

Once you have done the DFFP you can then do the coil training for the IUD letters of competence and the implant training.

The syllabus and logbook can be viewed on the faculty website (www.ffprhc. org.uk/) (under general training committee).

> Faculty of Family Planning and Reproductive Health
> 19 Cornwall Terrace, London NW1 4QP
> Tel. 020 7935 7196/7149

DCH (Diploma of Child Health)

This is a detailed diploma involving practical-based sessions as well as the exam. These sessions may be possible to do whilst in your paediatric job.

Only a few practices seem to be requesting this diploma, but as with all things, it may be something that tips the balance in your favour when applying for the post of your choice.

> Royal College of Paediatrics and Child Health
> 50 Hallam Street, London W1W 6DE
> Tel. 020 7307 5600
> www.rcpch.ac.uk/

Courses to Consider
Advanced life support (ALS)

Ensure this is up-to-date before your registrar year and that you have a signed form confirming that you are qualified in ALS. If you are thinking of taking the nMRCGP® you have to have proof of basic life support competency, which the ALS training incorporates.

Most trusts give this training free of charge for trust employees.

Acupuncture

Many hospital trusts will fund acupuncture courses. Acupuncture is as relevant to general practice as you want to make it. The courses tend to be held at weekends, which means getting study leave is not part of the ordeal. A good basic course to ensure you are competent to practice would take around four days.

Information can be found in the BMJ advertisements. See also:

> BMAS (British Medical Acupuncture Society)
> Newton House, Newton Lane, Whitley, Warrington WA4 4JA
> Tel. 01925 730727
> www.medical-acupuncture.co.uk

Other courses

Some half-day release courses (or within your post-graduate region) will offer the following courses to GP registrars:

♦ alternative Medicine

- ENT
- ophthalmology
- dermatology
- GP management issues
- communication skills.

All of the above, and more, would be time well spent. It is all about developing your own interest and deciding what kind of a service you would like to be able to offer your patients.

Courses to consider through your registrar year
Minor Surgery
You can pay to go on a minor surgery course whilst doing your hospital training. GP registrars can usually go on the course without having to use any of their allowance.

If you want to be signed up by your PCT for minor surgery, so you can be eligible to perform minor surgery under your contract (which attracts a payment for each individual case), then you need to do this course.

The theoretical course is not how you will become competent in minor surgery. You will learn this through either your trainer or other colleagues (e.g. dermatologists, surgeons, rheumatologists, etc.) in hospital posts.

Child Health Surveillance
It is important to check your regional policy as to what is required and whether you have to be on a named list to carry out any surveillance work.

Child health protection (especially the recognition of problems) is an important part of work in primary care and if you have the opportunity to attend one of these courses it would be worthwhile.

Palliative Care
Most regions are now running palliative care courses. Again, usually no payment is required for GP registrars.

Although palliative care is unlikely to be a huge part of day to day life, it will be the one thing that, if you do it well, you will be remembered and respected for.

The courses teach the knowledge base as well as the practical issues (e.g. setting up a syringe driver).

After you qualify

Self-employment as a GP/locum

Good records are essential. Outgoings that are tax deductible are also essential to keep receipts for.

Because GPs provide a service (rather than receiving a contract of service as in other NHS professions), we have a self-employed, independent contractor status.

Once you have qualified as a GP you need to register with the Inland Revenue as being self-employed. If you do not register within three months of starting work, you will probably be fined. You will find some information as well as a selection of relevant publications at www.inlandrevenue.gov.uk and the helpline for the newly self-employed is: 08459 15 45 15 (this is to register. Alternatively, you can complete a form CWF1).

By registering as self-employed you will pay Class 2 National Insurance (NI). At the end of the tax year, when you send in your self-assessment, the amount of NI contributions you owe will be calculated. This is then payable as Class 4 NI at the same time as you pay your income tax bill.

You also have to ensure you are registered with a PCT on their supplementary list.

Expenses which will probably be tax deductible

- Professional subscriptions: GMC, BMJ, DRCOG, DFFP, Defence Union, etc.
- Mileage: for visits, not to and from work. As a locum, all mileage is tax deductible because you are working from home.
- Office at home: running costs, rates, electricity, gas, etc. are worked out as a proportion depending upon the number of rooms in your house/sq.footage.
- Computer: if you use it for work.
- Stationery: used for work (e.g. paper, envelopes, stamps/postage, acetates).
- nMRCGP® exam fees: this is necessary if you want to be involved in training.
- Courses: if you pay for them (if reimbursed you must declare this).
- Telephone expenses: if using your home phone for work, then ensure that you get an itemised bill to be able to calculate the amount. Alternatively, your accountant may use estimates.
- Internet: links from home and anti-virus packages.
- Miscellaneous: digital camera if used for work purposes/teaching/ publications, (if also used for home then a proportion of the cost); books and equipment if necessary for your job.

Keep up-to-date records of all incomings and outgoings.

Speak to your accountant or the business advisors at the Inland Revenue. You are self-employed as a GP, and they are an excellent source of information and will help you with your tax return if needed. If speaking to a revenue advisor it is prudent to remember who they work for!

Remember that you will have to declare all incoming monies (e.g. cremations fees, DS1500s) from private work. Even if you have not filled in a tax return whilst doing your hospital jobs you could still be investigated. This is especially likely if your first tax return is as a GP. Get used to doing them early, when the figures are easier! And always keep all your receipts.

Applying for locum jobs

+ Negotiate pay before doing a job; ask around and find out what other people are charging.
+ Negotiate what work is to be done (length of surgery, number of appointments, visits, etc.).
+ Once the job is complete, or on a weekly/monthly basis, invoice the practice.
  • If you don't, you are unlikely to get paid.
  • If you take the invoice with you on the final day, apart from it saving on postage, your records will be up-to-date, and there is less chance of forgetting what you have claimed for.
+ Locums can contribute to the superannuation scheme. Your PCT will have the relevant information. If you ask them, they will send you the forms (that you will need the practice you are temporarily working in to complete) to prove what your earnings have been.
+ Information is also available from the NHS Pensions Agency: Tel. 01253 774774, www.nhspa.gov.uk.
+ Try to save around 40% of your income in a high-interest account for:
  • Income tax
  • Class 4 National Insurance
  • Superannuation
  • Defence subscriptions for next year.

Considerations when looking for a GP post

When making any major decision it is important to work out the things that are fundamentally important to you and the things you would be prepared to compromise on.

Don't feel you have to rush into anything. There are always jobs and, in the interim, locum work is not only lucrative but may help you develop your idea of how you want to work.

Below are some of the things to consider when choosing a post.

+ Full time or part time.
+ PMS or GMS practice.
+ Salaried, partnership or retainer.

- Portfolio career options.
- Outside work:
  - clinical assistant post
  - family planning
  - private health screening
  - obesity clinics
  - LMC involvement
  - CT work
  - post marketing surveillance work
  - forensic work.
- If considering a partnership:
  - rural/inner city
  - where in the country?
  - how many partners would you be comfortable with?
  - how many sessions do you want to work?
  - do you want to be involved in training or with medical students?
  - do you want a dispensing practice?
  - how involved do you want to be in: antenatal care, child health, minor surgery, practice development?
  - do other members of the PCT have a base at the practice?
  - what computer system is used?
  - who does the auditing?
  - what role do the practice nurses have (is there a nurse practitioner, triage, etc)?
  - what are the premises like (owned, rented, new or aging)?
  - what is car parking like (small things can become very irritating)?
  - how do the appraisals work, who does them?
  - what are the local hospitals, educational meetings, out-patient waiting times like?
  - what security measures are there?
  - what meetings are there (weekly business, nurse, practice, in-house educational, etc)?
  - does the practice have social events?
- Other issues:
  - what are the local schools like: comprehensive and public?
  - what are house prices like in the area?
  - what are the road/motorway links like (remember your family and social commitments!)?

Partnership agreement

If you are a member of the BMA request a copy of *Medical Partnership under the NHS*. This should get you orientated as to what issues a practice agreement should cover. You should be thinking towards signing a written mutual agreement at the end of your period of mutual assessment. It is foolhardy to enter into a partnership with no written agreement in place. In such an instance this is a partnership at will, which can be brought to an end as quickly as it is formed.

It is advisable to take specialist independent legal (and accountancy) advice before signing. You need to protect yourself, no matter how well you think you know your partners.

What should it cover?
- All parties' names and addresses.
- Commencement date.
- Declaration relating to termination of partnership, retirement, a party wishing to move, gross misconduct, etc.
- Capital assets.
- Sale and purchasing of shares.
- Valuation methods especially in relation to cost rent scheme.
- Occupation of premises by non-owning partners.
- Expenses – individual and partnership.
- Income – individual and partnership, especially notional/cost rent income, outside work (is it to be pooled?).
- Schedule of profit shares from commencement date to parity.
- Partners' obligations to each other.
- Partnership accounts (drawings, tax reserve, year end, accountants).
- Superannuation.
- Holiday and study leave.
- Sickness, maternity and paternity entitlement.
- Effect of retirement or death – restrictive covenant.
- Arbitration of provisions.
- Declaration about patients.

Things to consider in detail, prior to accepting the partnership
There will be things to negotiate and this will involve compromise.
- Commitment to the practice:
  - number of sessions to be worked
  - earning from outside interests/work (will this be pooled?).
- Finances.
- Determine the cost of buying in and the time to parity.
- Profit share distribution.
- Voting rights.
- Some matters should only be acted on with a unanimous agreement (e.g. appointment of a new partner).
- One vote per partner is ideal.

- Part-time partners should have equal voting power as they buy into a share of the profits but are 'jointly' liable and have the same professional interest in the business.
- Maternity leave and paternity leave clauses – time allowed must be fair.
- Determine what will happen to drawings and who will cover the locum costs and what happens to funds reimbursed by the PCT.
- Expulsion clauses.
  - This may be important if you have any existing conditions. Don't presume it will never happen to you (e.g. lengthy incapacity, gross misconduct).
- Expenses
  - This includes all things (e.g. phones, subscriptions, courses and travel, equipment, books, etc.). It needs to be explicit about what will be covered in the practice and what will be paid for personally.

Accounts

When considering buying into a practice, it is necessary to look over and to understand (to a certain degree) the practice accounts.

I am not an accountant, and certainly make no claim to be expert on the subject. Having been through the process and having to put your name to the yearly accounts will make you learn quickly. I hope you find this Noddy-like guide a useful starting point.

What you are looking at is:
- is the practice solvent
- how much will you be drawing
- have there been any major changes from one year to the next, and why
- where could the practice potentially improve?

When you receive the accounts they will probably be in a summarised format (i.e. not include every single transaction but have sections lumped together).

Look at the year of the accounts that you are given. Some run from the 6 April to 5 April (i.e. the tax year), others run from 1 January to 31 December. It doesn't really matter. Be aware that you may be looking at accounts well over 12 months old.

In the accounts you should see two columns of figures – the current year and the previous year for easy comparison.

Look at each of the following.
- The layout – is it a logical format?
- Is it clear where the numbers are from? If not, ask.
- How were the figures calculated?
- How did performance compare with previous years?
- How does it compare with the national average (often represented graphically at the end of the accounts using information from MedEconomics)?

- What areas can be improved?
- Are the following shown clearly:
  - value and ownership of property
  - fixed assets (fixtures, fittings, computers, furniture, drug stock)
  - investments and running costs?
- Is seniority pay, etc. kept personally or pooled?
- Does the practice pay for GMC, Defence union and professional subscriptions, etc.?
- How much profit was made and was this shared fairly in line with the partnership agreement?
- Is there a partnership tax account?
- How much tax and National Insurance are you likely to pay?
- Is there an accountant's report (a summary of the important features of the accounts)?

Also consider:
- are partner's current accounts drawn up by the accountant (i.e. not a separate account, as if each partner had their own account within the business). It is likely to include things such as seniority pay areas where one partner may assume all responsibility, etc. It is recommended that these accounts are zeroed each year. If a substantial amount builds up, the practice could go into the red if a partner was to leave and want that money reimbursed.
- getting professional help to go through the accounts with you (a specialist in GP finance and accountancy).
- sources of private income (insurance certificates, medicals, sick notes, etc.).
- if a practice is doing well above average, or below, why is this? Remember if fraud is committed (i.e. incorrect claims) money will have to be reimbursed to the PCT and Inland Revenue. There may be criminal proceedings. In this situation, all partners are liable.

Useful websites and references

Royal College of General Practitioners
www.rcgp.org.uk

British Medical Association and Clinical Evidence
www.bma.org.uk
www.clinicalevidence.com

www.bmj.learning.com

General Medical Council
www.gmc-uk.org

Bandolier (useful evidence-based reviews)
www.ebandolier.com

Cochrane Library
www.cochranelibrary.com/cochrane

Centre for Evidence-based Medicine
www.cebm.net

British National Formulary
www.bnf.org.uk/bnf/

Drug Information
www.druginfozone.nhs.uk

Medicines and Healthcare products Regulatory Agency
www.mhra.gov.uk

TOXBASE
www.toxbase.org

Department of Health
www.dh.gov.uk

Health Protection Agency
www.hpa.org.uk

GP Website database
www.gpwebsites.net

National electronic Library for Health
www.library.nhs.uk/Default.aspx

Medical searches online
www.searchmedica.co.uk/
www.gpnotebook.co.uk

Index